Immunopharmacology of Infectious Diseases

Vaccine Adjuvants and Modulators of Non-Specific Resistance

PROGRESS IN LEUKOCYTE BIOLOGY

TITLES IN THE SERIES

Volume 1
Viral Mechanisms of Immunosuppression
Norbert Gilmore and Mark A. Wainberg, *Editors*

Volume 2
The Physiologic, Metabolic, and Immunologic Actions of Interleukin-1
Matthew J. Kluger, Joost J. Oppenheim, and
Michael C. Powanda, *Editors*

Volume 3
Genetic Control of Host Resistance to Infection and Malignancy
Emil Skamene, *Editor*

Volume 4
Macrophage Biology
Sherwood Reichard and Mizu Kojima, *Editors*

Volume 5
Leukocytes and Host Defense
Joost J. Oppenheim and Diane M. Jacobs, *Editors*

Volume 6
Immunopharmacology of Infectious Diseases:
Vaccine Adjuvants and Modulators of Non-Specific Resistance
Jeannine A. Majde, *Editor*

Immunopharmacology of Infectious Diseases
Vaccine Adjuvants and Modulators of Non-Specific Resistance

Proceedings of the International Symposium on Immunological Adjuvants and Modulators of Non-Specific Resistance to Microbial Infections, Held at Columbia, Maryland, June 30–July 3, 1986

Editor

Jeannine A. Majde
Biological Sciences Division
Office of Naval Research
Arlington, Virginia

Alan R. Liss, Inc., New York

Address all Inquiries to the Publisher
Alan R. Liss, Inc., 41 East 11th Street, New York, NY 10003

Printed in the United States of America

Library of Congress Cataloging-in-Publication Data

Immunopharmacology of infectious diseases.

(Progress in leukocyte biology ; v. 6)
Consists of 30 papers presented at a conference held in July 1986 in Columbia, Md. as a satellite to the Sixth International Congress of Immunology in Toronto, Ont.
Includes index.
1. Immunopharmacology—Congresses. 2. Communicable diseases—Immunological aspects—Congresses. I. Majde, Jeannine A. II. International Congress of Immunology (6th : 1986 : Toronto, Ont.) III. Series. [DNLM: 1. Adjuvants, Immunologic—pharmacodynamics—congresses. 2. Antigens—immunology—congresses. 3. Infection—prevention & control—congresses. W1 PR6703 v.6 / QW 800 I335 1986]
RM370.I463 1987 616.9'0461 87-27723
ISBN 0-8451-4105-8

Dedication

This volume is dedicated to the memory of Dr. Edgar E. Ribi, whose breadth of investigations on the chemical, physical, and biological properties of adjuvants over a thirty-year period has stimulated many scientists in this and related fields. His recent achievement in chemically modifying bacterial lipopolysaccharides such as to remove their toxicity while retaining their adjuvant action has been a true milestone in adjuvant research; it is now realistic to consider the use of these potent immunomodulators in man. His insight, persistence, and meticulousness in the laboratory were exemplary of a true scientist. A tragic accident that resulted in his death on August 31, 1986 has left a real void in the ranks of adjuvant researchers.

Contents

Contributors

Anthony C. Allison, Institute of Biological Sciences, Syntex Research, Palo Alto, CA 94304 **[17,191]**

Carl R. Alving, Department of Membrane Biochemistry, Walter Reed Army Institute of Research, Washington, DC 20307-5100 **[171]**

F. Audibert, Department of Pharmacology and Therapeutics, Unversity of South Florida, College of Medicine, Tampa, FL 33612 **[203]**

Ichiro Azuma, Institute of Immunological Science, Hokkaido University, Sapporo 060, Japan **[245]**

William R. Beisel, Department of Immunology and Infectious Diseases, The Johns Hopkins School of Hygiene and Public Health, Baltimore, MD 21205 **[51]**

Beth Bennett, Department of Pathology, Emory University, Atlanta, GA 30322 **[181]**

Robert H.R. Bomford, Department of Experimental Immunobiology, The Wellcome Research Laboratories, Beckenham, Kent BR3 3BS, England **[165]**

Helmut Brade, Forschungsinstitut Borstel, D-2061 Borstel, Federal Republic of Germany **[75]**

Lore Brade, Forschungsinstitut Borstel, D-2061 Borstel, Federal Republic of Germany **[75]**

Noelene E. Byars, Institute of Biological Sciences, Syntex Research, Palo Alto, CA 94304 **[191]**

Raymond Castagna, Department of Microbiology and Immunology, SUNY, Health Science Center at Brooklyn, Brooklyn, NY 11203 **[113]**

Louis Chedid, Department of Pharmacology and Therapeutics, University of South Florida Medical College, Tampa, FL 33612 **[1,213]**

John D. Clements, Department of Microbiology and Immunology, Tulane University School of Medicine, New Orleans, LA 70112 **[139]**

John P. Craig, Department of Microbiology and Immunology, SUNY, Health Science Center at Brooklyn, Brooklyn, NY 11203 **[113]**

Robert M. Crawford, Department of Immunology, Walter Reed Army Institute of Research, Washington, DC 20307-5100 **[27]**

Charles E. Davis, Department of Immunology, Walter Reed Army Institute of Research, Washington, DC 20307-5100 **[27]**

The numbers in brackets are the opening page numbers of the contributors' articles.

Peter Dukor, Research Department, Pharmaceuticals Division, CIBA-GEIGY Limited, CH-4002 Basel, Switzerland **[255]**

David S. Finbloom, Department of Immunology, Walter Reed Army Institute of Research, Washington, DC 20307-5100 **[27]**

Anne H. Fortier, Department of Immunology, Walter Reed Army Institute of Research, Washington, DC 20307-5100 **[27]**

Robert F. Garry, Department of Microbiology and Immunology, Tulane University School of Medicine, New Orleans, LA 70112 **[139]**

Micheal J. Gilbreath, Department of Immunology, Walter Reed Army Institute of Research, Washington, DC 20307-5100 **[27]**

Yoji Goto, Kitasato Institute, Minato-ku, Tokyo 108, Japan **[223]**

John W. Hadden, Program of Immunopharmacology, University of South Florida Medical College, Tampa, FL 33612 **[337]**

Kazuhiro Harada, Department of Bacteriology, Osaka Prefectural Institute for Public Health, Higashinari-ku, Osaka 537, Japan **[223]**

Wayne T. Hockmeyer, Department of Immunology, Walter Reed Army Institute of Research, Washington, DC 20307-5100 **[171]**

Robert L. Hunter, Department of Pathology, Emory University, Atlanta, GA 30322 **[181]**

Joji Iida, Institute of Immunological Science, Hokkaido University, Sapporo 060, Japan **[245]**

Takako Ikeda, Department of Microbiology and Oral Microbiology, Osaka University Dental School, Suita, Osaka 565, Japan **[223]**

Chiaki Ishihara, Institute of Immunological Science, Hokkaido University, Sapporo 060, Japan **[245]**

Masaaki Ishizuka, Institute for Chemotherapy, Microbial Chemistry Research Foundation, Numazu, Shizuoka, Japan 410-03 **[303]**

Arthur G. Johnson, Department of Microbiology, University of Minnesota, School of Medicine, Duluth, MN 55812 **[291]**

Eve W. Johnson, Department of Microbiology, University of Texas Medical Branch, Galveston, TX 77550 **[61]**

Michel Joseph, Institut Pasteur, 59019 Lille-Cedex, France **[267]**

Shozo Kotani, Department of Microbiology and Oral Microbiology, Osaka University Dental School, Suita, Osaka 565, Japan **[223]**

Shoichi Kusumoto, Department of Chemistry, Faculty of Science, Osaka University, Toyonaka, Osaka 560, Japan **[91,223]**

Phillippe Lagrange, Institut Pasteur, 75724 Paris-Cedex 15, France **[267]**

Edward R. Leake, Department of Microbiology and Immunology, The Medical College of Pennsylvania, Philadelphia, PA 19129 **[313]**

E. Lederer, Institut de Biochimie, Université Paris-Sud, 91405 Orsay, France **[155]**

G. Lemaire, Institut de Biochimie, Université Paris-Sud, 91405 Orsay, France **[155]**

K.N. Leung, Department of Biochemistry and Chinese Medicinal Research Center, The Chinese University of Hong Kong, Shatin, N.T., Hong Kong **[325]**

Frank L. Lyon, Department of Microbiology and Immunology, Tulane University School of Medicine, New Orleans, LA 70112 **[139]**

Jeannine A. Majde, Biological Sciences Division, Office of Naval Research, Arlington, VA 22217 **[xix]**

K. Noel Masihi, Robert Koch Institute, Federal Health Office, West Berlin, Federal Republic of Germany **[101]**

Kim W. McIntyre, Department of Pathology, University of Massachusetts Medical School, Worcester, MA 01605 **[41]**

Monte S. Meltzer, Department of Immunology, Walter Reed Army Institute of Research, Washington, DC 20307-5100 **[27]**

Robert I. Mishell, Department of Microbiology and Immunology, University of California at Berkeley, Berkeley, CA 94720 **[125]**

Page S. Morahan, Department of Microbiology and Immunology, The Medical College of Pennsylvania, Philadelphia, PA 19129 **[313]**

Carol A. Nacy, Department of Immunology, Walter Reed Army Institute of Research, Washington, DC 20307-5100 **[27]**

Robert J. Natuk, Department of Pathology, University of Massachusetts Medical School, Worcester, MA 01605 **[41]**

Keiko Nishimura, Institute of Immunological Science, Hokkaido University, Sapporo 060, Japan **[245]**

Tomohiko Ogawa, Department of Microbiology and Oral Microbiology, Osaka University Dental School, Suita, Osaka 565, Japan **[223]**

Haruki Okamura, Department of Bacteriology, Hyogo College of Medicine, Nishinomiya, Hyogo 663, Japan **[223]**

Monique A. Parant, Lab Immunopharmacologie, Centre National de la Recherche Scientifique, Institut Biomédical des Cordeliers 15, rue de l'Ecole-de-Médecine, 75270 Paris Cedex 06, France **[235]**

Marc Pascal, Laboratoires Fournier, Research Center, Daix, 21121 Fontaine les Dijon, France **[267]**

J.F. Petit, Institut de Biochimie, Université Paris-Sud, 91405 Orsay, France **[155]**

Edgar Ribi, Ribi ImmunoChem Research, Inc., Hamilton, MT 59840 **[101]**

Karen A. Richard, Department of Hypersensitivity Diseases Research, The Upjohn Company, Kalamazoo, MI 49001 **[279]**

Roberta L. Richards, Department of Membrane Biochemistry, Walter Reed Army Institute of Research, Washington, DC 20307-5100 **[171]**

Ernst Th. Rietschel, Forschungsinstitut Borstel, D-2061 Borstel, Federal Republic of Germany **[75]**

Gilles Riveau, Department of Pharmacology and Therapeutics, University of South Florida, College of Medicine, Tampa, FL 33612 **[213]**

Ulrich Schade, Forschungsinstitut Borstel, D-2061 Borstel, Federal Republic of Germany **[75]**

Robert D. Schreiber, Department of Immunology, Walter Reed Army Institute of Research, Washington, DC 20307-5100 **[27]**

Gebhard Schumann, Research Department, Pharmaceuticals Division, CIBA-GEIGY Limited, CH-4002 Basel, Switzerland **[255]**

Tetsuo Shiba, Department of Chemistry, Faculty of Science, Osaka University, Toyonaka, Osaka 560, Japan **[91,223]**

Hidetoshi Shimauchi, Department of Microbiology and Oral Microbiology, Osaka University Dental School, Suita, Osaka 565, Japan **[223]**

Mary Sit, Department of Microbiology and Immunology, The Medical College of Pennsylvania, Philadelphia, PA 19129 **[313]**

Eric M. Smith, Departments of Microbiology and Psychiatry and Behavioral Sciences, University of Texas Medical Branch, Galveston, TX 77550 **[61]**

Barnet M. Sultzer, Department of Microbiology and Immunology, SUNY, Health Science Center at Brooklyn, Brooklyn, NY 11203 **[113]**

Haruhiko Takada, Department of Microbiology and Oral Microbiology, Osaka University Dental School, Suita, Osaka 565, Japan **[223]**

Ichiro Takahashi, Department of Microbiology and Oral Microbiology, Osaka University Dental School, Suita, Osaka 565, Japan **[223]**

Takashi Takahashi, Kitasato Institute, Minato-ku, Tokyo 108, Japan **[223]**

Tomio Takeuchi, Institute for Chemotherapy, Microbial Chemistry Research Foundation, Numazu, Shizuoka, Japan 410-03 **[303]**

Toshihide Tamura, Department of Bacteriology, Hyogo College of Medicine, Nishinomiya, Hyogo 663, Japan **[223]**

Shigenori Tanaka, Tokyo Research Institute, Seikagaku Kogyo Co. Ltd., Higashiyamato, Tokyo 189, Japan **[223]**

Daniel J. Tenney, Department of Microbiology and Immunology, The Medical College of Pennsylvania, Philadelphia, PA 19129 **[313]**

J.P. Tenu, Institut de Biochimie, Université Paris-Sud, 91405 Orsay, France **[155]**

Daniel E. Tracey, Department of Hypersensitivity Diseases Research, The Upjohn Company, Kalamazoo, MI 49001 **[279]**

Masachika Tsujimoto, Department of Microbiology and Oral Microbiology, Osaka University Dental School, Suita, Osaka 565, Japan **[223]**

J. Terry Ulrich, Ribi ImmunoChem Research, Inc., Hamilton, MT 59840 **[101]**

Hamao Umezawa, Institute for Chemotherapy, Microbial Chemistry Research Foundation, Numazu, Shizuoka, Japan 410-03 **[303]**

William R. Usinger, Department of Microbiology and Immunology, University of California at Berkeley, Berkeley, CA 94720 **[125]**

Raymond M. Welsh, Department of Pathology, University of Massachusetts Medical School, Worcester, MA 01605 **[41]**

Robert A. Wirtz, Department of Entomology, Walter Reed Army Institute of Research, Washington, DC 20307-5100 **[171]**

Yuichi Yamamura, Osaka University, Suita 565, Japan **[245]**

H.W. Yeung, Department of Biochemistry and Chinese Medicinal Research Center, The Chinese University of Hong Kong, Shatin, N.T., Hong Kong **[325]**

Ulrich Zähringer, Forschungsinstitut Borstel, D-2061 Borstel, Federal Republic of Germany **[75]**

Foreword

This series of books, PROGRESS IN LEUKOCYTE BIOLOGY, and the *Journal of Leukocyte Biology* are published by Alan R. Liss, Inc., for the Reticuloendothelial Society.

The series focuses on the biology of granulocytes, lymphocytes, and mononuclear phagocytes. This includes topics relating to the origins and developmental biology of these cells, their mechanism(s) of interpopulation communication, and the means by which they destroy infectious organisms, foreign tissue, or neoplastic cells.

In order to maintain the highest quality possible, there is an advisory board that recommends and approves publications in this series. The Publication Committee of the RES Society serves as the core of the board. In addition, a small number of key people throughout the world have been invited who are recognized for their expertise in granulocyte, lymphocyte, and macrophage biology.

This is an exciting area and it is growing in importance. We hope to capture the essence of this dialogue and continue to provide state-of-the-art coverage of this unfolding story.

Sherwood M. Reichard

Preface

This volume focuses on two relatively new fields of immunopharmacology: vaccine adjuvants and modulators of non-specific resistance. While these fields may appear operationally distinct, they are combined here because they are functionally interlocking at several levels. Both are concerned with stimulating immune function: adjuvants are defined here as substances that stimulate immune responses to vaccines; immunomodulators, in the context of this volume, are substances that stimulate those host defense functions that permit an organism to more effectively resist invasion of pathogens or bring under control a successful invader. The concepts discussed here represent an apparent radical departure from traditional immunopharmacology, which is directed at blockade of the immune system in inflammatory diseases and tissue transplantation. However, as our awareness of immunoregulatory processes increases, it appears that some of the targets and key events in each of these aspects of immunopharmacology may be the same.

In this volume, however, we are addressing those immunoregulatory substances that are active in inducing resistance to infectious diseases; adjuvants in prophylaxis and immunomodulators in therapy. An emphasis is placed on advances in vaccine adjuvants for two reasons:

Firstly, the adjuvant concept is narrower and more readily defined. The very narrowness of the concept offers a window to pharmacologic manipulation of the immune system in general. By drawing upon practical experience with adjuvants we can deduce structural principles that have a much broader application in immunopharmacology.

Secondly, the ongoing revolution in vaccine design, combined with the urgent need for improved vaccine design in the context of the Acquired Immunodeficiency Disease Syndrome (AIDS) epidemic, makes advances in vaccine adjuvants a most timely subject. Developments in biotechnology offer exciting alternatives to crude, often toxic, killed vaccines or potentially treacherous attenuated ones by providing a means for economically producing pure peptide antigens for use in immunization. However, such elegant materials lack the intrinsic adjuvanticity of whole organisms and often require the use of Freund's complete adjuvant, a preparation too toxic for human use, in order to express protective immunogenicity. The development of a non-toxic vaccine adjuvant that can efficiently potentiate protective immunity to an associated antigen will have a profound impact on both human and animal health.

Drugs directed at stimulating non-specific resistance to invasive disease represent a relatively new direction in Western medicine, which has long focused on drugs that inhibit the microbe or cancer cell. In the mid-1970's immunomodulatory drugs were found that had broad-spectrum utility in animal models of cancer as well as viral, bacterial, and fungal infections. These drugs have to date proved disappointing in the clinics when compared to conventional antibacterials and antineoplastics. Indeed the term "immunomodulator" has evolved to more accurately describe the subtle, occasionally negative or neutral effects of many of these drugs. Yet employing the host's own defenses offers, in theory, an elegant (and potentially non-toxic) approach to dealing with those microbial pathogens (most viruses and fungi, many bacteria and parasites) that have resisted our best efforts at specific pharmacologic attack. Furthermore, if our conception of the role of the immune response in resistance to the lethal course of cancer is accurate, the same immunopotentiating drugs should offer a far less toxic approach to controlling this scourge. However, the principle of "stimulating the phagocyte," in the words of George Bernard Shaw, remains a tantalizing if elusive approach to control of the body's invaders.

With these considerations in mind, this book has been assembled to bring together recent advances in molecular aspects of vaccine adjuvants and to sample some of the work being conducted all over the world with immunomodulators that have been examined in infectious models. The first brief section consists of an historical perspective of both fields by a pioneer in molecular immunopharmacology, Dr. Louis Chedid. The second section looks at some of the potential targets of immunopotentiators less frequently examined in this context, including physiological responses. The next two sections address rather comprehensively developments in microbially-derived and synthetic adjuvants. Finally, a variety of candidate immunomodulators, both old and new, are discussed, including traditional Chinese medicinals. The volume ends with an overview of the field of immunomodulators by Dr. John Hadden.

The assembly of this material is intended not only to inform but to stimulate the formulation of much-needed hypotheses that appear to be required for breakthroughs in immunopotentiator research. The AIDS epidemic has disturbed our complacency regarding our ability to control infectious diseases in industrial nations. While the therapeutic thrust of the attack on AIDS continues along conventional antibiotic lines, the massive assembly of resources offers an opportunity to drive research in new directions as well. This is already apparent in vaccine design. We offer this body of knowledge on vaccine adjuvants and immunomodulators as a point of departure for innovative research on all of the infectious diseases, major and minor, left to conquer. The potential of immunopharmacology in this context is yet to be tapped.

Jeannine A. Majde

Acknowledgments

This volume consists of 30 papers presented at an international conference that was convened in July, 1986, to assess the status of basic research on vaccine adjuvants and modulators of non-specific resistance to infectious agents. The conference was held in Columbia, Maryland, as a satellite to the Sixth International Congress of Immunology in Toronto, Ontario, Canada. Nineteen countries were represented. If vigorous discussion can be considered an index of success, the conference was indeed successful.

We wish especially to thank the sponsors of the conference, the Office of Naval Research, the Army Medical Research and Development Command, and the Air Force Office of Scientific Research. The support of these U.S. Department of Defense research agencies made the conference a reality.

Appreciation is also due to the program committee, chaired by Dr. Jeannine Majde and consisting of Dr. Louis Chedid, Dr. Arthur Johnson, and Dr. Shozo Kotani, who developed the essential structure of the meeting. We are also grateful to Dr. Sherwood Reichard and his staff in the Reticuloendothelial Society for their expert handling of the conference logistics.

Dr. Reichard and the executives of the Reticuloendothelial Society were also responsible for arranging the publication of these proceedings with the cooperation of Ms. Paulette Cohen of Alan R. Liss, Inc. The focus of this conference is quite unique, and we feel that this publication, combined with that of the extended abstracts of the poster sessions (available from the editor), document a body of work that is otherwise difficult to access.

Finally, we wish to thank the speakers, poster presenters, and other participants in the conference who provided its substance. We trust they will draw upon their shared knowledge in the years to come.

Immunopharmacology of Infectious Diseases: Vaccine Adjuvants and Modulators of Non-Specific Resistance, pages 1–15

MODULATION OF NON-SPECIFIC RESISTANCE TO INFECTION: REPORT ON A PILGRIM'S PROGRESS

Louis CHEDID

Immunothérapie Expérimentale, Institut Pasteur, Paris, France

Medical concepts have always oscillated between the hippocratic and the magical poles. The view of Hippocrates was that health represented a harmonious balance between four elements: water, fire, air and earth, and that disease resulted from the loss of that equilibrium. The more ancient approach (which existed in prehistorical times and is still practised widely by witch doctors) considers disease as the consequence of evil spirits invading the host. Charles Nicole has written very stimulating pages on the influence of religion on microbiology and vice-versa. Disease as a punishment of our immoral deeds is still strongly embedded in certain of our present day attitudes towards herpes or AIDS. In Ancient Egypt, high priests were also sophisticated physicians and surgeons. One can speculate that religious rites such as shaving, washing and especially purifying their instruments by fire were incidentally very successful recipes which contributed largely to protecting them from epidemics and enabling them to perform safely delicate operations on the brain and on the eye. Interestingly, Louis Pasteur's studies are related to the magical concept since they were based on the invasion of the host by evil microorganisms. The "magic bullet" concept is supported even more strictly by the notion of a direct interaction between foreign agents and microorganisms. Pasteurs's microbiological discoveries were initiated by observations made during investigations for the wine industry, and later he often used the word "putrefaction" or "fermentation of the blood" to describe disease. Nevertheless, the hippocratic dream of restoring or increasing health by influencing the host has attracted during the ages many investigators who wished to enhance what we now call "nonspecific immunity".

Although based on fragile evidence it has often been assumed that one disease excludes another. One of the best examples is the theory that tuberculosis can decrease susceptibility to cancer. This has initiated the tremendous corpus of work which was built around the experimental use of BCG. Another most widely used immunostimulant has been our beloved endotoxin. In many experimental models, minute amounts of lipopolysaccharide (LPS) have so markedly protected mice against a broad spectrum of infections that it seems reasonable to believe that this approach would indeed have been developed had antibiotics not been discovered.

Since it is the privilege of a keynote speaker to be autobiographical, allow me to tell you how I started my career as an endocrinologist and how important it was for me to meet in succession Hans Selye and René Dubos. Selye, as you all know, is the father of the stress syndrome. The agent which he routinely used to stimulate the hypophysis-adrenal axis was formalin. For some obscure reason, I chose to use endotoxins. This was a very lucky choice since it allowed us to discover with Monique and Francine Parant that adrenalectomized mice were 100,000-fold more susceptible to endotoxin, whereas their resistance to exotoxins remained unchanged. The latter, as you know, are controlled by humoral antibodies. In contrast, cortisone or rather glucocorticoids, must be considered as major endogenous products regulating non-specifically our resistance to endotoxic shock (Chedid and Boyer, 1951). The endocrine system plays a major role in resistance to infections. There exist innumerable examples of variations of morbidity and mortality related to hormonal factors such as diabetes or hypothyroiditis. Of course, we must not forget the influence of sex and admit with humility that in regard to disease, like in most other aspects of life, males represent the weaker sex not only during adult life but also after or even before birth. Curiously, nature seems to compensate this weakness by producing a greater number of male foetuses.

There exists a bizarre tendency to overlook also the role of the central nervous system as a major factor of immunity. The brain was only "discovered" 2500 years ago. Historically, the heart, the liver, the lungs, the abdomen have been most favored seats of the soul. In Ancient Egypt, when the Pharaoh was embalmed, great care was taken to place his heart in a separate sacred urn and only one organ was disdainfully removed and thrown away into the sands of the desert. This organ was the brain. Until recently, immunologists have adopted this same disrespectful attitude. Today, we are becoming overwhelmed by the number of bridges which exist between the central nervous and the immune systems and one can predict that the existing dichotomy will fade away. I have always been astonished by the fact that nobody was surprised to find that the best antigen for production of theta-antiserum was the brain. Even more astonishing is the fact that during the past 50 years fever has been regarded mostly as an adverse reaction. Should not the elevation of body temperature rather be considered as one of the host's most primitive and potent nonspecific immune response? Yet, as early as 2400 years ago Hippocrates (460-375 BC) wrote: "Those who have quartan fever (malaria) rarely have convulsions; those who have convulsions and later catch quartan fever are cured of their convulsions" (Aphorisms V, 70). The beneficial role of fever has been stated repeatedly during the centuries which have elapsed between Hippocrates and Wagner-Jauregg, who received the Nobel Prize in 1927 because of the therapeutic use of malarial pyrexia. Several decades previously, Louis Pasteur had recognized the role of fever in resistance to *Anthrax*. He assumed that birds' refractoriness to *Anthrax* was related to their normally higher temperature which inhibited the proliferation of this bacillus. He showed by heating rabbits that they became more resistant, whereas fowls became more susceptible if their temperature was lowered. He did not hesitate to write in his memorable report that "if this discovery is fully substantiated we could hope to cure a man infected by *Anthrax*... by elevating his temperature" (see in Chedid *et al.*, 1982). A century later, similar experiments with various animal species have shown that pyrexia does enhance resistance to infection in a very large number of species. For instance, following inoculation of microbial organisms, ectotherms will select a warmer environmental temperature and therefore fever can be developed by this process in many nonmammalian vertebrates. Thus, goldfish whose lower temperature preference is 28°C will survive after being infected with *Aeromonas hydrophila* if they maintain themselves at 33°C, whereas they will die at 25.5°C (Covert and Reynolds, 1977). Similar experiments have been performed in mammals. When rabbits were infected with *Pasteurella multocida*, a beneficial effect was observed if their temperature was increased about 2°C, whereas a statistically higher mortality rate was observed when it was lowered by administration of sodium salicylate (Vaughn *et al.*, 1980). It seems rather paradoxical that selection should have retained such a costly process as fever if it were not extremely important for survival. (It is calculated that a rise in body temperature of 3°C will result in approximately 25% of increased energy expenditure). Temperature elevation can enhance resistance to infection by a general increase of metabolism and by ridding the host of thermosensitive bacterial and viral agents. In harmony with this view are the insistent warnings of A. Lwoff against antipyretic drugs and their paradoxical use and abuse in certain viral infections (Lwoff, 1959). It is probably most unfortunate that aspirin, besides being antipyretic, relieves discomfort and headache, leading people to believe that its use is more beneficial than it really is during infectious diseases.

More recently, a great deal of interest has been devoted to macrophage factor/s responsible for production of fever, of acute phase reactants and also of lymphocyte-activating factor (LAF). As a matter of fact, a consensus developed stating that several monokines previously identified as being separate entities represented different facets of the same molecule which was called therefore Interleukin-1 (IL-1). Other monokines playing an important role in the host's natural resistance, such as interferon or tumor necrotizing factor (TNF), are also markedly increased by incubating cells with bacteria or viruses. As cloning experiments have shown, these last two agents are clearly different from LAF or LP, although under certain conditions they can be produced simultaneously by immunostimulants such as LPS. In contrast, it is possible to induce both LAF and LP without interferon by incubating cells with MDP and even LAF without LP by using an analog of MDP. As will be described later, muramyl peptides were at first identified and studied as adjuvants. Yet very soon they were also found to be capable of enhancing nonspecific resistance to infection.

The ability of MDP and some of its derivatives to stimulate nonspecific resistance of animals has been demonstrated against pathogenic microorganisms including *Klebsiella pneumoniae*, *Salmonella*, *Streptococcus pneumoniae*, *Pseudomonas aeruginosa*, *Candida albicans*, *Listeria monocytogenes* as well as *Toxoplasma gondii*, *Trypanosoma cruzii* (see in Chedid *et al.*, in press). More recently, certain muramyl peptides have been shown to prevent and even to cure several viral infections (Dietrich *et al.*, 1983; Acevedo *et al.*, 1985). In contrast to BCG or other bacterial products such as lipopolysaccharides (LPS) which are effective only when administered by the parenteral route, the protective effects of MDP and its derivatives have been observed when given by several routes including orally. Most interesting is the fact that, in mice immunodepressed by chemotherapy or radiotherapy, muramyl peptides have also increased nonspecific resistance to a challenge with *Klebsiella pneumoniae*, a common pathogen in immunocompromised cancer patients. Equally noteworthy is the finding that MDP could exhibit protective effects even against organisms rendered resistant to antibiotics, in the infectious model of mouse neonates which are known to have a poor immune status and to be highly susceptible to infections. Finally, beneficial effects of MDP and some of its derivatives have been demonstrated in mice previously splenectomized at 7 days of age and rendered therefore extremely susceptible as adults to *Klebsiella* or *Pneumococcus* challenge (Chedid *et al.*, in press). These data are of special relevance to human conditions where patients undergo splenectomy, e.g. auto-immune disorders, leukemias and lymphomas including Hodgkin's diseases.

How does the capacity of MDP to activate macrophages and to produce fever relate to resistance to infection? Kluger showed that fever protected rabbits infected with *Pasteurella multocida* (Kluger and Vaughn, 1978). *In vitro* studies allowed him to demonstrate that concomitant increase of temperature and decrease of iron and zinc levels in the blood could check the growth without killing the organisms (Kluger and Rothenberg, 1979). This inhibition is related to the influence of temperature on the "iron pump" which being blocked can no longer actively concentrate these ions. Low internal iron level allows the organisms to survive but hinder several of the syntheses required for production of virulence structures. We have been able to obtain similar results using *Klebsiella* and the serum of rabbits pretreated by either LPS or by MDP at dosages which produce very high fever. In rabbits the minimal pyrogenic dose of MDP is 25 μg/kg, and during the febrile response circulating LP can be detected. Besides, its capacity to elicit fever LP can produce hypoferremia, hyper-cupremia and an increase in the synthesis of serum acute-phase proteins by the liver (Dinarello, 1984). Our *in vitro* experiments showed that Klebsiella organisms proliferated much less when they were incubated at high temperature in serum samples obtained from rabbits pretreated with MDP (and which had a 50% reduction of its iron content). The morphology of these organisms is changed and so is their virulence if they are administered to normal mice.

At this stage, one could assume that the rapid production of LP by activated macrophages is capable of modifying the virulent phenotype by the combined action of fever and lowered metal concentration in the blood. These organisms would become more susceptible to phagocytosis and lysis by the RES. It can be easily assumed that several other factors such as acute-phase reactants must also be engaged in such a process. However, the above explanation (temperature increase and iron decrease) cannot explain that a non-pyrogenic derivative of MDP, Murabutide, can still enhance nonspecific resistance to Klebsiella.

As stated previously, MDP is a strong but selective macrophage activator. Thus, it is possible to induce separately LAF or LP by incubating phagocytic cells with certain MDP derivatives. By using certain MDP derivatives such as Murabutide it has been possible to selectively produce *in vivo* and *in vitro* LAF in the absence of LP (Damais *et al.*, 1982) and also without altering the circulating metal levels. Incidentally, these results also suggest that LAF production may be independent for MDP-induced hypoferremia and hypercupremia (Riveau *et al.*, 1986). Therefore, Murabutide is not pyrogenic, does not produce hypoferremia or endogenous pyrogen in rabbits, and yet can protect mice against *Klebsiella*. There must therefore exist, besides these mechanisms, one or several other nonspecific factors. An interesting candidate could be tumor necrotizing factor (TNF). As mentioned, macrophage activation produces several monokines other than IL-1 such as TNF. Indeed, recent experiments have shown us that cloned TNF increases resistance to bacterial and fungal infections (Parant *et al.*, 1986). Moreover, we have preliminary evidence that Murabutide can produce *in vitro* TNF and LAF without producing LP.

Since this Meeting is entitled also Immunological Adjuvants, I would like to share with you some personal views and to recall certain findings which have been very rewarding in this field.

I believe that it is fair to consider Ramon (1925) as the inventor of adjuvants (Ramon, 1925). He observed that the sera of horses he had immunized with diphtheria toxin had a greatly increased antitoxic titer if they had abscesses at the inoculation site. He then intentionally administered the toxin with pus or with "suppuration microbes". Again, the antitoxic capacity of the serum was enhanced. Later, he substituted other inflammatory agents such as bread crumbs or even tapioca and found that they were very effective enhancers of the immune response. Moreover, Ramon predicted that: "However interesting they may be for application, they are at least as valuable because of the investigations that they may generate in order to understand the intimate mechanisms of the production of antitoxins".

Most bacterial or viral products can enhance or down-modulate the immune response to an associated antigen. Endotoxins, as was discovered by Arthur Johnson, are most powerful immunological adjuvants (Johnson *et al.*, 1956). However, special attention must be given to Mycobacteria.

Independently from Ramon, Lewis had injected various antigens to guinea pigs which he had infected with virulent tuberculosis bacilli (Lewis and Loomis, 1924). He noticed that during this "allergic irritability" they produced high titers of antibodies. In the following years, Dienes reported that the response to ovalbumin was increased if the antigen was injected directly into tuberculous lesions (Dienes and Schoenheit, 1926). He also reported for the first time, I believe, the state of delayed sensitivity. It still remained to be shown that the same results could be obtained with killed Mycobacteria. Many years earlier (1897), Rabinowitsch had observed that saprophytic *M.butyricum*, if injected in butter, produced a lesion identical to virulent Mycobacteria (Rabinowitsch, 1897). This result inspired Coulaud and prompted him in 1934 to administer killed Mycobacteria in paraffin and to observe that this mixture produced a positive reaction to tuberculin (Coulaud, 1934). Freund in 1937, as a spin-off from serum complement studies, noticed that a guinea pig which had been injected with killed Mycobacteria a year earlier still presented positive tuberculin reactions (Freund *et al.*, 1937). However, such a recipe did not induce any effect vis-à-vis another antigen administered with killed Mycobacteria in mineral oil. It was in 1942 that he obtained the desired result by injecting antigens with killed bacteria in a water-in-oil emulsion. This preparation called Freund's complete adjuvant (FCA) is probably the most powerful adjuvant existing in our laboratories (Freund and McDermott, 1942). Its use has opened the avenues to many important discoveries such as autoimmunity, modulation of isotypes, and, of course, cell-mediated immunity. However, FCA is too toxic for use outside of the laboratory, mainly because it contains non-metabolizable mineral oil, and because the mycobacterial elements elicit severe granulomatous reactions.

Interestingly, Freund wrote in 1947 that: "It would be of great interest to identify the fraction or fractions which exert the adjuvant effect of Mycobacteria, and to know whether the effect could be produced without sensitization to tuberculin" (Freund, 1947). This question has been answered successfully: the component has been identified and does not sensitize to tuberculin. These studies have also led to the discovery of a most interesting family of molecules which are endowed with many other interesting immunopharmacological activities. I must add that personally they have rewarded me tremendously, scientifically and otherwise, since they made me meet with Edgar Lederer and work with him for many years.

After Freund's discovery, a progressive series of biochemical studies attempting to purify the active adjuvant components gradually succeeded in isolating ever smaller compounds. The search culminated with the discovery by Lederer's team of a natural monosaccharide-tripeptide (Ellouz *et al.*, 1974), and a synthetic monosaccharide dipeptide (Merser *et al.* 1975). Thus, the smallest structure possible that still resulted in adjuvant activity was N-acetylmuramyl-L-alanyl-D-isoglutamine or muramyl dipeptide (MDP). Very shortly after, Kotani and his colleagues (1975) achieved the same result. A family of similar compounds was rapidly synthesized and tested for adjuvant and other biological properties. Several investigators then examined the relationship between chemical structure and adjuvanticity (Chedid *et al.*, 1976; Azuma *et al.* 1976). Since that time MDP and MDP derivatives have been studied intensively and demonstrated to have numerous, potent, diverse and interesting properties. While many immunopharmacological activities may be clinically undesirable, they can often be dissociated from one another through the use of MDP derivatives. This allows selection of compounds that are adjuvant-active, yet non-toxic.

A most exciting finding was that certain pyrogenic derivatives of MDP are also capable of enhancing slow-wave sleep (SWS). Krueger, Pappenheimer and Karnovsky had previously isolated and purified slow-wave sleep factor from human urine and from brains of sleep-deprived animals, and shown it to be a muramyl peptide of a molecular weight close to 1000 (Krueger *et al.*, 1982a). This discovery led the investigators to study the influence of synthetic adjuvant-active muramyl peptides (Krueger *et al.*, 1982b). After icv perfusion of MDP or MDP-Lys in rabbits and in other animal species, a significant increase of SWS was observed. The somnogenic activity of MDP was also demonstrated in rabbits by parenteral and even by oral administration. Other authors have also reported that in rats iv injections of LPS or bacterial peptidoglycans and more recently of MDP (Masek and Kadlec, 1983) could produce various sleep modifications.

Inactive stereoisomers and certain adjuvant-active derivatives of MDP, which are nonpyrogenic, such as Murabutide, are also devoid of somnogenic activity. Nevertheless, pyrogenic and somnogenic activity of MDP can be dissociated. Thus, previous treatment of rabbits by acetaminophen inhibits the febrile response to MDP without changing its somnogenic activity (Krueger *et al.*, 1982b). Stereotactic lesions and studies on 5-hydroxytryptamine (5HT) metabolism suggest the involvement of neuromediators in modifications of sleep and thermoregulation by peptidoglycans. It has been shown that supernatants of MDP-treated macrophages or even purified IL-1 can also enhance both fever and slow-wave sleep (Krueger *et al.*, 1984). However, mechanisms by which MDP affects SWS and the consequence of this enhancement are still unknown. The possible role of SWS as a factor in immunity may constitute an important new area for future neuro-immunopharmacological studies.

Now let us open another chapter of this talk. The most effective way to influence infectious diseases has been prevention by vaccines and we are now entering into the Second Century of Louis Pasteur. Instead of conventional vaccines we are producing constructs with totally synthetic adjuvants and antigens.

Synthetic vaccines containing viral, bacterial, parasitic and hormonal synthetic antigens have been described and constitute a very rapidly expanding field of research. Although it can be safely predicted that the next modern vaccines will most likely be obtained by recombinant DNA methods, the "synthetic" approach still has certain theoretical superiorities vis-à-vis the "genetic" one. Thus, molecules containing less than 40 residues should be easier and cheaper to produce by synthesis and their safety and purity easier to control. Besides, these methods have the unique capacity of designing artificial sequences more immunogenic than the natural molecules. Today, the success of such a strategy has been repeatedly demonstrated in the field of hormones or other natural substances. A great deal of effort is now being devoted to the development of malarial vaccines employing synthetic antigens or fusion proteins since it has not been possible to produce effective malarial vaccines by conventional means. Recently, the structure of the *Plasmodium falciparum* circumsporozoite protein (considered as being the best candidate for a vaccine) was described (Dame *et al.*, 1984; Enea *et al.*, 1984). A copy of this protein was genetically engineered in *Escherichia coli* and synthetic peptides were constructed copying this structure. Both approaches have produced antigens which induced biologically active antibodies in experimental models (Balou *et al.*, 1985; Young *et al.*, 1985) and are being evaluated in human trials. The aim of these studies was to design models of synthetic vaccines presenting as few limitations as possible and capable of producing protective antibodies. These results also demonstrated that since synthetic structures can enhance the induction of biologically active antibodies (which are end-products) they are also able to stimulate the required previous sequences of nonspecific responses. They, therefore, allow us to find our way in view of identifying peptide sequences and conformational requirements of adjuvant-antigen constructs. In a way, these studies may some day represent a Rosetta Stone showing us that a small number of elements differently combined can confer a very large variety of signals. Although we are still groping in the dark, we may be entering an era which will give us a powerful tool and a better understanding of cell biology. In this respect, some exciting metaphorical knowledge may be gained by considering the analogies existing between immunology and language, and particularly the phonetic rules of English (see in Farb, 1975).

Noam Chomsky, the father of generative grammar, has written: "The central fact to which any significant linguistic theory must address itself is this: a mature speaker can produce a new sentence of his language on the appropriate occasion, and other speakers can understand it immediately, though it is equally new to them... Grammar is a device that specifies the infinite set of well-formed sentences and assigns to each of these one or more structural descriptions. Perhaps we should call such a device a *generative grammar*... which should, ideally, contain a central syntactic component..., a phonological component and a semantic component" (Chomsky, 1964). For a better understanding of "immuno-linguistics", there remains at least two difficult problems to solve. For Jerne, who quotes this passage in a most interesting article, it seems hard to find the equivalents of meaningful and meaningless antibodies (Jerne, 1984). Could we not suggest, however, that the equivalent of a semantic component would be the protective antibody which has risen during the most ancient dialogue between the host and the infectious agent? The second difficult problem would be to find the equivalent of the immune nonspecific language. Could the phonological equivalents of nonspecific immunity be comparable to the phonetic signals of animals which are by themselves a sentence rather than combinatory subunits of sounds? (see in Farb, 1975). Some findings indicate that we are not so distant from microbes and that messenger molecules which they contain could indeed be the ancestors of several vertebrate hormones and other mediators (Le Roith *et al.*, 1983). We are also finding more and more recognition by anti-peptide antibodies of foreign natural proteins, not to mention the astonishing cross-reactivity of monoclonals.

I feel bold enough to make the following predictions. We may some day be able to build constructs containing regions of peptides copying both bacterial and endogenous mediator structures in order to manipulate our specific and our non-specific immunity. We will become more and more aware that such a field will embrace newer and less doctrinal immunological systems. There exists for the future the potential use of several new approaches such as cellular engineering by repairing the defective bone marrow cells or introducing certain resistance-enhancing genetic materials. Certainly, today one sees much more clearly the relationship between the neuroendocrine factors and the immune system. Thus, LPS can induce leukocyte-derived corticotropin and endorphins (Harbour-McMenamin *et al.*, 1985). Interestingly, the cell which seems to be the most involved, this is the macrophage, appears to be a good connection between all these factors. We are all aware that this cell produces one or several monokines which elicit fever, and enhance slow-wave sleep. More recently, Blalock has shown that IL-1 and particularly a neuromonokine, hepatocyte-stimulating factor (HSF), can release ACTH as efficiently or even better than the hypothalamic corticotropin-releasing factor (Woloski *et al.*, 1985). We can expect a great future for HSF. Let us add in passing that TNF, another macrophage factor, can also induce fever and enhance SWS. The evidence showing that MDP is the minimal pyrogenic structure of peptidoglycans producing fever, SWS, and an increased antibody response has given us exquisite tools for future experiments involving the immune and the central nervous systems.

You will therefore forgive me if in concluding I say that muramyl peptides may become most valuable for a better understanding of the relationships between both systems, since they are the minimal structures of peptidoglycans for adjuvant activity and for pyrogenicity. Theoretically, fever could enhance resistance by two possible mechanisms: 1) inhibition of proliferation of thermosensitive organisms, and 2) production by exogenous pyrogens of monokines and/or other mediators which stimulate more directly the immune system.

It has been postulated that a macrophage factor (IL-1) could be responsible for both fever production and for lymphocyte activation. A consensus developed stating that several monokines previously identified as being separate entities represented different facets of the same molecule. However, it seems that different activities attributed to IL-1 such as pyrogenicity or lymphocytic activation can be selectively produced. Interestingly, pyrogenic IL-1 can lower the concentration of plasma iron which in turn can influence bacterial proliferation during fever. Acute-phase proteins have also a role in nonspecific resistance as indicated by studies concerned with leukocytic endogenous mediator (LEM), a soluble mediator which may be identical to endogenous pyrogen. Phenotypic alteration of bacterial cell wall could render the organisms more sensitive to certain other serum factors.

There likely exist other factors since resistance can be enhanced by agents, or under conditions which do not produce temperature elevation or hypoferremia. One of these factors could be TNF which has been shown to enhance resistance to bacterial infections. Our experiments were performed with crude preparations. Since TNF has recently been cloned and identified, it would be most interesting to see whether this molecule is endowed with both antitumor and antibacterial activities, or whether another molecule is responsible of the latter effect.

REFERENCES

Acevedo HF, Raikow RB, Acevedo HO, Delgado TF, Pardo M (1985).

Prevention of oncogenic viral infections in mice with CGP 11637, a synthetic muramyl dipeptide analog. Antimicrob Agents Chemother 28:589.

Azuma I, Sugimura K, Taniyama T, Yamawaki M, Yamamura Y, Kusumoto S, Okada S, Shiba T (1976). Adjuvant activity of mycobacterial fractions: immunological properties of synthetic N-acetylmuramyl dipeptide and related compounds. Infect Immun 14:18.

Ballou WR, Rothbard J, Wirtz RA, Gordon DM, Williams JS, Gore RW, Schneider I, Hollingdale MR, Beaudoin RL, Maloy WL, Miller LH, Hockmeyer WT (1985). Immunogenicity of synthetic peptides from circumsporozoite protein of *Plasmodium falciparum*. Science 228:996.

Chedid L, Audibert F, Lefrancier P, Choay J, Lederer E (1976). Modulation of the immune response by a synthetic adjuvant and analogs. Proc Natl Acad Sci USA 73:2472.

Chedid L, Boyer F (1951). Action antitoxique de la cortisone. CR Acad Sci Paris 233:1232.

Chedid L, Parant M, Parant F, Riveau G (1986). Nonspecific effects of LPS on bacterial infections. In Szentivanyi A, Nowotny A, Friedman H (eds): "The Immunobiology and Immunopharmacology of Bacterial Endotoxins, Basic and Clinical Aspects", New York: Plenum Press, in press.

Chedid L, Parant M, Riveau G (1982). Immunopharmacological activities of MDP. In Webb DR (ed): "Immunopharmacology and the Regulation of Leukocyte Function", New York: Marcel Dekker Inc., p.159.

Chomsky N (1964). "Current Issues in Linguistic Theory" Janua Linguarum, Series Minor, Mouton, The Hague.

Coulaud E (1934). Etat allergique durable obtenu chez les animaux de laboratoire par injection sous-cutanée de bacilles tuberculeux morts enrobés dans la paraffine solide. Rev Tuberc 2:830.

Covert JB, Reynolds WW (1977). Survival value of fever in fish. Nature 267:43.

Damais C, Riveau G, Parant M, Gerota J, Chedid L (1982). Production of lymphocyte-activating factor in the absence of endogenous pyrogen by rabbit or human leukocytes stimulated by a muramyl dipeptide derivative. Int J Immunopharmac 4:451.

Dame JB, Williams JL, McCutchan TF, Weber JL, Wirtz RA, Hockmeyer WT, Maloy WL, Haynes HD, Schneider I, Robert D, Sanders GS, Reddy EP, Diggs CL, Miller LH (1984). Structure of the gene encoding the immunodominant surface antigen on the sporozoite of the human malaria parasite *Plasmodium falciparum*. Science 225:593.

Dienes L, Schoenheit EW (1926). Local hypersensitiveness in tuberculous guinea pigs. Proc Soc Exp Biol Med 24:32.
Dietrich FM, Lukas B, Schmidt-Ruppin KH (1983). Prophylactic and therapeutic effects of MTP-PE, a synthetic muramyl peptide in experimental virus infections. In Proc 13th Int Congress Chemotherapy 91:50.
Dinarello CA (1984). Interleukin-1 and the pathogenesis of the acute-phase response. New Engl J Med 311:1413.
Ellouz F, Adam A, Ciorbaru R, Lederer E (1974). Minimal structural requirements for adjuvant activity of bacterial peptidoglycan derivatives. Biochem Biophys Res Com 59:1317.
Enea V, Ellis J, Zavala F, Arnot DE, Asavanich A, Masuda A, Quakyi I, Nussenzweig RS (1984). DNA cloning of *Plasmodium falciparum* circumsporozoite gene: amino acid sequence of repetitive epitope. Science 225:628.
Farb P (1975). Word Play. What happens when people talk? New York: Alfred A Knopf.
Freund J (1947). Some aspects of active immunization. Ann Rev Microbiol 1:291.
Freund J, Casals J, Hismer EP (1937). Sensitization and antibody formation after injection of tubercle bacilli and paraffin oil. Proc Soc Exp Biol Med 37:509.
Freund J, McDermott K (1942). Sensitization to horse serum by means adjuvants. Proc Soc Exp Biol Med 49:548.
Harbour-McMenamin D, Smith EM, Blalock JE (1985). Bacterial lipopolysaccharide induction of leukocyte-derived corticotropin and endorphins. Infect Immun 48:813.
Jerne LK (1985). The generative grammar of the immune system. The EMBO J 4:847.
Johnson AJ, Gaines S, Landy M (1956). Studies on the O antigen of *Salmonella typhosa*. V. Enhancement of the antibody response to protein antigens by the purified lipopolysaccharide. J Exp Med 103:225.
Kluger MJ, Rothenberg BA (1979). Fever and reduced iron: their interaction as a host defense response to bacterial infection. Science 203:374.
Kluger MJ, Vaughn LK (1978). Fever and survival in rabbits infected with *Pasteurella multocida*. J Physiol 282:243.
Kotani S, Watanabe Y, Kinoshita F, Shimono T, Morisaki I, Shiba T, Kusumoto S, Tarumi Y, Ikenaka K (1975). Immunoadjuvant activities of synthetic N-acetylmuramyl peptides or aminoacids. Biken J 18:105.
Krueger JM, Pappenheimer JR, Karnovsky ML (1982a). The composition of sleep-promoting factor isolated from human urine. J Biol Biochem 257:1664.
Krueger JM, Pappenheimer JR, Karnovsky ML (1982b). Sleep-

promoting effects of muramyl peptides. Proc Natl Acad Sci USA 79:6102.

Krueger JM, Walter J, Dinarello CA, Wolff SM, Chedid L (1984). Sleep-promoting effects of endogenous pyrogen (Interleukin-1). Am J Physiol 246:R994.

Le Roith D, Shiloach J, Berelowitz M, Frohman LA, Liotta AS, Krieger DT, Roth J (1983). Are messenger molecules in microbes the ancestors of the vertebrate hormones and tissue factors? Fed Proc 42:2602.

Lewis PA, Loomis D (1924). Allergic irritability. The formation of anti-sheep hemolytic amboreceptor in the normal and tuberculous guinea pig. J exp Med 40:503.

Lwoff A (1959). Factor influencing the evolution of viral disease at the cellular level and in the organism. Bact Rev 23:109.

Masek K, Kadlec O (1983). Sleep factor, muramyl peptides and the serotoninergic system. Lancet 1:1277.

Merser C, Sinay P, Adam A (1975). Total synthesis and adjuvant activity of bacterial peptidoglycan derivatives. Biochem Biophys Res Com 65:1316.

Parant M, Parant F, Vinit MA, Chedid L (1986). Tumor necrosis factor, an endotoxin-induced monokine, as mediator of non-specific antimicrobial immunity. EOS J Immunol Immunopharmac 6:S234.

Rabinowitsch L (1897). Zür Frage des Vorkommens von Tuberkelbazillen in Marktbutter. Zeit Hygiene 26:90.

Ramon G (1925). Sur l'augmentation anormale de l'antitoxine chez les chevaux producteurs de sérum antidiphtérique. Bull Soc Centr Med Vet 101:227.

Riveau G, Parant M, Damais C, Parant F, Chedid L (1986). Dissociation between muramyl peptide-induced fever and changes in plasma metal levels. Am J Physiol 250:C572.

Vaughn LK, Veale WL, Cooper KE (1980). Antipyresis: its effects on mortality rate of bacterially infected rabbits. Brain Res Bull 5:69.

Woloski BMRNJ, Smith EM, Meyer III WJ, Fuller GM, Blalock JE (1985). Corticotropin-releasing activity of monokines. Science 230:1035.

Young JF, Hockmeyer WT, Gross M, Ballou WR, Wirtz RA, Trosper JH, Beaudoin RL, Hollingdale MR, Miller LE, Diggs CL, Rosenberg M (1985). Expression of *Plasmodium falciparum* circumsporozoite proteins in *Escherichia coli* for potential use in human malaria vaccine. Science 228:958.

Immunopharmacology of Infectious Diseases: Vaccine Adjuvants and Modulators of Non-Specific Resistance, pages 17–26

AN OVERVIEW OF HOST DEFENSE MECHANISMS

Anthony C. Allison

Institute of Biological Sciences, Syntex Research

3401 Hillview Avenue, Palo Alto, CA 94304

INTRODUCTION

Many cell types and humoral mediators interact in resistance to infectious agents (Fig. 1). Since a comprehensive review of host defense mechanisms cannot be given in the space available, I shall focus attention on the elicitation of antibodies of various isotypes and of T-lymphocyte-mediated immune responses to infectious agents. The examples chosen are drawn largely from my personal experience, but they serve to illustrate the principles involved. Understanding the main effector mechanism of protective immunity in any combination of host and infectious agent provides the conceptual basis for the development of the novel vaccines that contemporary technology makes possible: the production of virus subunit and other antigens by recombinant DNA technology or peptide synthesis. These antigens elicit protective immunity only in the presence of adjuvants, as discussed elsewhere in this volume.

Some adjuvants elicit antibodies but not cell-mediated immunity, whereas others elicit both. The choice of an adjuvant for any vaccine should be determined by the relative importance of antibody formation and cell-mediated immunity, which has to be defined for each combination of host and infectious agent. Fortunately, general principles emerge from studies of experimental animals and humans with selective immunodeficiencies. Defects of antibody formation are associated with increased susceptibility to certain infections, whereas defects of cell-mediated immunity are associated with increased susceptibility to other infections.

SELECTIVE DEFICIENCIES

Rodents with T-lymphocyte deficiency can be obtained by genetic manipulation (nude mice and rats) or neonatal thymectomy. T-cell-defined mice show increased susceptibility to polyoma virus-induced tumors, which can be prevented by transfers of immune T-lymphocytes long after infection (Allison, 1980). They also succumb to infections with herpesviruses, poxviruses, Mycobacterium bovis BCG and malaria (Clark and Allison, 1974).

Selective deficiencies of T-lymphocytes in humans are rare, associated with hypoparathyroidism (Di George syndrome) and sometimes with deficiency of purine nucleoside phosphorylase and cartilage-hair hypoplasia (see Hayward, 1982). Children with these defects have died of generalized disease following herpes simplex virus infection or following vaccination with BCG or vaccinia virus.

Selective deficiency of antibody formation in mice can be produced by repeated inoculations of anti-μ serum during the neonatal period. Such mice have been used, for example, to show that recovery from the malaria parasite, Plasmodium chabaudi adami, is due to cell-mediated immunity rather than antibody formation (Grun and Weidanz, 1981). Cyclophosphamide treatment following antigen administration markedly suppresses antibody formation to the antigen used, and may, in fact, induce unresponsiveness to subsequent challenge with the same antigen. This treatment greatly increases susceptibility of animals to arthropod-borne viruses and influenza virus, for example. Mice can be passively protected by circulating antibodies against variant-specific determinants of influenza virus hemagglutinin (Virelizier, 1975).

Humans with defects of antibody formation are relatively common. About 1 in 500 lacks IgA, but only about one third of these show increased susceptibility to infections. Selective defects of IgG are rare, but associated with increased susceptibility to acute bacterial infections, paralytic poliomyelitis from vaccine strains and echovirus meningoencephalitis. Passive protection with immunoglobulins is effective.

Defects of C3 or of the capacity of leukocytes to kill micro-organisms also increase risk of acute and subacute bacterial infections, showing that antibodies, complement and leukocytes act together to protect against these organisms (Lachmann and Peters, 1982). It is therefore desirable to elicit antibodies of subclasses that interact well with complement and antibody-dependent effector cells (IgG_1 and IgG_3 in humans and IgG_{2a} in rodents).

I have elsewhere reviewed defects in neutrophils and monocytes that result in increased susceptibility to infection (Allison, 1982). These defects lie in the microbicidal mechanism itself, often in the cytochrome b_{-245} which we defined and showed to be abnormal in most families with chronic granulomatous disease (Segal et al., 1978). Alternatively, the cells may respond poorly to chemotactic mediators, so that they are not recruited to sites of infection.

ROLE OF T-LYMPHOCYTES IN HOST PROTECTION

A subset of helper T-lymphocytes (T_H1) produces interleukin-2,a 15,000 relative molecular mass glycoprotein (Mossman et al., 1986). In vitro studies show that antigen-activated precursors of the cytotoxic subset of T-lymphocytes (CTL) express receptors for IL-2. Binding of IL-2 is followed by proliferation of CTL and possibly their differentiation into cytotoxic effectors, although another factor may participate in the latter process (Wagner et al., 1982). IL-2 can also be used to produce clones of helper and of cytotoxic T-cells, which are useful for analysis of the role of such cells in host defense.

Figure 1 is a diagram of some of the cells and mediators interacting in host defense. The mechanisms by which T-lymphocytes terminate infections are complex. The best known is lysis of virus-infected target cells by CTL in a genetically restricted fashion (Zinkernagel and Doherty, 1979). However, this can apply also to cells infected with protozoan parasites, as we showed in the case of Theileria parva, which transforms lymphocytes into proliferating cell lines (Allison and Eugui, 1980).

When clones of CTL make contact with virus-infected cells having the same major histocompability (MHC) type, they liberate interferon-γ (IFN-γ, Morris et al., 1982) which can have direct antiviral effects on target cells, can increase expression of MHC antigens, which enhances specific cytotoxicity, and can activate macrophages (see below) and natural killer (NK) cells, which are thought to play a role in recovery from herpesvirus and some other virus infections (Lopez, 1984).

Immunity to herpes simplex virus (HSV) can be taken as an example of the complexity of host defense mechanisms. There is little doubt that T-lymphocytes play a major role: we showed that immunosuppressed mice can be protected from the lethal effects of HSV-1 infection by transfer of sensitized T-lymphocytes, not immune serum (Rager-Zisman and Allison, 1976). Neonates are prone to severe HSV-2 infections, and we showed that macrophages recovered from newborn mice are defective in their capacity to kill HSV (Hirsch et al., 1970). IFN-γ is a major activator of macrophages, and IFN-γ production is deficient in T-lymphocytes from neonates (Taylor and Bryson, 1985); in fact, the functionally immature monocytes of newborns show defective co-operation with T-lymphocytes in IFN-γ production. Other interferons also contribute to defense against HSV, since antibodies against IFN-α/β aggravate such infections in mice (Gresser et al., 1976). There is also evidence for a role of Lyt-1+ immune T-lymphocytes, which elicit delayed type hypersensitivity, in recovery from herpesvirus infections (Nash and Gell, 1983; Nagafuchi et al., 1982).

REACTIONS OF T-LYMPHOCYTES WITH CORE ANTIGENS OF VIRUSES

To neutralize, antibodies have to be directed against critical epitopes on the surface of the virus. These may undergo antigenic variation, as in the case of influenza virus, and certain individuals may not respond well to the epitopes because of their immune response genes. To obtain broader protection it would be desirable to elicit immune responses against more widely represented determinants. We showed that influenza virus nucleoprotein (NP), an internal component of the virus, is present on the surface of infected cells (Virelizier et al., 1976). Subsequent studies have shown that many clones of T-lymphocytes taken from infected animals have receptors for NP in the context of self MHC, and similar T-lymphocyte responses can also be demonstrated in humans (Townsend et al., 1986).

Chimpanzees can be protected against hepatitis B virus infection by eliciting antibodies against the surface antigen or by immunization with the core antigen of the virus (Murray et al., 1984). Presumably immune responses against core antigens on the surface of virus-infected cells are able to protect the host by lysing the infected cells or other mechanisms outlined above.

Thus core antigens of viruses, cloned and used with adjuvants that can elicit cell-mediated immunity, are attractive and novel candidates for vaccine strategies. For example, there is concern about variations in the surface antigen of the AIDS-related retrovirus LAV/HTLVIII, and the use in vaccines of the core antigen, product of the gag gene, as well as a construct of the envelope antigen, might be desirable.

ACTIVATION OF MACROPHAGES BY T-LYMPHOCYTES

This process, and the role of IFN-γ, has already been discussed in the context of HSV. We were also able to show that IFN-γ increases the capacity of macrophages to prevent the multiplication of influenza virus (Virelizier et al., 1977). Another T-lymphocyte product which is reported to activate macrophages, as well as stimulate their formation, is GM-CSF (Moore et al., 1981). T-lymphocyte-dependent activation of macrophages to limit multiplication of protozoan parasites and to kill metazoan parasites is discussed by Meltzer elsewhere in this volume.

The importance of macrophage-type cells in defense is shown by genetic differences in susceptibility to virus infections. Cultures of macrophages from strains of mice susceptible to a given strain of virus (e.g. yellow fever virus or murine hepatitis virus-3) support replication of the virus whereas cultures of macrophages from strains resistant to the virus do not (Allison and Burns, 1972). However, cultures of macrophages from resistant strains, taken during the prenatal period, do support virus replication, showing that resistance has both genetic and acquired components. Formation of IFN-γ and GM-CSF by activated T-lymphocytes is part of the acquisition of maturation.

INTERACTIONS OF ANTIBODIES AND EFFECTOR CELLS

As mentioned already, antibodies interact with complement and effector leukocytes to terminate infections. Circulating antibodies are sufficient to prevent passage of some viruses from primary sites of infection to secondary sites where they produce disease (e.g. poliovirus in the central nervous system). For example, circulating antibodies prevent damaging infections by Coxsackieviruses of the heart and pancreas. In young animals this mechanism is ineffective because the microbicidal capacity of macrophages to which antibodies carry viruses, has not yet matured.

Non-neutralizing antibodies can actually enhance infections of monocytes or macrophages by increasing uptake of virus through Fc receptors. We showed this for denguevirus, an important mosquito-borne virus in Asia and the Caribbean area. There are four serotypes; antibodies against heterologous strains bind the virus but do not neutralize. They actually increase denguevirus replication in human monocytes (Halstead et al., 1977). Such enhanced infections may give rise to complications such as the dengue shock syndrome, in which there is a generalized increase in vascular permeability. We have recently found that monocytes with enhanced denguevirus infections produce substantial amounts of peptidoleukotriene permeability-inducing factors, which may explain the shock syndrome. Clearly vaccination strategies will have to ensure that they do not increase the risk of such complications. Raising antibodies against all four serotypes of denguevirus should be feasible and should reduce the risk of complications.

Antibodies play other roles in protection. For example, they neutralize toxins and act against protozoa as well as bacteria and viruses. Examples are antibodies directed against the variant-specific glycoproteins of African trypanosomes and against the circumsprozoite protein of malaria sporozoites. Antibodies against the latter can prevent sporozoite-induced infections (Nussenzweig and Nussenzweig, 1985). However, even in such a well-studied situation there is evidence that cell-mediated immunity can substitute for antibodies. Mice unable to make antibodies following neonatal injections of anti-μ serum can be immunized by X-irradiated sporozoites against mosquito challenge (Chen et al., 1977).

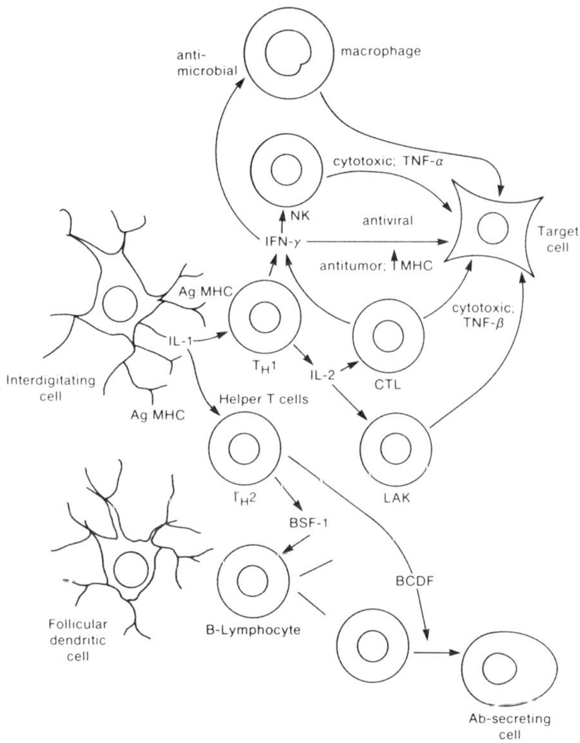

Figure 1. Interactions of various cell types in cell-mediated immunity (above) and antibody formation (below). Defined mediators include IL-1 and IL-2, IFN-γ and tumor-necrosis factors (TNF-α and TNF-β, the latter produced by T-lymphocytes and formerly known as lymphotoxin).

CONCLUSIONS RELEVANT TO VACCINATION

Some types of immunization, e.g. against tetanus and diphtheria toxoids, are reasonably satisfactory by current methods, which elicit antibodies but little or no cell-mediated immunity. However, it would clearly be advantageous to increase antibody formation of children during the first two years of life to bacterial polysaccharides and of old persons to influenza virus antigens. To develop effective inactivated virus or subunit vaccines against retroviruses such as LAV/HTLVIII or herpesviruses cell-mediated immunity is probably required. That is why an adjuvant formulation that increases cell-mediate as well as humoral immune responses to a wide range of antigens, including inactivated viruses and their subunits, could have practical value.

REFERENCES

Allison AC (1980) Immune responses to polyoma virus and polyoma virus-induced tumors. In Klein G ed. "Viral Oncology" New York: Raven Press, p. 481.

Allison AC (1982) Macrophages and neutrophils. In Lachmann PJ, Peters DK eds. "Clinical aspects of immunology. Oxford: Blackwell Scientific Publications 1:101.

Allison AC, Burns WH (1972) Immunogenicity of animal viruses. In Borek F ed. "Immunogenicity" Amsterdam: North Holland Press, p. 155.

Allison AC, Eugui EM (1980) Theileriosis: cell-mediated and humoral immunity. Am. J. Path. 102:114.

Clark IA, Allison AC (1974) Babesia microti and Plasmodium berghei yoelii infections in nude mice. Nature 252:328.

Gresser I, Tovey MG, Moury C, Bandu M-T (1976) Role of interferon in the pathogenesis of virus diseases of mice as demonstrated by the use of anti-interferon serum. J. Exp. Med. 144:1316.

Grun JL, Weidanz WP (1981) Immunity to Plasmodium chabaudi adami in the B-cell deficient mouse. Nature 290:143.

Halstead SB, O'Rourke EJ, Allison AC (1977) Dengue viruses and mononuclear phagocytes. II. Identity of blood and tissue leukocytes. J. Exp. Med. 146:218.

Hayward A (1982) Immunodeficiency. In Lachmann PJ, Peters DK, eds. "Clinical Aspects of Immunology" Oxford: Blackwell Scientific Publications 2:1658.

Hirsch MS, Zisman B, Allison AC (1970) Macrophages and age-dependent resistance to herpes simplex virus in mice. J. Immunol. 104:1160.

Lachmann PJ, Peters DK (1982) Complement. In Lachmann PJ, Peters DK eds. "Clinical Aspects of Immunology" Oxford: Blackwell Scientific Publications 1:18.

Lopez C (1984) Natural resistance mechanisms against herpesviruses in health and disease. In Rouse BT, Lopez C eds. "Immunobiology of herpes simplex virus infection" Boca Paton FL: CRC Press, p. 45.

Moore RN, Hoffeld JT, Farrar JJ, Shadduck RK (1981) Role of colony stimulating factors as primary regulators of macrophage functions. In Pick E ed. "Lymphokines" New York: Academic Press, 3:119.

Morris AG, Lin Y-L, Askonas BA (1982) Immune interferon release when a cloned cytotoxic T-cell line meets its correct influenza-infected target. Nature 295:150.

Mossmann TR, Cherivinski H, Bond MW, Giedlin MA, Coffman RL (1986) Two types of murine helper T-cell clone. 1. Definition according to profiles of lymphokine activities and secreted proteins. J. Immunol. 136:2348.

Murray K, Bruce SA, Hinnen A, Wingfield P van Erd PM, de Reus A, Schellekens H (1984) Hepatitis B virus antigens made in microbial cells immunize against viral infection. EMBO J. 3:645.

Nagafuchi S, Oda RH, Moni R, Taniguchi RT (1982) Role of Lyt-1 positive immune T-cells in recovery from herpes simplex virus infection in mice. Microbiol. Immunol. 26:359.

Nash AA, Gell PHG (1983) Membrane phenotype of murine effects and suppressor cells involved in delayed hypersensitivity and protective immunity to herpes simplex virus. Cell. Immunol. 75:348.

Nussenzweig V, Nussenzweig RS (1985) Circumsporozoite proteins of malaria parasites. Cell 42:401.

Rager-Zisman B, Allison AC (1976) Mechanism of immunologic resistance to herpes simplex virus (HSV-1) infection. J. Immunol. 116:35.

Segal AW, Jones OT, Webster D, Allison AC (1978) Absence of a newly described cytochrome b from neutrophils of patients with chronic granulomatous disease. Lancet 11:446.

Townsend ARM, Rothbard J, Gotch FM, Bahader G, Wraith D, McMichael AJ (1986) Cell 44:959.

Virelizier JL (1975) Host defenses against influenza virus: the role of anti-hemagglutinin antibody. J. Immunol. 115:434.

Virelizier JL, Allison AC, de Maeyer E (1977) Production by mixed lymphocyte cultures of a type II interferon able to protect macrophages against virus infections. Infect. Immun. 17:282.

Wagner H, Hardt C, Rouse BT, Rollinghoff M, Scheurich P, Pfitzennmaier K (1982) Dissection of proliferative and differentiative signals controlling murine cytotoxic T-lymphocyte responses. J. Exp. Med. 155:1876.

Zinkernagel RM, Doherty PC (1979) MHC-restricted cytotoxic T-cells: studies on the biological role of polymorphic major transplantation antigens determining T-cell restriction specificity, function and responsiveness. Advances Immunol. 27:52.

Immunopharmacology of Infectious Diseases: Vaccine Adjuvants and Modulators of Non-Specific Resistance, pages 27–39
Published 1987 by Alan R. Liss, Inc.

LYMPHOKINE REGULATION OF NONSPECIFIC MACROPHAGE CYTOTOXICITY AGAINST NEOPLASTIC AND MICROBIAL TARGETS

Monte S. Meltzer, Robert M. Crawford, Micheal J. Gilbreath, David S. Finbloom, Charles E. Davis, Anne H. Fortier, Robert D. Schreiber and Carol A. Nacy

Department of Immunology, Walter Reed Army Institute of Research, Washington, DC 20307-5100

Macrophages activated by components of the immune response are potent cytotoxic effector cells against neoplastic and microbial targets. Activated macrophages acquire extraordinary cytotoxic responses that are immunologically induced and not normally present in tissue macrophages during the steady-state or in cells that accumulate at reaction sites during acute inflammation. These unique effector cells are able to kill any of an enormous range of diverse targets (Table 1). Over the years, one of the more controversial areas of immunology concerns identification of immune signals that regulate the activated macrophage. At one moment, macrophage migration inhibition factor or MIF was the only lymphokine (LK) that affected macrophage function. This simple situation slowly evolved into an almost hopeless tangle of ill-defined, lymphokine activities with acronyms that included MAF, SMAF, MCF, MCIF and others. Recent reports document that interferon-gamma (IFN) is a macrophage activation factor (MAF) in both human and murine systems (Schreiber and Celada, 1985). Indeed, macrophages treated with recombinant IFN alone are activated to kill each of the targets listed in Table 1. Moreover, LK adsorbed with monoclonal anti-IFN antibody fails to activate macrophages for cytotoxicity against certain tumor and microbial targets

TABLE 1. Macrophage-mediated nonspecific cytotoxicity against neoplastic and microbial targets.

Tumor cells	Brucella abortus
	Chlamydia psittaci
Schistosoma mansoni	Francisella tularensis
	Listeria monocytogenes
Giardia lamblia	Mycobacterium tuberculosis
Leishmania major	Nocardia asteroides
Plasmodium falciparum	Pneumophilia legionella
Toxoplasma gondii	Rickettsia tsutsugamushi
Trypanosoma cruzi	Salmonella typhimurium
Aspergillus fumagatus	Cryptococcus neoformans
Blastomyces dermatitidis	Histoplasma capsulatum
Candida albicans	

TABLE 2. IFN-induced macrophage-mediated nonspecific cytotoxicity against tumor and schistosomula targets.

Macrophages treated *in vitro* with:	Macrophage-mediated cytotoxicity against: Tumor cells	Schistosomula
Recombinant murine		
IFN (100 IU/ml)	65%**	95%**
monoclonal anti-IFN	12%	0%
LK (100 IU/ml IFN)	68%**	97%**
monoclonal anti-IFN	23%	6%

(Table 2); mice treated with monoclonal anti-IFN antibody die from an otherwise nonlethal *L. monocytogenes* infection (Buchmeier and Schreiber, 1985). Despite the attractive fact that IFN as MAF fulfills Occam's razor [the simplest explanation among many is the best explanation], macrophage activation is not that simple. We review evidence in this report that shows regulation of macrophage effector function is controlled by multiple MAF, including but not limited to IFN, and fine-tuned by still other accessory activation factors for ultimate cytotoxic activity (Meltzer, 1981; Meltzer et al., 1982; Meltzer et al., 1986).

A number of years ago, we screened more than 20 murine continuous T cell lines for production of MAF after stimulation with several mitogens (Meltzer et al., 1982). Most T cell lines were inactive. LK from one subline of the EL-4 thymoma released MAF for cytotoxicity against tumor cell targets. This EL-4 derived MAF was not produced constitutively nor after treatment with the mitogens phytohemagglutinin or concanavalin A. Phorbol myristic acetate treated cells, however, released MAF in high titer. Of special interest was the repeated observation that under all treatment conditions, EL-4 culture fluids had little or no IFN activity by antigenic (ELISA) or functional (antiviral activity) analysis. Active EL-4 culture fluids were not directly toxic to either macrophage or tumor cells. Dose-response and time course for onset and loss of macrophage tumoricidal activity of cells treated with IFN or EL-4 derived MAF were comparable. Moreover, macrophages from strains of mice that were unresponsive to IFN for induction of tumoricidal activity also failed to respond to EL-4 derived MAF (Occhionero et al., 1984). Physicochemical characterization of the EL-4 MAF showed clear differences from IFN. Unlike IFN, the EL-4 derived MAF is stable to dialysis against pH 2 buffer and elutes from Sephadex G-100 with an apparent molecular weightof 25Kd. Recent reports, however, document discrete functional domains within the IFN molecule that separate sites for induction of antiviral activity from those that induce macrophage-mediated nonspecific tumor cytotoxicity (Schreiber et al., 1985). Thus, the EL-4 derived MAF may represent a breakdown product or otherwise altered fragment of IFN. We examined this possibility with a panel of hamster monoclonal or rabbit polyclonal anti-IFN antibodies. The hamster monoclonal antibodies, H1 and H21, are directed against different IFN epitopes. Both antibodies inhibit IFN-induced antiviral activity; H21 but <u>not</u> H1 also inhibits IFN-induced macrophage-mediated tumor cytotoxicity. Neither antibody, however, has any effect on macrophage tumoricidal activity induced by EL-4 derived MAF throughout a broad dose-response (Fig.

1). Active EL-4 culture fluids mixed with monoclonal or polyclonal anti-IFN antibodies and passed through a staphylococcal protein A column remained active. Identical treatment of spleen cell derived LK removed all activity for induction of macrophage cytotoxicity against tumor target cells. Results with these antibodies clearly show that the EL-4 derived MAF and IFN are antigenically distinct. Similar studies with monoclonal antibodies against recombinant LK or with the recombinant and/or highly purified LK themselves show that the EL-4 derived MAF is not CSF-1, GM-CSF, IL-1, IL-2 or IL-3.

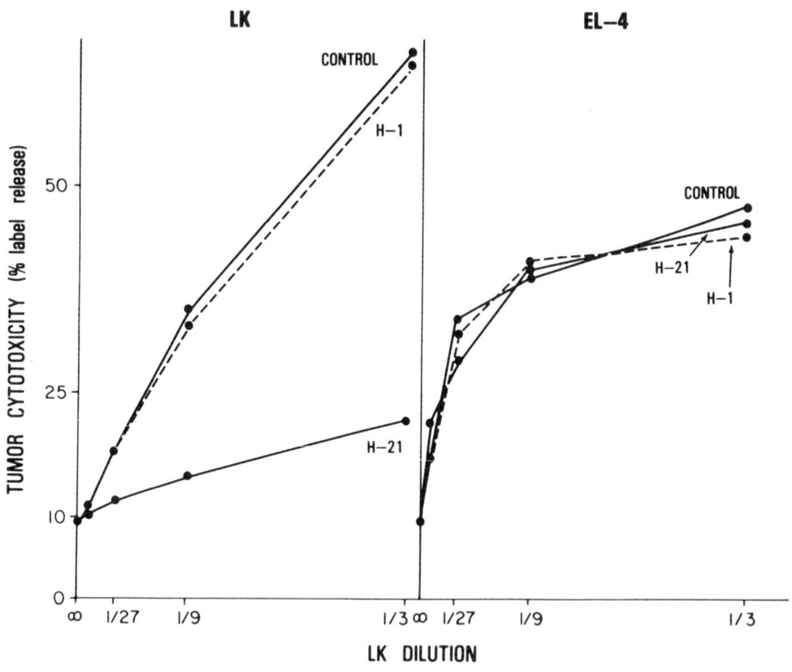

Fig. 1. EL-4 derived MAF: effect of H1 and H21 hamster monoclonal anti-IFN antibodies.

Perhaps the most interesting feature of the EL-4 derived MAF is its selective range of action: EL-4 derived MAF induces some, but not all reactions induced by IFN. EL-4 derived MAF and IFN each induce macrophage cytotoxicity against extracellular tumor cell targets and skin-stage schistosomula of S. mansoni. Unlike IFN, the EL-4 derived MAF does not activate macrophages to kill intracellular amastigote forms of L. major, does not induce fibroblast antiviral activity and does not increase macrophage Ia antigen expression (Nacy et al., 1983). In the long term, one would like to exploit this selective effect on macrophage function for immunotherapeutic intervention in neoplastic or infectious disease.

The preceding data clearly document a murine MAF physicochemically, antigenically and physiologically distinct from IFN. Further insight into the molecular regulation of macrophage activation derives from studies on microbicidal activity against intracellular parasites. Macrophage microbicidal activity consists of at least 2 reactions that can be modified by LK. Firstly, the relative susceptibility of macrophage populations to initial infection by any one of several parasites is decreased by prior exposure to LK (LK-induced resistance to infection). Secondly, cells that do become infected kill the intracellular parasite after LK treatment (LK-induced intracellular killing). The first LK-induced reaction is of special interest. Macrophages treated with LK cannot be infected with any of several obligate intracellular parasites, e.g. certain leishmania, rickettsia, chlamydia, mycobacteria and others. A similar phenomenon also occurs with macrophages activated in vivo during M. bovis, strain BCG infection or after treatment with killed Propionibacterium acnes (Corynebacterium parvum) (Nacy et al., 1984). It is important to note that LK-induced resistance to infection is microbe specific: phagocytosis of inert particles such as latex beads or red blood cells or even dead parasites remains unaffected. It is interesting that this LK-induced resistance to infection is not very much different in concept from the phenomenon of viral interference, the first described activity for interferons in general. Thus the most likely molecular candidate in LK for resistance to infection is IFN. This is not the case. LK activity that induces resistance to in-

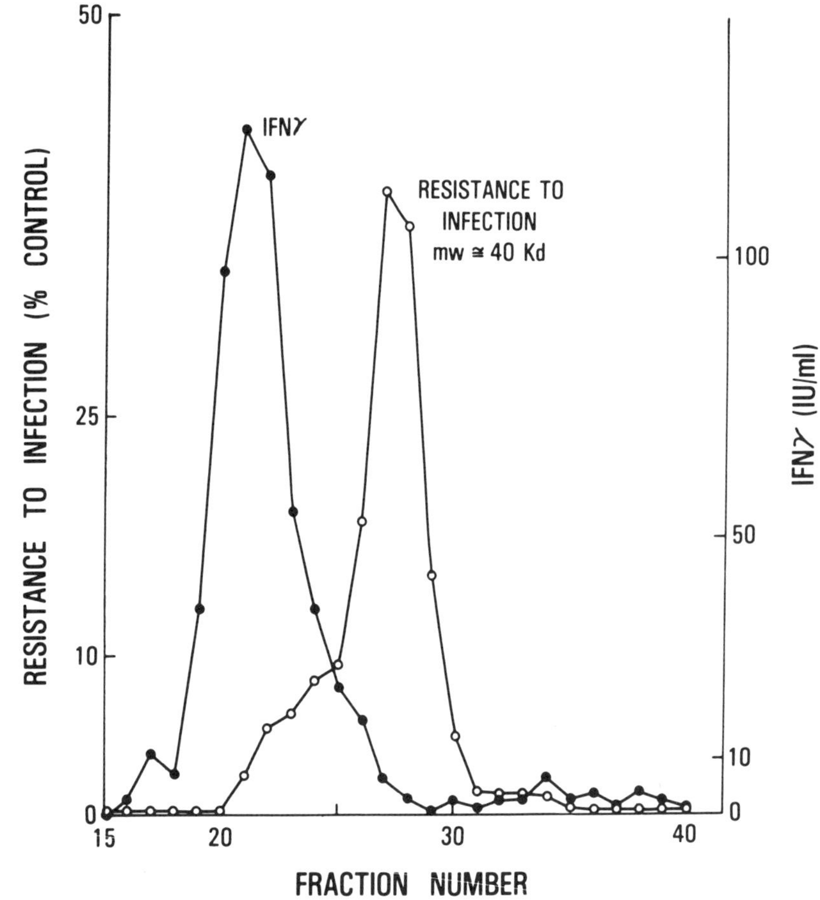

Fig. 2. LK-induced macrophage resistance to infection against L. major: separation of IFN and LK for induction of resistance to infection by gel chromatography

fection elutes from gel chromatography with an apparent molecular weight of about 40 Kd (Fig.2). This molecular weight is not very much different from that of IFN which fractionates in the 45 to 55 Kd region. However, peak LK activity for resistance to infection is reproducibly separated from the peak IFN activity. The question of whether or not IFN can induce resisance to infection was addressed directly with recombinant murine IFN (Table 3). No activity for resistance to infection was detected in macrophages treated with recombinant

TABLE 3. Macrophage microbicidal activity against *L. major*: LK-induced resistance to infection.

Macrophages treated *in vitro* with:	% infected macrophages	Resistance to infection
MEDIUM	63	0%
LK (100 IU/ml IFN)	12	81%**
monoclonal anti-IFN	56	11%
Recombinant murine IFN (100 IU/ml)	59	6%
monoclonal anti-IFN	62	2%
EL-4 derived MAF	18	71%**

IFN throughout a broad dose-response ($\leq$200 IU/ml) and time course ($\leq$24 hrs). Surprisingly, experiments with monoclonal anti-IFN antibodies raised an apparent paradox: even though recombinant IFN at all concentrations tested failed to induce resistance to infection, the high titers of activity in spleen cell-derived LK were completely abrogated by treatment with anti-IFN antibodies. We resolved this paradox in the following manner. Active spleen cell-derived LK with about 100 IU/ml IFN was treated with anti-IFN immunoaffinity chromatography. All IFN activity was removed in the eluate and the once active LK now failed to induce resistance to infection. The inactive LK was fractionated by gel chromatography and all fractions were inactive (Fig. 3). To each inactive fraction, we then added 5 IU/ml recombinant IFN. Addition of low concentrations of IFN completely restored LK activity for resistance to infection so that the elution pattern of IFN-depleted LK (Fig. 3) and that of control LK (Fig. 2) were now identical. Thus, induction of macrophage resistance to infection by intracellular parasites is absolutely dependent upon the interaction of 2 different MAF:

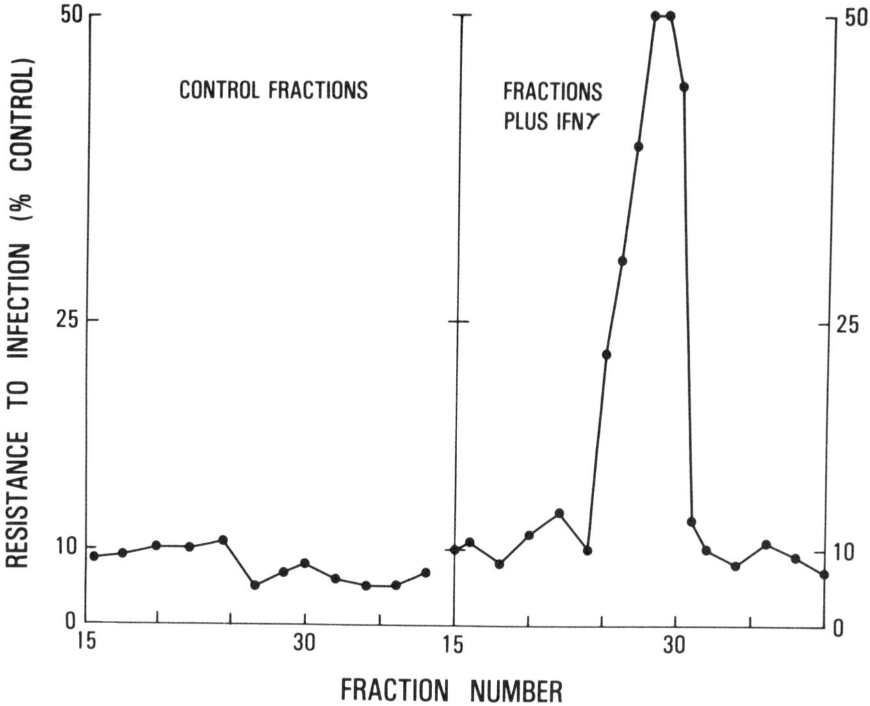

Fig. 3. LK-induced macrophage resistance to infection against L. major: activity of gel chromatography fractions with and without IFN.

neither act alone. One MAF is IFN; the other factor is antigenically and physicochemically distinct.

A similar interaction of MAF can be documented for induction of intracellular killing of parasite targets by activated macrophages. Macrophages treated with recombinant IFN develop potent cytotoxic activity against intracellular amastigotes of L. major (Nacy et al., 1985). In contrast, the EL-4 derived MAF fails to induce this microbicidal activity throughout an extensive dose-response and time course. Cells treated with IFN and the EL-4 derived MAF show 5-to 10-fold more microbicidal activity than macrophages exposed to either factor

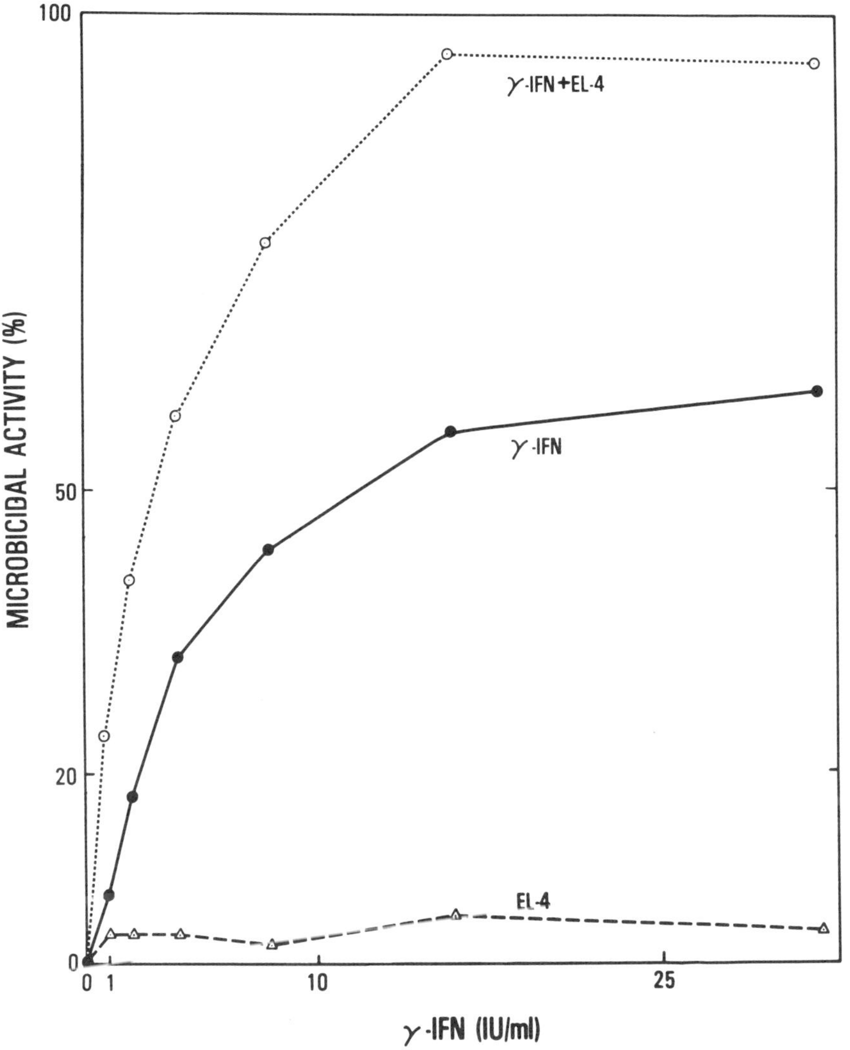

Fig. 4. Synergistic interaction of IFN and EL-4 derived MAF for induction of macrophage microbicidal activity against L. major.

alone (Fig 4). This EL-4 derived MAF is not directly toxic to leishmania, is unaffected by

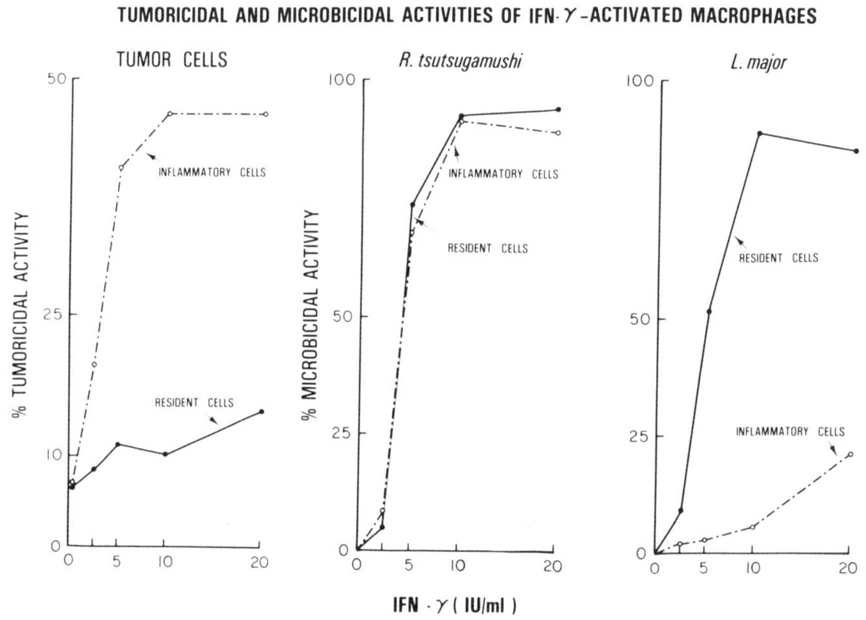

Fig. 5. Tumoricidal and microbicidal activities of IFN-activated macrophages: cytotoxicity by equal numbers of inflammatory and resident peritoneal macrophages.

polymyxin B and is physicochemically (apparent molecular weightof 25 Kd) and antigenically (activity persists after anti-IFN immunoaffinity chromatography) unrelated to IFN. Thus, once again we document multisignal control of macrophage function.

The preceding examples amply document complex but integrated control of macrophage effector function by multiple LK. Even with a single defined stimulus, however, the ultimate reaction may not always be predictable: macrophage response to a single activation signal for induction of cytotoxicity changes with cell maturation and/or differentiation (Fig. 5) (Meltzer et al., 1986). For example, the level of IFN-induced tumoricidal activity with inflammatory macrophages is more than 10-

fold greater than that induced with equal numbers of resident peritoneal cells given identical treatment. Interestingly, differences in macrophage response are not related to number of IFN receptors: and resident macrophages are comparable. An entirely different phenomenon occurs with IFN-induced macrophage microbicidal activity. The number of macrophages infected with R. tsutsugamushi in resident and inflammatory cell populations are equal. Small amounts of IFN ($\leq$10 IU/ml) added to infected cell cultures activates macrophages to kill the intracellular bacteria. In contrast to tumoricidal activity, no difference in IFN dose-response is detected between resident and inflammatory cell populations for induction of microbicidal activity. Similarly, macrophages infected with amastigotes of L. major also respond to IFN and develop microbicidal activity. In this case, microbicidal activity induced in the resident macrophage population is more than 10-fold greater than that induced in inflammatory macrophages. Thus we easily document changes in macrophage response to a single activation stimulus with cell differentiation. We also document striking system specificity: for any particular target, resident macrophages may be more, less, or equally responsive to an activation signal than equal numbers of inflammatory cells.

In many ways, regulation of nonspecific macrophage cytotoxicity is analogous to operation of a radio. The initial response is selection of an appropriate AM or FM radio. By analogy, the initial reaction in macrophage activation is accumulation of the appropriately responsive cell: for certain reactions, tissue macrophages are adequate or even optimal; other reactions are dependent upon inflammatory cells (Fig. 5). The second response is turning the radio on. For the activated macrophage this is the priming reaction and for many cytotoxic effector functions the priming signal is IFN. Macrophages exposed to a priming signal enter into a receptive state in which they are not yet cytotoxic but are then able to respond to certain trigger signals and develop full tumoricidal or microbicidal activity. Trigger signals may be either endogenous (LK) or exogenous (bacterial endotoxic lipopolysaccharides) stimuli. This trigger reaction is analogous to selection of an appropriate radio frequency or station. The final response for operation of the radio is volume control. The "volume" of the activated macrophage is regulated by certain accessory activation factors. These signals either amplify (Fig. 4) or suppress cytotoxic reactions of activated macrophages (Gilbreath et al., 1985; Nacy1984). The interactions of each of the preceding signals form an integrated regulatory network for the initiation and fine control of macrophage effector function.

REFERENCES

Buchmeier NA and Schreiber RD (1985). Requirement of endogenous interferon-γ production for resolution of Listeria monocytogenes infection. Proc Nat Acad Sci 82:7404-7409.

Gilbreath MJ, Nacy CA, Hoover DL, Alving CR, Swartz GMJr and Meltzer MS (1985). Macrophage activation for microbicidal activity against Leishmania major: inhibition of lymphokine activation by phosphotidylcholine-phosphotidylserine liposomes. J Immunol 134:3420-3424.

Meltzer MS (1981). Tumor cytotoxicity by lymphokine-activated macrophages: development of macrophage tumoricidal activity requires a sequence of reactions. Lymphokines 3:319-343.

Meltzer MS, Benjamin WR and Farrar JJ (1982). Macrophage activation for tumor cytotoxicity: induction of macrophage tumoricidal activity by lymphokines from EL-4, a continuous T-cell line. J Immunol 129:2802-2807.

Meltzer MS, Occhionero M and Ruco, LP (1982). Macrophage activation for tumor cytotoxicity: regulatory mechanisms for induction and control of cytotoxic activity. Fed Proc 41:120-127.

Meltzer MS, Hoover DL, Gilbreath MJ, Schreiber RD and Nacy CA(1986). Experimental variables for induction of activated cytotoxic macrophages.

Ann Inst Pasteur/Immunol 137C:191-198.

Nacy C.A (1984). Macrophage activation to kill Leishmania tropica: characterization of a T cell-derived factor that suppresses lymphokine-induced intracellular destruction of amastigotes. J Immunol 133:448-453.

Nacy CA, James SL, Benjamin WR, Farrar JJ, Hockmeyer WT and Meltzer MS (1983). Activation of macrophages for microbicidal and tumoricidal effector functions by soluble factors from EL-4, a continuous T-cell line. Infect Immun 40:820-824.

Nacy CA, Oster CN, James SL and Meltzer MS (1984). Microbicidal effector reactions of activated macrophages against intracellular and extracellular parasites. Cont Topics Immunobiol 14: 147-170.

Nacy CA, Fortier AH, Meltzer MS, Buchmeier NA and Schreiber RD (1985). Macrophage activation to kill Leishmania major: activation of macrophages for intracellular destruction of amastigotes can be induced by both recombinant interferon-γ and non-interferon lymphokines. J Immunol 135:3505-3511.

Occhionero M, Leonard EJ and Meltzer MS (1984). Functional characterization of lymphokines from the EL-4 cell line that activate macrophages for nonspecific tumor cytotoxicity. J Leuk Biol 35:405-414.

Schreiber RD and Celada A (1984). Molecular characterization of γ interferon as a macrophage activating factor. Lymphokines 11:87-113.

Schreiber R D, Hicks LJ, Celada A, Buchmeier NA and Gray PW (1985). Monoclonal antibodies to murine γ-interferon which differentially modulate macrophage activation and antiviral activity. J Immunol 134:1609-1614.

Immunopharmacology of Infectious Diseases: Vaccine Adjuvants and Modulators of Non-Specific Resistance, pages 41–50

INFILTRATION AND CHEMOTAXIS OF NATURAL KILLER/LARGE GRANULAR LYMPHOCYTES DURING VIRUS INFECTION

Robert J. Natuk, Kim W. McIntyre and Raymond M. Welsh
Department of Pathology, University of Massachusetts Medical School, 55 Lake Avenue North, Worcester, Massachusetts 01605

INTRODUCTION

Natural killer (NK) cells are large granular lymphocytes (LGL's), that is, large mononuclear lymphoid cells which contain cytoplasmic azurophilic granules and have a high cytoplasmic to nuclear ratio (Timonen, et al., 1979). During virus infection NK cell activity becomes greatly enhanced following the induction of interferon (IFN) production (Welsh, 1978). IFN, a biological response modifier (BRM), has been shown to regulate NK cell activity by increasing their lytic capability (Targan and Dorey, 1980) and inducing their blastogenesis (Biron et al., 1984). Augmented NK cell activity may be associated with liver, lung, spleen, meningeal exudate or peritoneal exudate cell (PEC) populations, depending on the route of virus inoculation (Welsh, 1978; Doherty and Korngold, 1983; Stein-Streilein, et al., 1983; Welsh et al., 1986).

NK cells may play roles in resistance to virus infection (Bukowski, et al., 1985) and prevention of malignant metastases (Wiltrout, et al., 1985). Therefore, it is important to understand how NK/LGL's are regulated in terms of their proliferation, activation, and distribution. If NK/LGL's play roles in combatting viral infections, there may be a mechanism to stimulate accumulation of NK cells at sites of virus infection. Whereas NK cell activity has been measured following virus infection, NK/LGL infiltration into sites of virus replication has not been previously studied. Certain BRM's, such as IFN and interleukin 2 (IL-2) would probably be synthesized at such sites and may influence NK/LGL migration. In this report, we show that NK/LGL's accumulate at sites of virus infection, and we analyze factors responsible for this accumulation.

MATERIALS AND METHODS

Male 4-10 wk old C57BL/6J or C3H/St mice were infected intraperitoneally (i.p.) or intravenously (i.v.) with 3 x 10^7 plaque forming units (pfu) of vaccinia virus, strain IHDJ (VV), 2-8 x 10^4 pfu of mouse hepatitis virus, strain A59 (MHV), 8 x 10^4 pfu of lymphocytic choriomeningitis virus, strain Armstrong (LCMV), or 4 x 10^4 pfu of murine cytomegalovirus, strain Smith (MCMV). Some mice were injected i.p. with 0.02 ml of rabbit anti-serum against asialo GM1 (AGM1, Wako Chemicals, Dallas, TX) 0-4 hr prior to infection in order to deplete NK cells.

Peritoneal exudate cells were prepared from mice as described previously (Natuk and Holowczak, 1985). Liver leukocytes were obtained by in situ perfusion with 0.05% collagenase and 0.05% dispase, essentially as described by David, et al., (1975). Leukocytes were separated from hepatocytes by metrizamide density gradient centrifugation (Wiltrout, et al., 1984). These effector cell populations were stained with Wright's-Giemsa and tested at effector-to-target ratios of 25:1 (PEC) and 10:1 (liver leukocytes) for NK cell activity in 4-5 hr cytotoxicity assays using ^{51}Cr-labeled YAC-1 cells. Spontaneous release was always under 12%.

Chemotaxis of NK/LGL's was assessed by employing a modification of the Boyden chamber technique (Boyden, 1962). Briefly, presumptive chemotactic factors were placed in the bottom chamber and PEC's from MHV-infected mice were placed in the top chamber. The two chambers were separated by two 5.0 μm polycarbonate filters. The cells which migrated to the bottom chamber after 6 1/2 or 12 hr of incubation were identified by Wright's-Giemsa staining of cytocentrifuge preparations. LGL migration was expressed as a percentage of the LGL migration measured using serum-free RPMI medium alone. A two-tailed Student's t-test was used to determine the significance of differences (P values) between experimental groups and controls. Peritoneal washout fluids were collected from mice after peritoneal lavage with 4.0 ml of serum-free RPMI medium. Cells were removed by centrifugation, and the supernatant fluids (peritoneal washout) were stored at -70°C. Human recombinant IL-2 (Amgen Biologicals, Thousand Oaks, CA) and mouse Cytimmune IFN-beta (Lee Biomolecular Research Laboratories, Inc., San Diego, CA) were tested as chemotactic agents.

RESULTS

Accumulation of NK/LGL'S in vivo During Virus Infection

Very low NK cell activity and LGL numbers were associated with PEC's collected from control unmanipulated mice (Table 1). NK cell activity and LGL numbers were considerably higher in liver leukocytes from control mice. Intraperitoneal but not i.v. inoculation with VV, MHV, LCMV, or MCMV resulted in a 4- to 20-fold augmentation of the NK cell activity and a 3- to 40-fold increase in LGL number associated with PEC populations harvested from mice at 3 days postinfection (p.i.) (Table 1). Injection of LCMV, MHV, or MCMV resulted in 2- to 10-fold augmentation of NK cell activity and a 2- to 10-fold increase in LGL number associated with liver leukocytes at 3 days p.i. (Table 1).

TABLE 1. Virus-Induced Augmentation of NK Cell Activity and LGL Cell Number

	PEC's		Liver Leukocytes	
Treatment	LGL Number	% YAC-1 Lysis	LGL Number	% YAC-1 Lysis
Control	1.8	2.3	22.	5.8
LCMV-ip	17.	51.	52.	16.
LCMV-iv	1.2	4.4	-	-
MCMV-ip	6.9	10.	210.	43.
MCMV-iv	<1.4	3.5	-	-
MHV-ip	69.	24.	50.	22.
MHV-iv	2.9	6.4	180.	54.
MHV ip + iv	3.8	18.	120.	48.
VV-ip	70.	22.	-	-
VV-iv	1.7	5.4	-	-

Liver leukocytes and PEC's were harvested from mice infected i.v. or i.p. with the indicated virus at 3 days p.i. NK cell activity and the number of LGL's ($x10^4$) were determined as described in Materials and Methods.
(-) = not determined.

Injection of antiserum to asialo GM1 reduced the NK cell activity by greater than 85% and the number of LGL's by greater than 75% in either cell population from both control and virus-infected animals (data not shown). The LGL's found in PEC's at 3 days p.i. were nonadherent to plastic, asialo GM1$^+$, Thy 1.2$^{+/-}$, Lyt 2$^-$ and J11d$^-$ (Table 2). Liver LGL's found at 3 days p.i. were similarly nonadherent, asialo GM1$^+$, Thy 1.2$^{+/-}$ and J11d$^-$ (Table 2). These LGL's were therefore of the NK cell antigenic phenotype. Microscopic analyses of Wright's-Giemsa stained cell preparations indicated that 20 to 50% of the liver and PEC NK/LGL's in virus-infected mice had blast cell morphology.

TABLE 2. Characterization of Virus-Induced NK/LGL's in Liver Leukocyte and PEC Populations at 3 Days p.i.

Cells	Treatment	% Reduction NK Activity	% Reduction LGL Number
Nonadherent PEC's	Anti-asialo GM1	89.	85.
	Anti-Thy 1	61.	59.
	J11d	4.5	0
	Anti-Lyt 2	9.0	0
Liver Leukocytes	Anti-asialo GM1	97.	83.
	Anti-Thy 1	24.	50.
	J11d	3.	0

Liver leukocyte or nonadherent PEC populations were prepared from mice at 3 day p.i. and were treated with various antisera and complement. NK cell activity and LGL number were determined and expressed as the % reduction as compared to cells treated with complement alone.

The accumulation of NK/LGL's in the liver and peritoneal cavity was studied under conditions of virus inoculation at two different sites (i.p. and i.v.) (Table 1). A correlation existed between the number of visible liver lesions in MHV-infected mice and accumulation of liver NK/LGL's at 3 days p.i (data not shown). High numbers of liver lesions were obtained when the virus was administered i.v., or i.v. plus i.p. In contrast, a strong PEC NK/LGL response required an i.p., administration of MHV. In several experiments a pattern emerged that suggested a competition for NK/LGL's occurred between the two sites of virus replication, as mice inoculated simultaneously at both sites failed to develop a significant peritoneal infiltrate when the liver was severely inflamed.

Chemotactic Factors for LGL at Sites of Virus Infection

Peritoneal washout fluid collected from virus-infected mice was demonstrated to contain chemotactic factors which attracted NK/LGL's. MHV-elicited nonadherent PEC's treated with rabbit complement and monoclonal J11d antibody, which eliminates B cells, neutrophils and eosinophils (Bruce, et al., 1981), were used as a source of NK/LGL, which represented 20 to 35% of the remaining cell population.

Washout fluids collected from mice at 3 days p.i. from MHV-and VV-infected mice both served to attract NK/LGL's *in vitro* (Table 3). The attraction was directionally oriented and was not due to increased randomized cellular motility, as the concentration of the washout fluid had to be greater in the bottom chamber than in the top chamber. Peak numbers of PEC's accumulated in the peritoneal cavity at 3-4 days following i.p. infection with MHV but declined significantly by 7 days p.i. MHV-PEC washout fluids collected at both 7 and 10 days p.i. had a diminished ability to attract NK/LGL's as compared to washout fluid collected at 3 days p.i. (Table 3). A different pattern of accumulation of LGL's and chemotactic factors was observed during LCMV infection. Here, both the LGL's and the chemotactic factors were at higher levels in the peritoneal cavity at 7 than at 3 days p.i.

TABLE 3. Virus-Induced Peritoneal Washout Fluids Contain Chemotactic Factors for NK/LGL's.

Source of Peritoneal Wash	LGL Number	% YAC-1 Lysis	Chemotactic Activity	P Value
uninfected	1.8	1.7	190	<0.2
3 day MHV	69.	24.	350	<0.01
7 day MHV	14.	13.	200	<0.05
10 day MHV	3.3	7.1	110	NS
3 day VV	110.	46.	340	<0.05
3 day LCMV	14.	23.	100	NS
7 day LCMV	150.	7.3	240	<0.01

Peritoneal cavities of uninfected or virus-infected mice were washed with serum-free RPMI at the time indicated p.i. The number of LGL ($x\ 10^4$) and the NK cell activity were determined as described in Materials and Methods. The cell-free peritoneal washout fluids were then assayed for NK/LGL chemotactic activity as described in Materials and Methods.

Effects of IL-2 and IFN-Beta Preparations on LGL Chemotaxis

IL-2 and IFN are molecules likely to be found at sites of virus replication and were therefore examined for chemotactic activity. Preparations containing human recombinant IL-2 were found to have chemotactic activity for NK/LGL's (Table 4) as well as for non-LGL-lymphocytes. IL-2 did not enhance NK/LGL migration when added to the cells in the top of the Boyden chamber, indicating that chemokinetic activity was not stimulated by IL-2 (Table 4). Preparations containing mouse IFN-beta at a concentration of 10^5 units/ml were also found to attract NK/LGL's (Table 4), non-LGL-lymphocytes, and macrophages. This enhancement of NK/LGL mi-

TABLE 4. Preparations Containing Interleukin 2 and Interferon-Beta are Chemotactic for NK/LGL's

Assay Time (HR)	Number Units/ml IL-2 IFN in Chambers Bottom	Top	Migrated NK/LGL's % of Control	P Value
6 1/2	50 IL-2	-	250.	<0.01
	25 IL-2	-	250.	<0.001
	12 IL-2	-	140.	<0.1
	6 IL-2	-	120.	NS
	-	50 IL-2	120.	NS
	-	25 IL-2	110.	NS
	25 IL-2	25 IL-2	120.	NS
6 1/2	10^5 IFN	-	190.	<0.1
	-	10^5 IFN	100.	NS
	10^5 IFN	10^5 IFN	79.	NS
12	10^5 IFN	-	430.	<0.001
	-	10^5 IFN	250.	<0.05

IL-2 and IFN-beta were tested for chemotactic activity at the indicated concentrations in either the bottom chamber or top chamber (with cells) or in both chambers.

gration could be detected following 6 1/2 hr incubation, but was more prominent after 12 hrs. In the short (6 1/2 hr) assays no chemokinetic effect was observed, but with longer incubation periods a chemokinetic effect was observed (Table 4). Resuspension of cells in 10^5 units/ml of IFN-beta did not increase the responsiveness of these cells to IL-2 preparations (data not shown). These data suggest that both IL-2 and IFN-beta may be chemotactic for LGL, but they do not rule out the possibility that contaminants in these preparations may be responsible for the chemotactic activity.

DISCUSSION

Here we demonstrated that accumulation of NK/LGL's occurs at sites of virus replication and at sites of virus-induced pathological lesions in vivo. Up to 40-fold more LGL's were recovered from the peritoneal cavity or the livers of infected mice as compared to unmanipulated mice. These LGL's found within the first 3 days of infection have an NK cell phenotype, and between 20-50% of these NK/LGL's have blast cell morphology. This suggests that upon arrival, the inflammatory NK/LGL can undergo at least one round of cell division which could serve to increase the localized NK/LGL cell number.

Simultaneous inoculation of high doses of MHV i.p. and i.v. resulted in extensive liver lesions and a marked increase in the number of liver NK/LGL's. The accumulation of peritoneal NK/LGL's did not occur following the dual inoculation of high doses of MHV, suggesting that the total number of responding inflammatory NK/LGL's may be limited in vivo and that the inflammatory cells present in infected liver and PEC populations may arise from the same pool of precursor NK/LGL's.

The site from which these inflammatory NK/LGL's come remains to be identified. Biron and Welsh (1982) demonstrated that NK/LGL blastogenesis occurs in spleens of virus-infected mice. However, splenectomy does not prevent the induction of NK/LGL responses in either the liver or peritoneal cell populations (unpublished results). Bone marrow and perhaps even the liver remain as potential sources for these inflammatory NK/LGL's.

NK/LGL's responded to chemotactic factors present in peritoneal washout fluids collected from virus-infected mice inoculated i.p. (Table 3). These factors may be responsible for the measured accumulation of peritoneal NK/LGL's following i.p. viral infections. The amount of chemotactic activity associated with the peritoneal washout fluid from MHV-infected mice closely paralleled the kinetics of LGL recruitment to the peritoneal cavity during infection. In MHV-infected mice, the greatest amount of chemotactic activity was measured at 3 days p.i., which coincided with the peak number of NK/LGL's found in the peritoneal cavity. Both the total number of LGL's in the peritoneal cavity and the amount of chemotactic activity associated with the peritoneal washout fluid decreased with time p.i. (Table 3). In contrast, peritoneal washout fluid obtained from LCMV-infected mice at 7 days p.i. contained more chemotactic activity then did washout fluids collected at 3 days p.i. During this virus infection, greater numbers of LGL's were found at 7 days rather than 3 days p.i. This large increase in LGL cell number appears to be the result of an accumulation of many Lyt 2^+ LGL's (75% of total LGL population), which are not NK cells but appear to be cytotoxic T lymphocyte (CTL)/LGL (Biron, et al., 1986). This suggests that factors found in the peritoneal cavity of LCMV-infected mice which may be responsible for the accumulation of CTL/LGL's can also attract NK/LGL's.

Preparations containing either IL-2 or IFN-beta (both which presumably would be synthesized at sites of virus replication) were demonstrated to have some chemotactic activity for NK/LGL's as well as for other cell types. Other studies have indicated that NK/LGL's recovered from normal human donors did not respond to IL-2 as a chemotactic factor (Pohajdak, et al., 1986). A possible explanation for this descrepancy may be that the human study employed normal non-activated NK/LGL's while our study employed activated NK/LGL's which may have recently responded to chemotactic factors *in vivo*. These cells may interact with IL-2 differently than nonactivated NK/LGL's.

IFN-beta has been suggested by Pohajdak, et al. (1986) to have chemotactic activity for human NK/LGL's, whereas Bottazzi, et al. (1985) have suggested that IFN-beta only stimulated chemokinetic movement of human NK/LGL's. IFN-beta in our hands was only chemotactic at very high concentrations ($1x10^5$ unit/ml). In long but not short assays, IFN-beta appeared to also have a chemokinetic effect on NK/LGL's. Cautious interpretation of the chemotactic effects of IFN *in vivo* is needed because of the high concentration required to demonstrate chemotactic effects *in vitro*.

SUMMARY AND CONCLUSIONS

NK/LGL's accumulate at sites of virus infection *in vivo*. Factors localized at these sites have chemotactic activity for virus-induced NK/LGL's *in vitro*. IL-2 and IFN preparations have chemotactic activity for NK/LGL's and may be partly responsible for the accumulation of NK/LGL's.

ACKNOWLEDGEMENTS

This research was supported by USPHS grants AI-17672, CA-34461, and AI-07272. We thank Ms. Dottie Walsh for preparation of the manuscript.

REFERENCES

Biron CA, Natuk RJ, Welsh RM. (1986). Generation of large granular T lymphocytes *in vivo* during viral infection. J Immunol 136:2280.

Biron CA, Sonnenfeld G, Welsh RM (1984). Interferon induces natural killer cell blastogenesis *in vivo*. J Leuk Biol 35:31.

Botazzi B, Introna M, Allavena P, Villa A, Mantovani A (1985). *In vitro* migration of human large granular lymphocytes. J Immunol 134:2316.

Boyden S (1962). The chemotactic effect of mixtures of antibody and antigen on polymorphonuclear leukocytes. J Exp Med 115:453.

Bruce J, Symington FW, McKearn TJ, Sprent J (1981). A monoclonal antibody discriminating between subsets of T and B cells. J Immunol 127:2496.

Bukowski JF, Warner JF, Dennert G, Welsh RM (1985). Adoptive transfer studies demonstrating the antiviral effect of natural killer cells *in vivo*. J Exp Med 161:40.

David GB, Galbraith W, Geyer SB, Koether A McD, Palmer NF, Pixler J (1975). Improved isolation, separation and cytochemistry of living cells. Prog Histochem Cytochem 7:1.

Doherty PC, Korngold R (1983). Characteristics of poxvirus-induced meningitis: Virus-specific and non-specific cytotoxic effectors in the inflammatory exudate. Scand J Immunol 18:1.

Natuk RJ, Holowczak JA (1985). Vaccinia virus proteins on the plasma membrane of infected cells. III. Infection of peritoneal macrophges. Virol 147:354.

Pohajdak B, Gomez J, Orr FW, Khalil N, Talgot M, Greenberg AH (1986). Chemotaxis of large granular lymphocytes. J Immunol 136:278.

Stein-Streilein J, Bennett M, Mann D (1983). Natural killer cells in mouse lung: surface phenotype, target preference, and response to local influenza virus infection. J Immunol 131:2699.

Targan S, Dorey F (1980). Interferon activation of "pre-spontaneous killer" (PRE-SK) cells and alteration in kinetics of lysis of both "PRE-SK" and active SK cells. J Immunol 124:2157.

Timonen T, Ranki A, Saksela E, Hayry P (1979). Human natural cell-mediated cytotoxicity against fetal fibroblasts. III. Morphological and functional characterization of the effector cells. Cell Immunol 48:121.

Welsh RM, Jr (1978). Cytotoxic cells induced during lymphocytic choriomeningitis virus infection of mice. I. Characterization of natural killer cell induction. J Exp Med 148:163.

Welsh RM, Biron CA, Bukowski JF, McIntyre KW, Natuk RJ, Yang H (1986). Regulation of viral infections by large granular lymphocytes. In JJ Oppenheim, DM Jacobs (eds): "Leukocytes and Host Defense". New York: Alan R. Liss, p 403.

Wiltrout RH, Mathieson BJ, Talmadge JE, Reynolds CW, Zhang S-R, Herberman RB, Ortaldo JR (1984). Augmentation of organ-associated natural killer activity by biological response modifiers. Isolation and characterization of large granular lymphocytes from the liver. J Exp Med 160:1431.

Immunopharmacology of Infectious Diseases: Vaccine Adjuvants and Modulators of Non-Specific Resistance, pages 51–60

NUTRITIONAL AND METABOLIC FACTORS IN HOST RESPONSES TO INFECTION

William R. Beisel

Department of Immunology and Infectious Diseases, The Johns Hopkins School of Hygiene and Public Health, Baltimore, Maryland 21205

INTRODUCTION

Malnutrition and infectious diseases are closely linked in Third World populations as well as in our most modern medical centers. In combination, malnutrition and infection account for far more deaths each year than any other cause. This linkage between malnutrition and infection is complex, and one that involves many variables and interactions (Scrimshaw et al., 1968).

Various forms of malnutrition and their accompanying changes in body composition and cellular metabolism can have a profound effect on the ability of the body to resist infection. Malnutrition can disrupt the funtion of the immune system and other non-specific (i.e., antigen independent) forms of host defense against infection. These secondary changes usually lead to a weakening of host resistance and an increased susceptibility to infection. But paradoxically, some forms of malnutrition cause certain infections to be less severe than usual.

These complex interactions must also be viewed from the other direction. Infectious diseases are accompanied by a plethora of changes in host metabolism (Beisel, 1985; Powanda and Canonico, 1981). These metabolic changes, in turn, can deplete the body of many important nutrients and induce secondary changes in immunological functions. The combination of interactions between infection and malnutrition can thus produce a vicious cycle or a downhill spiral leading to death (Keusch and Scrimshaw, 1986).

EFFECTS OF MALNUTRITION ON INFECTION

Generalized malnutrition, as seen clinically, is usually associated with an inadequate intake of dietary protein as well as calories, and commonly is termed Protein-Energy Malnutrition (PEM). Although animal models can be produced with deficits of protein, energy, or of both in combination, the PEM seen in clinical settings typically includes multiple deficiencies of other essential single nutrients, such as the vitamins and trace elements. Varying combinations of deficits, or an isolated deficit of certain single essential nutrients, can impair the function of the immune system and reduce host resistance against infection (Suskind, 1977; Chandra and Newberne, 1977; Beisel, 1982; Stinnett, 1983; Watson, 1984; Gershwin et al., 1985).

The likelihood that an infection will occur in a malnourished individual is dependent on the type and duration of malnutrition. Isolated deficiencies of single nutrients produce different effects on the immune system and on host resistance. Further, simple starvation in the absence of intercurrent disease produces markedly different changes in metabolism and body composition than the changes caused by disease-induced cachexia (Beisel, 1985). These differences are outlined in Table 1.

Starvation in the Absence of Disease

With simple uncomplicated starvation, metabolic adaptation is rapid, and mechanisms are employed by the body to conserve protein nitrogen to a maximum degree. This is accomplished by reducing basal metabolic rates, by lowering glucose production and metabolism, and by employing fatty acids and/or ketones as the principal sources of cellular energy. Even the brain adapts to a ketone economy within several days (Cahill, 1970).

By conserving protein in this manner the body can maintain the competence of the immune system and other defensive mechanisms for long periods of time. Individuals who totally reject all food intake will die of inanition, not infection. Similarly, patients with anorexia nervosa may exhibit minor changes in immunologic functions, but they rarely experience severe problems due to infectious disease. On the other hand, if partial

Table 1. A Comparison of Alterations in Metabolism, Physiology and Body Composition, as Seen in Simple (Uncomplicated) Starvation versus Disease-Induced Cachexia.

	Starvation-Induced Cachexia	Disease-Induced Cachexia
Body Metabolisn	Decreased	Increased
Body Temperature	Decreased	Often High
Body Nitrogen	Conserved	Lost
Somatic Protein	Conserved	Catabolized
Acute Phase Proteins	Not Induced	Synthesized
Body Water	Reduced	Expanded
Glucose Synthesis	Reduced	Stimulated
Ketone Synthesis	Increased	Inhibited
Urea Synthesis	Reduced	Increased
Branched-Chain Amino Acid Oxidation in Muscle	Reduced	Increased
Insulin secretion	Markedly Reduced	Increased
Defensive Mechanisms:		
- in early cachexia	Normal	Activated
- in chronic cachexia	May be Impaired	Severely Impaired
Secondary Infections	Rare	Common
Terminal Events	Inanition	Infection, Multi-organ Failure

starvation lasts for long periods of time (many months to years) immune system disfunctions will occur and secondary infections will develop (Winick, 1979).

Disease Induced Cachexia

The cachexia induced by disease is characterized by rapid changes in body composition, a hightened cellular metabolism, catabolism of somatic body proteins and stored nutrients, losses of many nutrients via increased excretion and a decrease in nutrient intake because of anorexia, in combination with an altered ability of the gut to digest and absorb dietary nutrients (Beisel, 1985; Keusch and Scrimshaw, 1986). Because of the rapid depletion of body nitrogen reserves and the dependence of all host defensive mechanisms on protein synthesis, disease induced cachexia leads rapidly to immunoincompetence and a weakening of the non-specific host defense mechanisms as well.

If an acute infection or other severe disease occurs in a patient with the marasmic form of PEM (dry cachexia), the further wasting of body nutrients and an accumulation of body water will convert the PEM to the very dangerous wet form, kwashiorkor.

The Acute-Phase Response and Cachexia

Any severe disease process or trauma that produces an inflammatory response can lead to body wasting and cachexia through the same common mechanism. This mechanism involves the initiation of a generalized acute-phase response by Interleukin-1 which is secreted by blood monocytes, tissue macrophages, and certain other cells when they are activated (Beisel, 1985; Kluger et al, 1985; Editorial, 1985). Interleukin-1-secreting cells can be activated by engaging in phagocytic activity, or by being stimulated by any of a large variety of substances, such as bacterial endotoxins, antigen-antibody complexes, polynucleotides, lymphokines, and tissue debris.

Despite its complexity and multiple components (see Table 2), the acute-phase reaction is a typical phenomenon in many different forms of infection, trauma, or other disease process including metastatic malignancy and advanced heart disease. The various components of the acute-phase reaction are now believed to each be of some

Table 2. Aspects of the Generalized Acute-Phase Response that Appear to be Initiated by Interleukin-1 (IL-1).

Central Nervous System Responses to IL-1
- Fever, with accompanying generalized hypermetabolism
- Anorexia, with diminished food and fluid intake
- Somnolence

Skeletal Muscle Responses to IL-1
- Activation of proteolytic enzymes in skeletal muscle
- Degradation of contractile proteins
- Release of free amino acids into plasma
- Myalgia

Hepatic Responses to IL-1
- Accelerated uptake of free amino acids, zinc, and iron
- Accelerated gluconeogenesis
- Accelerated ureagenesis
- Accelerated lipogenesis
- Reduced ketogenesis
- Accelerated synthesis of many proteins
  - For intracellular use:
    - Multiple enzymes (such as tryptophan oxygenase, tyrosine transaminase)
    - Metallothionein (for binding zinc)
  - For secretion into plasma:
    - Acute-phase reactants (haptoglobin, alpha-1-antitrypsin, ceruloplasmin, fibrinogen, C-reactive protein, serum amyloid A protein, alpha-1-acid globulin, i.e., orosomucoid)
    - Lipoproteins

Pancreatic Islet Cell Responses to IL-1
- Accelerated release of insulin into plasma
- Accelerated release of glucagon into plasma

Bone Marrow Responses to IL-1
- Leukocytosis
- Activation of neutrophils

Immune System Actions of IL-1
- Lymphocyte Activation
- Stimulation of lymphocytes to produce Interleukin-2

potential benefit in terms of host survival, healing of damaged tissue, and elimination of the disease process.

Despite its benefits, the acute-phase response incurs large costs in terms of the losses of body nutrients that lead rapidly to cachexia. The IL-1 stimulation of hypermetabolism, muscle protein breakdown, gluconeogenesis, and ureagenesis all help to deplete body stores of nitrogen, vitamins and minerals. The endotoxin-induced release from macrophages of another closely related mediator, variously termed cachectin or tumor necrosis factor (Beutler et al, 1985), also contributes to alterations in fat metabolism. Although the acute-phase response includes an IL-1-induced stimulation of the immune system, this stimulation can be rendered ineffective if the nutritional losses incurred during prolonged disease prevent optimal function by the lymphocytes and other defensive body cells.

The febrile and inflammatory responses, the mobilization of phagocytic cells, the sequestration of iron, zinc, and often sodium, the production of acute-phase reactant proteins, interferons, monokines, lymphokines, and immunoglobulins, and the activation of the kinin, complement, and coagulation systems also serve to distinguish disease induced cachexia from that due to simple starvation.

SYNERGISM VERSUS ANTAGONISM

If malnutrition causes an infection or other disease process to become more severe, as it often does, the interaction is said to be synergistic (Scrimshaw et al, 1968). A lack of various nutrients, alone or in combination, can have important detrimental effects on the immune system as well as on other host defensive mechanisms. These dysfunctions will be described in greater detail in subsequent paragraphs. Nutritionally induced immunoincompetence can readily explain synergistic interactions between malnutrition and infection.

On the other hand, if malnutrition causes an infectious process to be less severe than normally anticipated, the interaction is considered to be an antagonistic one. Antagonistic interactions have generally been demonstrated in animal models (Scrimshaw et al, 1968), where they often occur in systemic viral, helminthic, or protozoal diseases.

In contrast to the frequent occurrence of synergistic interactions in human infections, instances of antagonism are relatively rare, but are best documented in patients with severe iron deficiency (Beisel, 1982).

Antagonistic interactions between malnutrition and an infectious illness have been explained by an obligate dependence of invading microorganisms on enzyme systems and metabolites of host cells, or a higher organism requirement than the host for a particular dietary nutrient (Scrimshaw et al, 1968). Additional mechanisms may contribute to antagonism, as listed in Table 3.

Table 3. Mechanisms by Which Malnutrition May Cause an Infection to Be (or to Appear) Less Severe.

1. By reducing, slowing, or eliminating metabolic processes within host cells that are used by microorganisms for growth and replication.

2. By reducing the availability of specific nutrients or host metabolites that are essential for microorganism replication or the production of toxins.

3. By creating functional imbalances within the immune system (such as an inhibition of suppressor cells in the presence of normal helper cell function) that could serve to enhance the production of antibodies.

4. By inhibiting major signs of illness, such as fever, leucocytosis, or inflammatory or granulomatous reactions, and thereby to mask the presence of an infection.

EFFECTS OF MALNUTRITION ON THE IMMUNE SYSTEM

Generalized Malnutrition

As seen clinically, generalized malnutrition usually involves a multiplicity of nutrient deficiencies of varying severities. Depending on their severity and duration, these deficiencies can lead to widespread secondary effects on the immune system. These effects can include both anatomical derangements of lymphoid tissues as well as abnormalities in cellular functions. Non-specific defense mechanisms can also be impaired.

Virtually all lymphoid tissues become atrophic. The thymus involution is most severe, and lymphoid elements may be replaced widely by fibrous stroma. In lymph nodes, T-cell areas show greater defects than B-cell loci, and in the blood, T-cell counts are also lowered the most. These anatomical changes can best be assessed clinically by examining the tonsils, which may be reduced to mere traces.

The adverse effects of malnutrition on cell mediated immunity is also the most pronounced during clinical or laboratory testing. Anergy may be demonstrated by the lack of delayed dermal hypersensitivity reactions using skin tests with common antigens (such as tuberculin, monilia, trichophytin, candida, streptokinase-streptodornase, and mumps). Malnourished patients may not become sensitized to a new test antigen such as keyhole limpet hemocyanin, and they may fail to exhibit an inflammatory response to dermal application of a nonspecific chemical irritant such as 2,4-dinitrofluoro (or chloro) benzene. Because of dysfunction of killer T-cells, allografted tissues may not be rejected by severely malnourished patients or animals (Suskind, 1977; Chandra and Newberne, 1977; Stinnett, 1983).

T-lymphocyte blastogenic transformation studies in vitro show defective responses to both nonspecific mitogens and familiar antigens. T-cells also fail to respond in mixed lymphocyte cultures (Suskind, 1977).

In contrast to the abnormalities in cell mediated immunity during generalized malnutrition, humoral immunity is generally retained, and some tests may suggest that humoral immunity may even be enhanced. Plasma cells which produce immunoglobulins are rarely involved in the atrophy of lymphoid tissues, and serum concentrations of all classes of immunoglobulins may be increased. Malnourished children may develop antibodies to many food antigens (Chandra and Newberne, 1977). In contrast to elevations of total IgM or total IgG in serum, the primary humoral responses of specific IgM and IgG to some vaccines is depressed in malnourished patients (Gershwin et al, 1985). Secretory IgA is consistently depressed also.

Malnourished patients retain their ability to produce acute-phase reactant proteins (Suskind, 1977), but the synthesis of interferon, complement system proteins, lymphokines, and monokines may all be impaired. Other non-specific defenses may be weakened: tissue barriers may become atrophic; mucosal surfaces secretions may be diminished (e.g., lysozyme, gastric HCl); febrile and inflammatory reactions may not be generated; neutrophilic functions may be impaired; and eosinophiles may disappear (Beisel, 1985; Winick, 1979). Allergic illnesses may also disappear during prolonged malnutrition (Winick, 1979).

Essential Single Nutrient Malnutrition

Although studies are far from complete, a lack of an essential nutrient can often have severe immunological consequences (Beisel, 1982). Deficiencies of protein, essential amino acids, vitamin A, pyridoxine, folic acid, iron, or zinc lead to impairments of T-cell functions and cell mediated immunity. Deficiencies of zinc are the most dramatic in either animals or in man. The congenital defect in zinc absorption, acrodermatitis enteropathica, produces extensive immunological defects and early death. Oral zinc therapy can return these patients to good health.

Although the immunologic effects are less pronounced, deficiencies of protein, essential amino acids, thiamin, or riboflavin can interfere with humoral immunity. Vitamin C deficiency, on the other hand, has little apparant effect on lymphocytes, but can interfere dramatically with neutrophil mobility and mobilization. Iron deficiencies also induce neutrophil enzyme defects. Immunological changes begin to appear when hemoglobin values fall below 10 g/dl (Srikantia et al, 1986).

Nutritional Rehabilitation Therapy

Because they are acquired as a secondary consequence of nutritional deficiencies, immunological problems due to malnutrition are not as severe as those due to genetic defects in the immune system. These secondary immunologic defects can be prevented or reduced in severity if a good nutritional status can be maintained during infection or other forms of illness and trauma (Keusch and Scrimshaw, 1986). Further, immunologic dysfunctions associated with even severe malnutrition can generally be reversed almost completely if the malnutrition is corrected.

REFERENCES

Beisel WR (1982). Single nutrients and immunity. Am J Clin Nutr 35:417-468.

Beisel WR (1985). Nutrition and infection. pp 369-394, in Linder MC (Editor) Nutritional Biochemistry and Metabolism. Elsevier, New York.

Beutler BA, Milsark IW, Cerami A (1985). Cachectin/Tumor necrosis factor: production, distribution, and metabolic fate in vivo. J Immunol 135:3972-3977.

Cahill GG Jr (1970). Starvation in man. N Eng J Med 282:668-675.

Chandra RK, Newberne PM (1977) Nutrition, Immunity, and Infection. Plenum Press, New York.

Editorial (1985). Interleukin-1 in defense of the host. Lancet 2:536-537.

Gershwin ME, Beach RS, Hurley LS (1985). Nutrition and Immunity. Academic Press, Orlando.

Keusch GT, Scrimshaw NS (1986). Selective primary health care: Strategies for control of disease in the developing world. XXIII. Control of infection to reduce the prevalence of infantile and childhood malnutrition. Rev Infect Dis 8:273-287.

Kluger MJ, Oppenheim JJ, Powanda MC (1985): The Physiologic, Metabolic, and Immunologic Actions of Interleukin-1. Alan R. Liss, Inc., New York.

Powanda MC, Canonico PG (1981). Infection: The Physiologic and Metabolic Responses of the Host. Elsevier/North Holland Biomedical Press, Amsterdam.

Scrimshaw NS, Taylor CE, Gordon JE (1968). Interactions of Nutrition and Infection. World Health Organization, Geneva.

Srikantia SG, Siva Prasad J, Bhaskaram C, Krishnamachari KAVR (1986). Anaemia and immune response. Lancet 1: 1307-1309.

Stinnett JD (1983). Nutrition and the Immune Response. CRC Press, Boca Ratan.

Suskind RM (1977). Malnutrition and the Immune Response. Raven Press, New York.

Watson RR (1984). Nutrition, Disease Resistance, and Immune Function. Marcel Dekker, Inc., New York.

Winick M (1979). Hunger Disease. John Wiley & Sons. New York.

Immunopharmacology of Infectious Diseases: Vaccine Adjuvants and Modulators of Non-Specific Resistance, pages 61–73

LEUKOCYTE PRODUCTION AND SENSITIVITY TO NEUROENDOCRINE HORMONES INDUCED BY INFECTIOUS AGENTS OR THEIR PRODUCTS

Eve W. Johnson and Eric M. Smith

Departments of Microbiology, (E.W.J., E.M.S) and Psychiatry & Behavioral Sciences, (E.M.S), University of Texas Medical Branch, Galveston, TX 77550.

INTRODUCTION

That the neuroendocrine and immune systems comprise a functionally integrated unit is an idea which is rapidly gaining support and momentum. The foundations of this new field, neuroimmunoendocrinology (psychoneuroimmunology, neuroimmunomodulation) are in documented observations of neuroendocrine influences on immunologic function via "hard-wired" (nerve endings and neurotransmitters) and humoral (hormones and lymphokines) pathways. Direct communication between the central nervous system and organs of the immune system is indicated by innervation of the spleen, thymus, lymph nodes, gut-associated lymphoid tissue (GALT), and bone marrow (for review see Felten et al., 1985). Neural regulation of immune responsiveness is witnessed in both positive and negative effects of various brain lesions on immune functions (Cross et al., 1980; Brooks et al., 1982). Classical Pavlovian conditioning has been shown to exert alterations in immune responses (for review see Ader and Cohen, 1981), and the effect of "stress" on immunity has been reviewed (Riley, 1981). Not only is this link through "hard-wiring" but soluble substances such as neuroendocrine hormones and neurotransmitters have profound immunomodulating activities. This includes pituitary hormones and adrenal steroids (for review see Blalock et al., 1985b). That this intercommunication is not one-way, but is reciprocal, has been hinted at by the observation that antigenic challenge yields an increase in the firing rate of neurons in the hypothalamus (Besedovsky et al., 1977). Also, bona fide immune products such as interleukin-1 (IL-1)(Woloski et al.,

1985) and thymosin (Healy et al., 1983) can transmit signals to cells of the hypothalamic-pituitary axis. Thus, the immune system is regulated by the neuroendocrine system and, in turn, neuroendocrine function seems to be subject to influence by the immune system.

It is the working hypothesis of this laboratory that there are important homeostatic reasons for this bidirectional regulation to take place, and the mechanisms involved can be understood on a molecular and cellular level by defining a set of signal molecules and their specific receptors which are common to cells of both systems. In the following review, our findings are emphasized with regard to neuroendocrine substances produced by cells of the immune system in response to infectious agents or their products, and the effect of peptide hormones, mediated probably via cell surface receptors, on specific leukocyte functions. Additionally, the implications for an immune-neuroendocrine circuit are discussed.

LEUKOCYTE PRODUCTION OF NEUROENDOCRINE HORMONES IN RESPONSE TO INFECTIOUS AGENTS OR THEIR PRODUCTS.

Initial investigations revealed the coordinate expression of interferon α (IFN α), corticotropin (ACTH) and endorphins by human peripheral blood leukocytes infected with Newcastle Disease Virus (NDV)(Blalock and Smith, 1980; Smith and Blalock, 1981). Subsequently, interferon inducers such as tumor cells (Smith and Blalock, 1981) and bacterial lipopolysaccharide (LPS) (Harbour-McMenamin et al., 1985) were shown to induce production of these same peptide hormones. Leukocyte-derived ACTH and endorphins have since been shown to be identical to their pituitary counterparts in terms of antigenicity, molecular weight, bioactivity, and retention time on reverse-phase HPLC (for review see Blalock, 1984). Very recently it has been reported that NDV-infected splenocytes express the proopiomelanocortin (POMC) gene (Westly et al., 1986); the product of this gene, POMC, is the precursor molecule that is cleaved <u>in situ</u> into ACTH and endorphins in the anterior pituitary. Furthermore, POMC has also been detected in macrophages (Lolait et al., 1986) and preproenkephalin mRNA in helper T lymphocytes (Zurawski et al., 1986). POMC appears to be similarly processed into ACTH and endorphins in leukocytes (Harbour-MeMenamin, unpublished observations). Thus, it appears that leukocytes express the same POMC gene as that in the pituitary.

Human peripheral blood mononuclear cells also produce thyrotropin (TSH) when stimulated with staphylococcal enterotoxin A (SEA) (Smith, et al., 1983), and human chorionic gonadotropin (hCG) when stimulated by alloantigen in mixed lymphocyte culture (Harbour-McMenamin et al., 1986). Significantly, ACTH, TSH and endorphins are synthesized *de novo* rather than passively acquired since these molecules could be intrinsically radiolabeled with tritiated amino acids during *in vitro* induction. Published evidence for other leukocyte hormones exists for vasoactive intestinal peptide (VIP) (Giachetti et al., 1978; O'Dorisio et al., 1980) and somatostatin (Lygren et al., 1984). Preliminary evidence indicates that human and mouse leukocytes can produce growth hormone (GH), follicle-stimulating hormone (FSH), and leutinizing hormone (LH) (Smith, Blalock and Bost, unpublished observations). It has been speculated that the immune system may produce many more, if not all, of the peptide hormones classically considered to be products of the neuroendocrine system (Blalock et al., 1985a).

Some important concepts, with regard to control of leukocyte hormone production, emerge from the observations summarized above. First and most obvious, the particular hormone induced seems to vary with the stimulus employed. As illustrated in Table 1, virus infection (Smith and Blalock, 1981; Jordan et al., unpublished observations) and LPS stimulation (Harbour-McMenamin et al., 1985) yielded the *de novo* synthesis of ACTH and endorphins, while a mixed lymphocyte reaction (MLR) elicited hCG production (Harbour-McMenamin, et al., 1986) and SEA induced TSH production (Smith et al., 1983). Thus, the stimulus selected seems, in part, to determine the hormonal response. In addition, the particular cell type (for instance, B cell, T cell or macrophage) responsible for hormone production represents an added variable which is currently under investigation. For example, LPS appears to induce production of ACTH and endorphins in a subpopulation of murine B lymphocytes (Harbour-McMenamin, unpublished observations). Lolait and coworkers (1984) have reported the presence of β-endorphin in a subpopulation of mouse splenic macrophages. That leukocyte populations can differentially perceive immunostimulants (virus, bacteria, tumor cells, mitogens) implies that cells of the immune system function in a sensory capacity to detect these noncognitive stimuli (Blalock et al., 1985a). Finally, leukocyte production of hormones occurs not only in the presence of infectious agents and immunogens but seems also to be centrally controlled (like their pituitary-derived counterparts) through the production of hypothalamic releasing factors. For example, corticotropic releasing factor (CRF) and argenine vasopressin (AVP) work separately or in concert to induce synthesis of leukocyte ACTH and endorphins (Smith et al., 1986). GH, LH, FSH and TSH all appear to be inducible in leukocytes by treatment with the appropriate hypothalamic releasing factors (Smith, Harbour-McMenamin, Bost and Blalock, unpublished observations).

TABLE 1. Leukocyte production of neuroendocrine hormones in response to different infectious or immune stimuli.

Stimulus	Immunoreactive hormone	Reference
NDV, HSV	ACTH endorphins	Smith and Blalock, 1981; Jordan et al., unpublished observations
LPS	ACTH endorphins	Harbour-McMenamin et al., 1985
SEA	TSH	Smith et al., 1983
MLR	hCG	Harbour-McMenamin et al., 1986
Tumor Cells	ACTH endorphins	Smith and Blalock, 1981

What is the physiologic relevance of leukocyte-derived peptide hormones? To date, these seem to function both in a neuroendocrine capacity and, as discussed in a later section of this review, in an immunomodulatory capacity. In terms of their in vivo neuroendocrine activity, leukocyte-derived ACTH and endorphins are probably the most extensively investigated. Experiments utilizing hypophysectomized (pituitaryless) mice showed that NDV infection resulted in a time-dependent increase in serum corticosterone (Smith et al., 1982). Immunoreactive ACTH was found in the spleens of these mice. Thus, sufficient extra-pituitary ACTH was produced to elicit products of a classical stress response, and spleen cells proved to be at least one source of this ACTH. Splenocyte ACTH production was also shown in this study to be subject to the same feedback control as pituitary ACTH. Leukocyte-derived endorphins are thought to be components of LPS-induced endotoxic shock (Harbour-McMenamin et al., 1985). Endogenous opioids, or endorphins, have long been implicated in the pathophysiology of gram-negative sepsis and endotoxic shock, since naloxone, an opiate antagonist, relieves the hypotension and hypothermia associated with these trauma. Because in vitro LPS-stimulated leukocytes synthesize endorphins that are functionally and biochemically identical to pituitary endorphins (Harbour-McMenamin et al., 1985), and because leukocyte depletion in vivo has been shown to alleviate some of the same symptoms as naloxone treatment (Bohs et al., 1979), it has been postulated that leukocytes are an important source of the endorphins involved in the manifestations of endotoxic shock. These experiments and observations substantiate the notion that cells of the immune system can sense a stressor, in the form of infectious agents or tumors, and respond by producing signal molecules that can be interpreted by cells of the neuroendocrine system (and ultimately the central nervous system).

LEUKOCYTE SENSITIVITY TO NEUROENDOCRINE HORMONES.

Several laboratories have been interested in the effects of neuroendocrine hormones on the immune system. Our initial interest lay in demonstrating whether those hormones produced by leukocytes might function in an immunoregulatory capacity. The list of hormones able to modulate experimentally-defined immune responses is rapidly expanding and now includes ACTH, the endorphins, TSH, VIP, oxytocin, insulin, growth hormone, and AVP. In several cases, immunoregulatory activity is reinforced by the discovery of specific leukocyte receptors for the ligand of interest.

Immunoregulatory Functions of Neuroendocrine Hormones.

Perhaps the best-characterized neuroendocrine mediator of immune responses is ACTH. As previously discussed, human lymphocytes stimulated with IFN inducers produce a peptide that is structurally and functionally identical to pituitary ACTH (Smith and Blalock, 1981). We have found that ACTH, in turn, can modulate a variety of in vitro correllates of immune function. For instance, pharmacologic doses of ACTH (0.5 μM to 2 μM) have been shown to dramatically suppress the antibody response to both a T cell dependent antigen (sheep red blood cells, SRBC) and a T cell independent antigen (dinitrophenyl-Ficoll, DNP-Ficoll) in a standard plaque-forming cell (PFC) assay. T cell function appeared to be more sensitive to ACTH than B cell function, since inhibition of the anti-SRBC response required only one-fourth the amount of ACTH needed to suppress the anti-DNP-Ficoll response (Johnson, et al., 1982b). In a later study, ACTH 1-39 was shown to inhibit leukocyte production of IFNγ in response to SEA (Johnson et al., 1984), again at pharmacologic doses. It is possible to demonstrate these inhibitory effects at physiologic ACTH concentrations if the culture medium is replenished daily. In contrast, the shorter, fully steroidogenic, ACTH 1-24 has no activity in these systems. Investigations in progress are examining the ability of ACTH to influence the generation of cytotoxic T cells in a one-way MLR. Preliminary results indicate a suppression of cytotoxic activity, at physiologic levels of ACTH (0.001 uM) in the absence of 2 mercaptoethanol (2 ME), which is a normal component of culture media used in this assay (Johnson, Klimpel and Smith, unpublished observations). Other authors have demonstrated further immunoregulatory roles for ACTH, including abrogation of the ability of IFNγ to activate mouse peritoneal macrophages to a tumoricidal state (Koff and Dunegan, 1985) and enhancement of B cell growth and differentiation (Alvarez-Mon et al., 1985). Thus, there is little doubt that ACTH can function in a lymphokine capacity.

TSH and endorphins, molecules also shown to be inducible in leukocytes, also act to alter in vitro immune responses. α endorphin, but not the related peptide β- or γ-endorphin, suppressed the number of antibody cells in a PFC assay (Johnson et al., 1982b). Heijnen et al. (1986) showed that α-endorphin inhibits the PFC response by both abrogating antibody secretion by B cells and inhibiting secretion of a T cell-derived T helper factor. In contrast to ACTH and α endorphin, TSH was shown in the PFC assay to enhance the B cell response, as would a B cell growth factor (BCGF) or B cell differentiation factor (BCDF)(Blalock et al., 1984), and enhancement required the presence of T cells

(Kruger and Blalock, 1986). Interestingly, some of the described BCGF have a molecular weight similar to that of the α or β chains of TSH (Blalock et al., 1985a). That leukocytes can both produce and respond to ACTH, TSH and endorphins implies that these peptides may function in an autocrine or paracrine fashion in intraimmune system regulation.

Still other products of the neuroendocrine system can influence immune responses. VIP acts to suppress T cell mitogenisis _in vitro_ (Ottaway and Greenberg, 1984) and to inhibit lymphocyte migration (O'Dorisio et al., 1985). AVP and oxytocin were demonstrated to replace the interleukin-2 (IL-2) requirement for IFN γ production (Johnson et al., 1982a). Growth hormone and insulin have both been shown to behave as growth factors in potentiating mitogenic and antigenic stimulation of lymphocytes (Snow, 1985). A recent report details the suppressive effect of insulin and insulin-like growth factor-1 (IGF-1) on IL-2-mediated lymphocyte proliferation and the generation of antibody-producing cells (Hunt and Eardley, 1986). These examples, and a host of others not reviewed here because of space limitations, support the contention that control of immune function can occur through these neuroendocrine peptides of either immune or neuroendocrine origin.

Leukocyte Receptors for Neuroendocrine Hormones.

That leukoctye function can be modulated by neuroendocrine peptides implies that the observed responses occur as a result of interactions between ligands and specific cell surface receptors. Leukocyte binding sites for a number of neuropeptides have been described and include those for ACTH (Johnson et al., 1982b), endorphins (Wybran et al., 1979; Hazum et al., 1979; Johnson et al., 1982b), VIP (Danek et al., 1983; Ottaway et al., 1983), insulin (Krug et al., 1972; Helderman and Strom, 1978), growth hormone (Arrembrecht, 1974; Lesniak et al., 1974).

Thus far, the most extensively investigated of the immunocyte hormone receptors is that for ACTH. Initial binding studies using ^{125}I-ACTH demonstrated the presence of both high- and low-affinity receptors for the peptide hormone on mouse splenocyte membranes. The development of a new methodology for the isolation of receptors (Bost et al., 1985) has permitted the purification of the adrenal ACTH receptor.

This 225,000 dalton molecule is comprised of 83,000, 64,000, 52,000 and 22,000 dalton subunits; the 83,000 dalton subunit has been shown to include the ACTH binding-site (Bost et al., 1986). Analogous experiments to purify mouse spleen and human peripheral leukocyte cells have demonstrated a similar, if not identical, ACTH receptor (Bost and Blalock, unpublished observation). Antibody to the adrenal ACTH receptor has since allowed direct examination of the distribution of cells bearing ACTH receptors by immunofluorescence analysis (Johnson et al., 1986) Our results indicate a differential and characteristic distribution of ACTH receptor-positive cells both at the level of the whole lymphoid organ and among purified cell populations. 47% of mouse spleen cells and 32% of mesenteric lymph node cells were shown to express ACTH receptors under resting conditions. In contrast, unstimulated thymocytes possess few or no surface ACTH receptors. Among purified leukocytes populations, 47% of B cells, 23% of T cells, and 47% of peritoneal macrophages possess ACTH receptors. Importantly, functions of all three of these leukocyte populations have been shown to be modulated in the presence of ACTH (discussed above). Of special interest, thymocytes will dramatically up-regulate surface ACTH receptors when stimulated with the mitogens phytohemagglutinin or concanavalin A: receptor up-regulation follows a dose responsive pattern and includes as much as 90% of cells within 48 hours post-stimulus (Johnson, Smith, Bost and Blalock, unpublished observations). Such receptor up-regulation in the presence of mitogen is reminiscent of IL-2 receptor activity (for review, see Smith, 1984), and implies important regulatory roles for the specific ligand, ACTH, in the ontogeny and/or function of T lymphocytes.

Leukocyte ACTH receptors, then, provide a prototype for specific neuropeptide receptors on cells of the immune system. It is possible that, just as leukocytes may produce many or all of the known neuroendocrine hormones, they may also express specific receptors for many or all of these signal molecules.

CONCLUSIONS

Clearly, the immune and neuroendocrine systems comprise a functionally integrated unit and at least one means of interaction seems to occur through a shared set of chemical mediators and their respective receptors. The structural characterization described above suggests, at least in the case of ACTH, that lymphocytes express the same POMC and ACTH receptor as cells of the pituitary and adrenal, respectively. Hypothetically then, cells of the immune system function in a sensory capacity to perceive "stress" signals (invading pathogens) not recognized by the central nervous system. In turn, they produce immunoreactive peptide hormones which can be recognized by cells of the neuroendocrine system and are then translated to yield homeostatic change. Conversely, central nervous system perception of cognitive stimuli results in the release of neuroendocrine peptides which influence leukocyte function via interaction with specific cell surface receptors. In addition, products of either the neuroendocrine or immune systems can function in intrasystem regulation. It is hoped that by further defining these molecules and receptors which link the systems together that a better understanding of neuroendocrine and psychologic diseases, as well as the pathophysiology of infectious diseases, may be gained. Furthermore, knowledge of these interrelationships may allow more effective use of lymphokines or hormones therapeutically with fewer negative side effects.

ACKNOWLEDGMENTS

We wish to acknowledge the excellent collaboration of Dr. J.E. Blalock on much of the work described herein. Also appreciated is the excellent typing of the manuscript by Gloria Collins. These studies were supported in part by the Office of Naval Research (#N00014-84-K-0486).

REFERENCES

Ader R, Cohen N (1981). Conditioned immunopharmacologic responses. In Ader R (ed): "Psychoneuroimmunology," Orlando: Academic Press, Inc., p 281-319.

Alvarez-Mon M, Kehrl JH, Fauci AS (1985). A potential role for adrenocorticotropin in regulating B lymphocyte functions. J Immunol 135:3823.

Arrembrecht S (1974). Specific binding of growth hormone to thymocytes. Nature 252:255.

Besedovsky HO, Felix D, Haas H (1977). Hypothalamic changes during the immune response. Eur J Immunol 7:323.
Blalock JE (1984). The relationship between neuroendocrine hormones and lymphokines. In Pick E (ed): "Lymphokines 9," New York: Academic Press, p 1.
Blalock JE, Harbour-McMenamin D, Smith EM (1985a). Peptide hormones shared by the neuroendocrine and immunologic systems. J Immunol 135(2) Suppl:8585.
Blalock JE, Johnson HM, Smith EM, Torres BA (1984). Enhancement of the in vitro antibody response by thryrotropin. Biochem Biophys Res Commun 30L30,
Blalock JE, Smith EM (1980). Human leukocyte interferon: structural and biological relatedness to adrenocorticotropic hormone and endorphins. Proc Natl Acad Sci USA 77:5972.
Blalock JE, Smith EM, Meyer WJ (1985b). The pituitary-adrenocortical axis and the immune system. In Besser GM, Rees LH (eds): "Clinics in Endocrinology and Metabolism," Philadelphia: W.B. Saunders Company, p 1021.
Bohs CT, Fish JC, Miller TH, Traber DL (1979). Pulmonary vascular response to endotoxin in normal and lymphocyte-depleted sheep. Circ Shock 6:13.
Bost KL, Blalock JE (1986). Molecular characterization of a corticotropin (ACTH) receptor. Mol Cell Endocrinol 44:1.
Bost KL, Smith EM, Blalock JE (985). Similarity between the corticotropin (ACTH) receptor and a peptide encoded by an RNA that is complementary to ACTH mRNA. Proc Natl Acad Sci USA 82:1372.
Brooks WH, Cross RJ, Roszman TL, Markesbery WR (1982). Neuroimmunomodulation: neural anatomical basis for impairment and facilitation. Ann Neurol 12:56.
Cross RJ, Markesbery WR, Brooks WH, Roszman TL (1980). Hypothalamic immune interactions. I. The acute effect of anterior hypothalamic lesions on the immune response. Brain Res 196:79.
Danek A, O'Dorisio TM, George JM (1983). Specific binding sites for vasoactive intestinal peptide on nonadherent peripheral blood lymphocytes. J Immunol 131:1173.
Felten DL, Felten SY, Carlson SL, Olschowka JA, Livnat S (1985). Noradrenergic and peptidergic innervation of lymphoid tissue. J Immunol 135:2.
Giachetti A, Goth A, Said SI (1978). Vasoactive intestinal polypeptide (VIP) in rabbit platelets and rat mast cells. Fed Proc 37:657.

Harbour-McMenamin D, Smith EM, Blalock JE (1985). Bacterial lipopolysaccharide induction of leukocyte-derived corticotropins and endorphins. Inf Immun 48:813.
Harbour-McMenamin D, Smith EM, Blalock JE (1986). Production of immunoreactive chorionic gonadotropin during mixed lymphocyte reactions: a possible selective mechanism for genetic diversity. Proc Natl Acad Sci USA (in press).
Hazum E, Chang K, Cuatrecasas P (1979). Specific non-opiate receptors for β-endorphin. Science 205:1033.
Healy DL, Hodgen GD, Schulte HM, Chrousos GP, Loriaux DL, Hall NR and Goldstein AL (1983). The thymus-adrenal connection: Thymosin has corticotropin-releasing activity in primates. Science 222:1353.
Heijnen CJ, Berers C, Kavelaars A, Ballieux RE (1986). Effect of α-endorphin on the antigen-induced primary antibody response of human blood B cells in vitro. J Immunol 136:213.
Helderman JH, Strom TB (1978). Specific insulin binding sites on T and B lymphocytes as a marker of cell activation. Nature 274:62.
Hunt P, Eardley DD (1986). Suppressive effects of insulin and insulin-like growth factor-1 (IGF-1) on immune responses. J Immunol 136:3994.
Johnson EJ, Bost KL, Smith EM, Blalock JE (1986). Distribution of ACTH receptors on murine mononuclear leukocytes. Submitted.
Johnson HM, Farrar WL, Torres BA (1982a). Vasopressin replacement of interleukin 2 requirement in gamma interferon production: lymphokine activity of a neuroendocrine hormone. J Immunol 129:983.
Johnson HM, Smith EM, Torres BA, Blalock JE (1982b). Neuroendocrine hormone regulation of in vitro antibody production. Proc Natl Acad Sci USA 79:4171.
Johnson HM, Torres BA, Smith EM, Dion LD, Blalock JE (1984). Regulation of lymphokine (γ-interferon) production by corticotropin. J Immunol 132:246.
Koff WC, Dunegan MA (1985). Modulation of macrophage-mediated tumoricidal activity by neuropeptides and neurohormones. J Immunol 135:350.
Krug U, Krug F, Cuatrecasas P (1972). Emergence of insulin receptors on human lymphocytes during in vitro transformation. Proc Natl Acad Sci USA 69:2604.
Kruger T, Blalock JE (1986). Cellular requirements for thyrotropin enhancement of in vitro antibody production. J Immunol: in press.

Lesniak MA, Gordon P, Roth J, Gavin JR (1974). Binding of ^{125}I-human growth factor to specific receptors on human cultured lymphocytes. J Biol Chem 249:1661.
Lolait SJ, Clements JA, Markwick AJ, Cheng C, McNally M, Smith AI, Funder JW (1986). Proopiomelanocortin messenger ribonucleic acid and posttranslational processing of endorphin in spleen macrophages. J Clin Invest 77:1776.
Lolait SJ, Lim ATW, Toh BH, Funder JW (1984). Immunoreactive β-endorphin in a subpopulation of mouse spleen macrophages. J Clin Invest 73:277.
Lygren I, Revhaug A, Burhol PG, Giercksy KE, Jenssen TG (1984). Vasoactive intestinal peptide and somatostatin in leukocytes. Scand J Clin Lab Invest 44:347.
Ottaway CA, Bernaerts C, Chan B, Greenberg GR (1983). Specific binding of vasoactive intestinal peptide to human circulating mononuclear cells. Can J Physiol Pharmacol 61:664.
Ottaway CA, Greenberg GR (1984). Interaction of vasoactive intestinal peptide with mouse lymphocytes: specific binding and the modulation of mitogen responses. J Immunol 132:417.
O'Dorisio MS, O'Dorisio TM, Cataland S, Blacerzak SP (1980). Vasoactive intestinal peptide as a biochemical marker for polymorphonuclear leukocytes. J Lab Clin Med 96:666.
O'Dorisio MS, Wood CL, O'Dorisio TM (1985). Vasoactive intestinal peptide and neuropeptide modulation of the immune response. J Immunol 135(2)Suppl:8025.
Riley V (1981). Psychoneuroendocrine influences on immunocompetence and neoplasia. Science 212:1100.
Smith EM, Blalock JE (1981). Human leukocyte production of ACTH and endorphin-like substances: association with leukocyte interferon. Proc Natl Acad Sci USA 78:7530.
Smith EM, Meyer WJ, Blalock JE (1982). Virus-induced corticosterone in hypophysectomized mice: a possible lymphoid adrenal axis. Science 218:1311.
Smith EM, Morrill AC, Meyer WJ, Blalock JE (1986). Corticotropin releasing factor induction of leukocyte derived immunoreactive ACTH and endorphins. Nature: in press.
Smith EM, Phan M, Kruger TE, Coppenhaver DH, Blalock JE (1983). Human lymphocyte production of immunoreactive thyrotropin. Proc Natl Acad Sci USA 80:6010.
Smith KA (1984). Interleukin 2. Ann Rev Immunol 2:319.
Snow EC (1985). Insulin and growth hormone function as minor growth factors which potentiate lymphocyte activation. J Immunol 135(2)Suppl:7735.

Westly HJ, Kleiss AJ, Kelley KW, Wong PKY, Yuen P-H (1986). Newcastle disease virus-infected splenocytes express the proopiomelanocortin gene. J Exp Med 163:1589.

Woloski BMRNJ, Smith EM, Meyer WJ, Fuller GM and Blalock JE (1985). Corticotropin-releasing activity of monokines. Science 230:1035.

Wybran J, Appelbroom T, Famaey J-P, Govaerts A (1979). Suggestive evidence for receptors for morphine and met-enkephalin on normal blood T lymphocytes. J Immunol 123:1068.

Zurawski G, Benedik M, Kamb BJ, Abrams JS, Zurawski SM, Lee FD (1986). Activation of mouse T-helper cells induces abundant preproenkephalin mRNA synthesis. Science 32:232.

Immunopharmacology of Infectious Diseases: Vaccine Adjuvants and Modulators of Non-Specific Resistance, pages 75–89

BACTERIAL ENDOTOXINS: RELATION OF CHEMICAL STRUCTURE TO BIOLOGICAL ACTIVITY

Ernst Th. Rietschel, Lore Brade, Ulrich Schade, Ulrich Zähringer and Helmut Brade

Forschungsinstitut Borstel, D-2061 Borstel, FRG

INTRODUCTION

Fever, changes in leukocyte counts, hypotension and diarrhea are symptoms of infections caused by gram-negative bacteria such as Escherichia, Pseudomonas, Vibrio and Bacteroides. In severe cases, the infection may lead to disseminated intravascular coagulation and irreversible shock. These acute pathophysiological effects can also be elicited by killed bacteria and their active principle was identified as a cell surface component which could later be isolated by suitable extraction procedures. Because of its tight association with the bacterial cell and its toxic properties this molecule has been termed **endotoxin** (see Westphal et al., 1986). The obvious similarity between symptoms of gram-negative bacteriemia and the biological effects of endotoxins has led to the assumption that endotoxin, released from multiplying or desintegrating bacteria, is an important causative agent in the manifestation of sepsis.

In more recent years it has been recognized that endotoxins, in addition to their toxic properties, are endowed with a wide spectrum of biological activities which may be considered beneficial for the host (Nowotny and Behling, 1982). Such activities include induction of nonspecific resistance against bacterial and viral infections, of resistance to irradiation, tumour necrosis and stimulation of the immune response to unrelated antigens. These beneficial activities have raised the possibility of a clinical application of endotoxin which, however, is hitherto hampered by the intrinsic toxic properties of the molecule.

Endotoxin effects, regardless whether detrimental or beneficial, are mediated phenomena. They are the result of the interaction of endotoxin with, notably, mononuclear host cells (Freudenberg et al., 1986), the secretion by these cells of endogenous mediators such as interleukin 1 (IL-1), tumour necrosis factor (TNF), metabolites of arachidonic acid (prostaglandins, leukotrienes), colony stimulating factor (CSF) and the subsequent action of these mediators on different organs and body sites (Schlessinger, 1980). This mediator concept is strongly supported by the recent findings that drugs interfering with mediator synthesis, mediator receptor antagonists or antisera to mediators suppress endotoxin-induced lethality (see eg. Hagmann et al., 1984; Beutler et al., 1985).

CHEMISTRY AND BIOLOGY OF ENDOTOXIN

In view of their biological significance it was of great theoretical and practical interest to elucidate the chemical structure of endotoxins and to characterize those substructures which determine their different biological properties. The investigations of numerous laboratories demonstrate that endotoxins of all gram-negative bacteria studied so far conform to a common structural principle: They consist of a hydrophilic **polysaccharide** component and a covalently linked hydrophobic lipid portion, termed **lipid A** (Lüderitz et al., 1982). Hence, chemically, endotoxins are **lipopolysaccharides** (LPS). In Enterobacteria the polysaccharide portion consists of two subcomponents which are under separate genetic control: The O-specific chain and the core.

The **O-specific chain** represents a polymer of identical oligosaccharides, the repeating units. The nature and type of linkage of the individual monosaccharide residues within a repeating unit is characteristic and unique for a given LPS and the parental bacterial strain. This chemotype classification is the molecular correlate of the known serotype classification which describes the antigenic properties of the O-chain (Kauffman-White scheme). Therefore, the O-specific chain shows great variability if LPS of different origin are compared.

The **core oligosaccharide** architecture exhibits, compared to the O-specific chain, less variability. Thus, for larger groups of bacteria (e.g. for all Salmonella species and some E.coli strains) the lipid A proximal portion of the core oligosaccharide (inner core) is identical or closely related in composition. Despite numerous studies, the structure of this inner core region is not yet known in all details. This is mainly due to the presence of various charged residues such as phosphoryl and phosphorylethanolamine groups and, in particular, of an unusual octulosonic acid, i.e. 2-keto-3-deoxyoctonic acid (KDO,

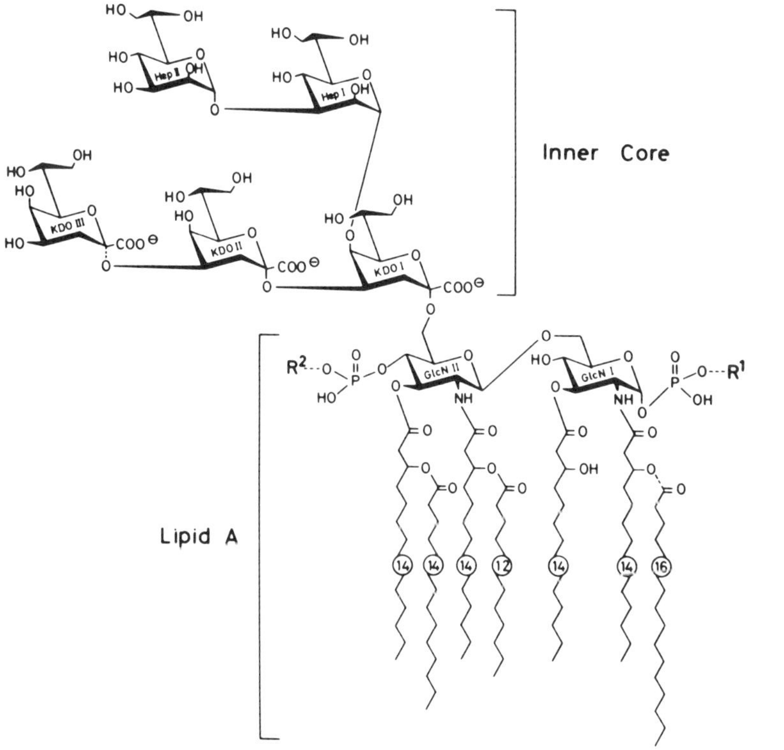

Fig. 1. Proposed chemical structure of the lipopolysaccharide of a Salmonella minnesota Rd$_1$P$^-$ mutant (strain R$_7$). The LPS regions inner core and lipid A are indicated. The lipid A structure was elucidated using S.minnesota Re LPS. Symbols R^1 and R^2 represent phosphorylethanolamine and 4-amino-4-deoxy-L-arabinose. Dotted lines indicate non-stoichiometric substitution and numbers in circles refer to numbers of carbon atoms in the acyl chains.

also termed 3-deoxy-D-manno-2-octulosonic acid, dOclA), the chemical and physicochemical analysis of which harbours great difficulties. Recently, however, significant advances have been made in the structural elucidation of the KDO-containing inner core region (Tacken et al., 1986). In these investigations enterobacterial rough-(R) mutants which synthesize LPS lacking the O-chain and part of the core and which have a phosphate-free saccharide portion (P^- mutants) proved to be most valuable. The structure of the enterobacterial lipid A proximal core region as proposed for a Salmonella minnesota Rd_2P^- mutant is shown in Fig. 1.

Accordingly, one KDO residue is present in the main core oligosaccharide chain (KDO I) being substituted in position 4 by an α-linked second KDO group (KDO II) which in turn carries, in nonstoichiometric amounts, a third α-linked KDO residue (KDO III) at position 4. At position 5, KDO I is substituted by L-glycero-D-manno-heptose (Hep I) to which a further Hep residue (Hep II) is linked at position 3. In LPS of higher mutants and wild type bacteria the saccharide chain extends from the hydroxyl group in position 3 of Hep II.

The KDO-containing inner core region and its chemical structure is recently receiving increasing attention for several reasons. i) Multiplying R-mutants whose LPS is devoid of KDO have not been isolated so far. This suggests that the KDO-comprising inner core region (together with lipid A, see below) plays a vital role for the growth of the bacterial cell. At present, however, it is not fully understood why KDO is essential for the survival of gram-negative bacteria (Osborn, 1980). ii) Enterobacterial R-mutants are assumed to be nonpathogenic and the core oligosaccharide (unlike the O-specific chain), therefore, appeared to be unimportant in bacterial virulence. In recent years, however, certain human pathogens such as Neisseria meningitidis, N.gonorrhoeae, Acinetobacter calcoaceticus, Campylobacter jejunii, Bordetella pertussis, and Haemophilus influenzae were recognized to synthesize an LPS lacking repeating units but containing a core-like oligosaccharide (for literature see Hitchcock et al., 1986). The core of LPS of Chlamydia trachomatis which are highly pathogenic obligate intracellular bacteria even resembles in composition that of enterobacterial deep rough mutants of the Re-chemotype in that it consists of mainly KDO (Brade et al., 1985). The role of the KDO-containing

LPS core in microbial pathogenicity should, therefore, be reevaluated. iii) The fact that the architecture of the inner core region appears, among different gram-negative bacteria, to be highly conserved renders this LPS domain an attractive target for studies concerning immunological cross-protection against pathogenic gram-negative bacteria and their endotoxins. Accordingly, polyclonal antisera and monoclonal antibodies (murine and human) against the inner core region are presently being produced and tested for cross-protecting activity in many laboratories (for literature see Jirillo et al., 1986). iv) Recently, the Hep I-KDO I disaccharide (Fig. 1) was recognized to be involved in a common determinant present in LPS of all gram-negative bacteria tested so far (Brade and Galanos, 1983). This common determinant interacts specifically with a nonimmunoglobulin factor which is present in high titers in sera of experimental animals and humans. In mice, this activity was characterized as a naturally occuring serum protein with a molecular weight of 28 kd (Brade and Brade, 1985). After interaction with LPS, the serum factor activates complement via the classical pathway (L. Brade and M. Loos, unpublished data). The physiological significance of these observations, the origin of the protein and the relevance of its interaction with LPS are presently under investigation in our laboratory. v) Finally, biological interest in the inner core region was greatly stimulated by the observation that synthetic (nonpyrogenic) or bacterial oligosaccharides such as the core-derived Hep II - Hep I - KDO I trisaccharide (see Fig. 1) induce the release of IL-1 from human mononuclear cells (Lebbar et al., 1986). The minimal structure required to trigger IL-1 secretion appears to reside in a disaccharide which comprizes a neutral sugar (eg. Hep) being linked to position 5 of KDO.

For any of these core related biological activities the exact structural prerequisites are not known. An understanding of the molecular basis of these phenomena presupposes knowledge on the core architecture thus justifying our present efforts of a further elucidation of the detailed chemical structure of this LPS region.

Lipid A represents the covalently linked lipid component of LPS (Rietschel et al., 1984). From enterobacterial LPS it can be isolated after mild acid hydrolysis. Free (polysaccharide-deprived) lipid A was found to induce, in experimental animals, all those pathophysiological effects (including fever, hypotension and lethality) that are known to be elicited by endotoxin (Galanos et al., 1977). In a now classical review it was indeed postulated already in 1954 that the endotoxic principle of LPS is embedded in the lipid A component (Westphal and Lüderitz, 1954). With the aim to define those structural features which make lipid A such a potent pyrogen and toxin, we and also other laboratories have studied its chemical structure. The architecture of enterobacterial lipid A is known today and that of S.minnesota lipid A is shown in Fig. 1. S.minnesota lipid A consists of a (ß1-6) linked **D**-glucosamine disaccharide which carries an ester-bound phosphoryl residue in position 4', an α-linked phosphoryl residue in position 1 and four (**R**)-3-hydroxymyristoyl groups in positions 2 and 3 (GlcN I) and in positions 2' and 3' (GlcN II, Fig. 1). The hydroxy fatty acids at positions 2' and 3' are, at their 3-hydroxyl groups, acylated by lauric and myristic acid, respectively, and that at position 2 by nonstoichiometric amounts of palmitic acid. The phosphoryl groups carry, also in nonstoichiometric amounts, phosphorylethanolamine and 4-amino-4-deoxy-**L**-arabinose (residues R^1 and R^2 of Fig. 1). Their exact location is presently under investigation (Rietschel et al., 1984; Strain et al., 1985). In free lipid A the hydroxyl groups in positions 4 and 6' are free. In enterobacterial LPS (Fig. 1) the latter primary hydroxyl group serves as the attachment site of KDO i.e. the core and polysaccharide component (for literature see Zähringer et al., 1985).

Lipid A's derived from endotoxically active LPS of different bacterial origin are structurally closely related. Thus, lipid A is characterized by a central 1,4'-bisphosphorylated, (ß1-6)-interlinked **D**-glucosamine disaccharide which carries two moles of ester- and two moles of amide-linked (**R**)-3-hydroxy fatty acids (in positions 2, 3, 2' and 3') of which, in general, two residues are 3-O-acylated. This structural principle is found in LPS of taxonomically remote bacteria and it, therefore, represents the most conservative structural element of LPS. A limited structural variability of lipid A from different bacteria is due to variations in the type and chain lengths of fatty acids, and to the presence of different polar headgroups bound to phosphate residues. In some cases, like in Escherichia coli and Salmonella, the acyl chains and headgroups are not present in stoichiometric amounts implying a certain microheterogeneity of lipid A preparations (Takayama et al., 1984). It should be noted that certain gram-negative bacteria (notably photosynthetic bacteria) form LPS which are endotoxically less or not active. Their lipid A component has been studied and shown to differ significantly in structure from those lipid A's described above (Mayer et al., 1984).

SYNTHETIC LIPID A

The recognition of the significance of lipid A for endotoxicity had already many years ago initiated investigations into the structural and conformational requirements which confer biological activity to this unusual molecule. Conclusions as to their nature had been predominantly drawn from comparative biological and structural studies on chemically degraded or modified LPS and lipid A's of different bacterial origin. Such studies proved to be most valuable in that they have pointed to certain biologically important lipid A components such as acyl and phosphoryl groups, but it was always felt that the unequivocal identification of important determinants of biological activity

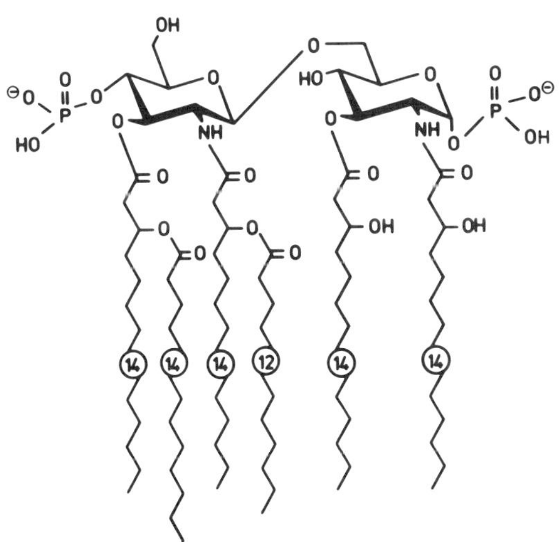

Fig. 2. Chemical structure of synthetic Escherichia coli lipid A (preparation 506 or LA-15-PP) (Imoto et al. 1985)

would only be possible by the physicochemical and biological analysis of chemically synthesized lipid A as well as part structures, analogues and derivatives thereof.

In 1984, Shiba, Kusumoto and their coworkers succeeded in the chemical synthesis of E.coli lipid A, the structure of which is shown in Fig. 2 (Imoto et al., 1985). It corresponds to the lipid A structure shown in Fig. 1 except that in the synthetic preparation (termed 506 or LA-15-PP) palmitic acid and phosphate substituents ($R^1 = R^2 = H$) are lacking. The structural identity of the 1'-monodephospho part structures of synthetic and bacterial free E.coli lipid A was demonstrated by ^{1}H-nuclear magnetic resonance, infrared spectroscopy, thin layer chromatography and other physicochemical methods. Synthetic E.coli lipid A (compound 506) was then analyzed for biological activity in the Max-Planck-Institut für Immunbiologie (Freiburg) and in our Institute (Borstel) in various endotoxin test systems *in vivo* and *in vitro*, in comparison with bacterial free E.coli lipid A and some of the results obtained are summarized in Table 1.

TABLE 1. Synthetic lipid A (preparation 506) and bacterial Escherichia coli free lipid A express identical endotoxic activities (Galanos et al., 1985)

Endotoxin Test System	Dose required to induce biological effect with	
	Synthetic Lipid A (Preparation 506)	Bacterial free Lipid A (E.coli)
	µg	
Lethality (LD_{50})[1]	0.01	0.01
Pyrogenicity (MPD-3)	0.004	0.005
Local Shwartzman Reaction[2]	6.2	6.2
Endotoxin Cross-Tolerance[3] (100% survival)	30	30
B-Lymphocyte Mitogenicity (Index of 10)	0.2	0.1
Macrophage Activation (Release of 10 ng/ml PGE_2)	1	1

1, In D-galactosamine-sensitized mice;

2, Preparative dose causing in rabbits a (+++)-reaction after challenge with synthetic or bacterial E.coli free lipid A (50 µg)

3, Dose inducing 100% survival of mice 4 days after tolerance induction to a LD_{100} challenge of S.arbortus equi lipopolysaccharide (200 µg)

We found that in all test systems employed including pyrogenicity, lethal toxicity, Shwartzman reactivity, induction of endotoxin cross-tolerance, B-lymphocyte mitogenicity, macrophage activation (prostaglandin E_2 release) and gelation of the Limulus amebocyte lysate the synthetic preparation 506 was, on a weight basis, of identical activity as its bacterial counterpart (Galanos et al., 1985). Similar results were also obtained by other groups (Kotani et al. 1985; Homma et al., 1985). In addition, synthetic lipid A exhibited identical immunogenic and antigenic properties as bacterial lipid A (Brade et al., 1985) and both preparations were equally effective in inducing IL-1 release from human mononuclear cells (Loppnow et al., 1986).

These results demonstrate that indeed lipid A represents the endotoxic center of LPS implicating that variable substituents of bacterial lipid A are not required for the expression of endotoxicity and that the structural proposal for lipid A, as derived from analytical work, is correct.

STRUCTURE-ACTIVITY RELATIONSHIPS

Synthetic lipid A has certainly closed that chapter of endotoxin research which dealt with the search for the endotoxic principle. At the same time, however, the availability of synthetic lipid A and part structures marks the beginning of a new era in which some of the still open questions in endotoxin research may be answered. Among these, the problem as to the minimal structural and conformational requirements for lipid A activity has recently been studied. The scope of this short review does not allow to present all relevant data in detail (for literature see Rietschel et al.; 1986, Kanegasaki et al., 1986). Rather, some key results and conclusions concerning lipid A structure-activity relationships will be summarized below.

Lipid A part structures containing one **D-glucosaminyl** residue, two or three acyl chains and one phosphoryl group at either position 1 or 4 (thus resembling the reducing or distal unit of lipid A) exhibit in vitro activities such as B-lymphocyte mitogenicity, macrophage activation and Limu-

---

Synthetic E.coli lipid A in now commercially available (Daiichi Pure Chemicals, Tokyo, Japan)

lus amebocyte lysate gelation. In contrast, these monosaccharide part structures lack endotoxic in vivo activities such as pyrogenicity and lethality. It, therefore, appears that the presence of a disaccharide is essential for the expression of endotoxicity.

The biological significance of **phosphoryl** groups was studied by analysing the 1'- and 4'-monodephospho part structures of synthetic lipid A and the tetraacyl lipid A precursor Ia (compound 406). It was generally found that the 1'- and 4-monodephospho derivatives are less active than the parent compounds as pyrogens, lethal toxins and, in the case of monophosphoryl lipid A part structures, in preparing for or in eliciting the local Shwartzman reaction. Individual monodephospho part structures were also generally less active in in vitro tests, only some compounds exhibiting similar activity as the corresponding bisphosphorylated compounds 406 and 506 (see eg. Loppnow et al., 1986). The phosphate-free part structures of synthetic lipid A and precursor Ia are insoluble in water and, as expected, essentially inactive in all parameters tested. These findings suggest that two phosphoryl groups are required for maximal expression of endotoxicity.

It had previously been documented that deacylated LPS samples are significantly less active in typical endotoxin test systems and **fatty acids**, therefore, were assumed to be essential for endotoxicity. It was not known, however, whether the number of fatty acids present, their nature, their type of linkage and their distribution or all these factors together were of importance. Recently, it was shown that among synthetic bisphosphorylated lipid A part structures containing the (ß1-6) linked D-glucosamine disaccharide such as de-O-acyl lipid A (containing two acyl groups), precursor Ia (four acyl groups), precursor Ib (five acyl groups), E.coli lipid A (six acyl groups) and heptaacyl S.minnesota lipid A (seven acyl groups) the structures containing five or six fatty acids expressed maximal endotoxic activity while molecules containing less or more acyl chains were of lower activity (for summary see Rietschel et al., 1986). It was further demonstrated that synthetic analogues containing five fatty acids, however, in a different arrangement as in E.coli lipid A exhibit only marginal endotoxicity (Tanamoto et al., 1984). Therefore, the location of fatty acids on the backbone as well as the quantitiy of acyl groups present (i.e. the hydrophobicity) are of importance for lipid A endotoxic activity.

In summary, the available evidence suggests that maximal endotoxicity is expressed by a molecule containing two (ß1-6) interlinked D-glucosamine residues, two phosphoryl groups and five (as in precursor Ib) or six (as in E.coli lipid A) fatty acids in a defined distribution. Molecules lacking only one component are, irrespective of the chemical nature of the component, endotoxically less active. This shows that slight modifications of the lipid A architecture result in a significant change of biological activity suggesting that endotoxicity is not dependent on one single or specific lipid A constituent, i.e. a toxophore group but rather is determined by several factors which may cause an equilibrated balance of hydrophilic and hydrophobic forces, resulting in an "endotoxic conformation". Being in this particular conformation, lipid A is watersoluble, bioavailable and endotoxically active.

CONCLUDING REMARKS

Endotoxins have, in the past, greatly contributed to the development of the field of immunological adjuvants and modulators of nonspecific resistance to microbial infections. Today we can define those structures within the complex endotoxin molecules which are capable of interacting with and thereby activating humoral and cellular components of the immune system. These structures are located in the most conservative regions of endotoxins i.e. the lipid A component and the KDO-containing inner core portion which both exhibit intrinsic biological activity. Lipid A induces typical endotoxic effects such as pyrogenicity and lethal toxicity and, in addition, it stimulates certain immune cells to secrete endogenous mediators which e.g. enhance the immune response to unrelated antigens. Inner core-derived oligosaccharides lack toxic activity. They trigger, however, mononuclear cells to the production of immunostimulating molecules such as interleukin 1. The overall chemical architecture of these immunoreactive LPS-regions is largely known. Future studies will now concentrate on the elucidation of the fine structure and, in particular, the conformation of these regions with the aim to understand, on a molecular basis, the mechanisms underlying their mode of action. The knowledge thus gained may finally bring about their application as immunological adjuvants in clinical medicine.

ACKNOWLEDGEMENTS

The financial support of the Deutsche Forschungsgemeinschaft (Br 731/4-1, Scha 402/1-1) and the Fonds der Chemischen Industrie (ETR) is gratefully acknowledged. We thank M. Lohs and B. Köhler for preparing illustrations and photographs and I. Bendt for typing this manuscript.

REFERENCES

Beutler B, Milsark IW, Cerami AC (1985). Passive immunization against cachectin / tumour necrosis factor protects mice from lethal effect of endotoxin. Science 229:869-871.

Brade L, Brade H (1985). A 28,000 Dalton protein of normal mouse serum binds specifically to the inner core region of bacterial lipopolysaccharide. Infect Immun 50:687-694.

Brade H, Galanos C (1982). Isolation, purification and chemical analysis of the lipopolysaccharide and lipid A of Acinetobacter calcoaceticus NCTC 10305. Eur J Biochem 122:233-237.

Brade L, Rietschel ETh, Kusumoto S, Shiba T, Brade H (1986). Immunogenicity and antigenicity of synthetic Escherichia coli lipid A. Infect Immun 51:110-114.

Freudenberg MA, Keppler D, Galanos C (1986). Requirement for lipopolysaccharide-responsive macrophages in galactosamine-induced sensitization to endotoxin. Infect Immun 51:891-895.

Galanos C, Lüderitz O, Rietschel ETh, Westphal O (1977). Newer aspects of the chemistry and biology of bacterial lipopolysaccharides, with special reference to their lipid A component. In: Goodwin TW (ed) International review of biochemistry, Biochemistry of lipids II. Vol 14, University Park Press, Baltimore, 239-335.

Galanos C, Lüderitz O, Rietschel ETh, Westphal O, Brade H, Brade L, Freudenberg MA, Schade U, Imoto M, Yoshimura H, Kusumoto S, Shiba T (1985). Synthetic and natural Escherichia coli free lipid A express identical endotoxic activities. Eur J Biochem 148:1-5.

Hagman W, Denzlinger C, Keppler D (1984). Role of peptide leukotrienes and their hepatobiliary elimination in endotoxin action. Circ Shock 14:223-235.

Hitchcock PJ, Leive L, Mäkelä PH, Rietschel ETh, Strittmatter W, Morrison DC (1986). A review of lipopolysaccharide nomenclature - past, present and future. J Bacteriol, in press

Homma JY, Matsuura M, Kanegasaki S, Kawakubo Y, Kojima Y, Shibukawa N, Kumazawa Y, Yamamoto A, Tanamoto K, Yasuda T, Imoto M, Yoshimura H, Kusumoto S, Shiba T (1985). Structural Requirements of lipid A responsible for the functions: a study with chemically synthesized lipid A and its analogues. J Biochem (Tokyo) 98:395-406.

Imoto M, Yoshimura H, Sakaguchi N, Kusumoto S, Shiba T (1985). Total synthesis of Escherichia coli lipid A. Tetrahedron Lett 26:1545-1548.

Jirillo E, Miragliotta G, Galanos C, Rietschel ETh, Michalek SM, McGhee JR (eds). Endotoxin: structural aspects and immunobiology of host responses. EOS - Riv Immunol Immunofarm 6:1-275 (Suppl.)

Kanegasaki S, Tanamoto K, Yasuda T, Homma JY, Matsuura M, Nakatsuka M, Kumazawa Y, Yamamoto A, Shiba T, Kusumoto S, Imoto M, Yoshimura A, Shimamoto T (1986). Stucture-activity relationship of lipid A: Comparison of biological activities of natural and synthetic lipid A's with different fatty acid compositions. J. Biochem (Tokyo) 99:1203-1210.

Kotani S, Takada H, Tsujimoto M, Ogawa T, Takahashi I, Ikeda T, Otsuka K, Shimanchi H, Kasai N, Mashimo J, Nagao S, Tanaka S, Harada K, Nagaki K, Kitamura H, Shiba T, Kusumoto S, Imoto M, Yoshimura H (1985). Synthetic lipid A with endotoxic and related biological activities comparable to those of a natural lipid A from an Escherichia coli Re-mutant. Infect Immun 49:225-237.

Lebbard S, Cavaillon JM, Caroff M, Ledur A, Brade H, Sarfati R, Haeffner-Cavaillon N (1986). Molecular requirement for Interleukin 1 induction by lipopolysaccharide - stimulated human monocytes: Involvement of the heptosyl-2-keto-3-deoxyoctulosonate region. Eur J Immunol 16:87-91.

Loppnow H, Brade L, Brade H, Rietschel ETh, Kusumoto S, Shiba T, Flad HD (1986). Lipid A-induced production of Interleukin 1 in human monocytes. Eur J Immunol, in press

Lüderitz O, Freudenberg MA, Galanos C, Lehmann V, Rietschel ETh, Shaw DH (1982). Lipopolysaccharides of gram-negative bacteria. In membrane lipids of prokaryotes. Razin S, Rottem S (eds) Current topics in membranes and transport. Academic Press Inc. New York, 17:79-151.

Mayer H, Salimath PV, Holst O, Weckesser J (1984). Unusual

lipid A-types in phototrophic bacteria and related species. Rev Infect Dis 6:542-545.
Nowotny A, Behling UH (1982). Studies of host defenses enhanced by endotoxins: A brief review. Klin Wochenschr 14:735-739.
Osborn MJ (1979). Biosynthesis and assembly of the lipopolysaccharide of the outer membrane. In Inouye M (ed). Bacterial outer membranes. New York: Wiley-Interscience Publications, 15-34.
Rietschel ETh, Wollenweber HW, Brade H, Zähringer U, Lindner B, Seydel U, Bradaczek H, Barnickel G, Labischinski H, Giesbrecht P (1984). Structure and conformation of the lipid A component of lipopolysaccharides. In: Proctor RA (ed), Handbook of endotoxin, Vol 1, Rietschel ETh (ed), Chemistry of endotoxin, Elsevier, Amsterdam, New York, Oxford, 187-220.
Rietschel ETh, Brade H, Brade L, Brandenburg K, Schade U, Seydel U, Zähringer U, Galanos C, Lüderitz O, Westphal O, Labischinski H, Kusumoto S, Shiba T (1986). Lipid A, the endotoxic center of bacterial lipopolysaccharide: relation of chemical structure to biological activity. 2nd International Conference on Endotoxins and their detection with the Limulus Amebocyte Lysate. (Watson S ed). Alan R Liss Inc, New York, in press
Schlessinger D (ed) (1980). Endogenous mediators in host response to bacterial endotoxin. Microbiology - 1980, Am Soc Microbiol, 2-167.
Strain SM, Armitage IM, Anderson L, Takayama K, Qureshi N, Raetz CRH (1985). Location of polar substituents and fatty acyl chains on lipid A precursors from a 3-deoxy-D-manno-octulosonic acid-deficient mutant of Salmonella typhimurium. J Biol Chem 260:16089-16098.
Tacken A, Rietschel ETh, Brade H (1986). Methylation analysis of the heptose / 3-deoxy-D-manno-2-octulosonic acid region (inner core) of lipopolysaccharide from Salmonella minnesota rough mutants. Carb Res, 148, in press
Takayama K, Qureshi N, Ribi E, Cantrell JL (1984). Separation and characterization of toxic and nontoxic forms of lipid A. Rev Inf Dis 6:439-443.
Tanamoto K, Zähringer U, McKenzie GR, Galanos C, Rietschel ETh, Lüderitz O, Kusumoto S, Shiba T (1984). Biological activities of synthetic lipid A analogues: Pyrogenicity, lethal toxicity, anticomplement activity, and induction of gelation of Limulus amebocyte lysate. Infect Immun 44:421-426.

Westpahl O, Lüderitz O (1954). Chemische Erforschung von Lipopolysacchariden Gram-negativer Bakterien. Angew Chem 66:407-417.

Westphal O, Lüderitz O, Galanos C, Mayer H, Rietschel ETh (1986). The story of bacterial endotoxin. Adv Immunopharmacol (Chedid L, Hadden JW, Ipreafico F, Dukor P, Willoghby D, eds) 3:13-34, Pergamon Press.

Zähringer U, Lindner B, Seydel U, Rietschel ETh, Naoki H, Unger FM, Imoto M, Kusumoto S, Shiba T (1985). Structure of de-O-acylated lipopolysaccharide from the Escherichia coli Re mutant F 515. Tetrahedron Lett 26:6321-6324.

Immunopharmacology of Infectious Diseases: Vaccine Adjuvants and Modulators of Non-Specific Resistance, pages 91–99

CHEMICAL SYNTHESIS OF LIPID A AND ITS ANALOGS FOR ELUCIDATION OF BIOLOGICAL ACTIVITIES OF ENDOTOXINS

Tetsuo Shiba and Shoichi Kusumoto

Department of Chemistry, Faculty of Science, Osaka University, Toyonaka, Osaka 560, Japan

INTRODUCTION

Since the first recognition of an endotoxin activity in *Vibrio cholerae* by R. Pfeiffer at the end of last century, chemical research has focused on an elucidation of the structure of an entity which was found in the outermost surface of the cell wall of Gram negative bacteria, particularly in view of its induction of multiple responses involved in self-defense mechanisms of the host.

Meanwhile the endotoxin activity has been found to be located in the lipid A part, which is linked to a polysaccharide moiety in lipopolysaccharide (LPS). Although a tentative chemical structure of lipid A responsible for the endotoxicity of either *Salmonella* type (Galanos et al., 1977), or *Escherichia coli* type lipid A (Rosner et al., 1979) were assumed, the exact linkage positions and nature of fatty acids attached to the β(1-6)-D-glucosamine disaccharide phosphorylated at the 1 and 4' positions remained ambiguous.

A decisive structure could not be derived at that time mainly because of the extreme heterogeneity of the samples of lipid A. With this in mind, we approached the true chemical structure of lipid A by preparation of many candidates of the active structure through chemical synthesis. Although we tested more than ten different kinds of synthetic compounds which were all acylated at 2,3,4,2', 6'-positions on β(1-6)-D-glucosamine disaccharide according to the earlier proposed structure, none of them exhibited the full activity of lipid A (Shiba and Kusumoto, 1984). Therefore, we turned to the reinvestigation of the structure of the natural lipid A molecule.

In collaboration with a German group, we obtained a chemically pure and single substance as the 1-dephospho-4'-dimethylphosphoryl derivative of natural E. coli type lipid A. From results of two-dimensional NMR (nuclear magnetic resonance) analysis, we could conclude the fatty acid linkage pattern as 2,3 2',3'-acyl disaccharide in contrast to the earlier one (Imoto et al., 1983). In order to confirm this newly proposed structure, we first synthesized a biosynthetic precursor of lipid A designated precursor Ia (1) which has been assumed to possess only four (R)-β-hydroxymyristic acids as fatty acid components (Imoto et al., 1984). The synthetic product obtained thruough twenty synthetic steps was found to be quite identical to the natural acidic precursor Ia in many biologicaltests, indicating the correctness of the new acid linkage positions (Galanos et al., 1984; Kotani et al., 1984).

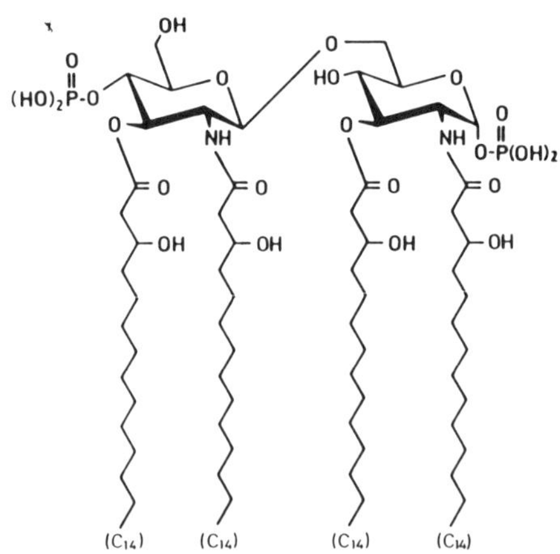

1

Concerning the whole structure of lipid A, we then applied FD-MS (field desorption mass spectrometry) to determine the linkage of the additional two fatty acids to the precursor Ia molecule. Finally we could propose structure 2 for E. coli lipid A (Imoto et al., 1985a).

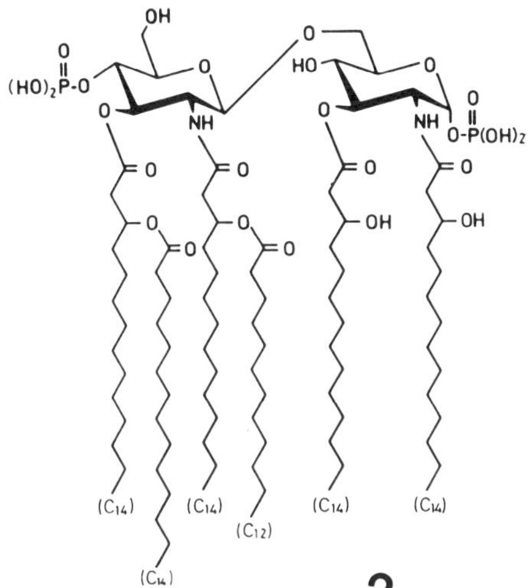

2

RESULT

After the proposal of a reliable structure of E. coli lipid A, the total synthesis of this compound (2) was achieved through twenty four synthetic steps, including the main paths shown in the scheme below (Imoto et al., 1985b). Thus, in order to construct the asymmetrically acylated disaccharide structure of 2, monosaccharide components which already contain most of the acyl groups and one of the phosphates at the correct positions were first prepared and then coupled together to form a β(1 6)-linked disaccharide. Only the β-lauroyloxymyristoyl group on the 2'-amino function was introduced after the formation of the disaccharide skeleton since this particular N-bound acyl group proved to be unstable under the conditions of the glycosidation reaction. The glycosidic phosphate had to be formed at the final stage of the synthesis because of its instability. Hydrogenolytic removal of the all protecting groups afforded the desired disaccharide 1,4'-bisphosphate acylated at 2,3,2',3'-positions (2).

The final synthetic product was identified to be the natural E. coli lipid A in every respect, not only in terms of physical properties, but also with respect to many biological activities. Physical properties covering elemental analysis, TLC and NMR gave satisfactory results.

Biological tests were performed mainly at the Max-Planck Institut für Immunbiologie, Freiburg, the Forschungsinstitut Borstel (Galanos et al., 1985), the Dental School, Osaka University (Kotani et al., 1985), the School of Pharmaceutical Science, Showa University, Tokyo, (Kasai et al., 1985), the Kitasato Institute, Tokyo (Kanegasaki et al., 1986) and so on. The biological activities tested so far involve lethal toxicity, pyrogenicity, local Shwartzman reaction, Limulus amoebocyte lysate gelating activity, tumor necrotizing activity, mitogenicity, induction of prostaglandin

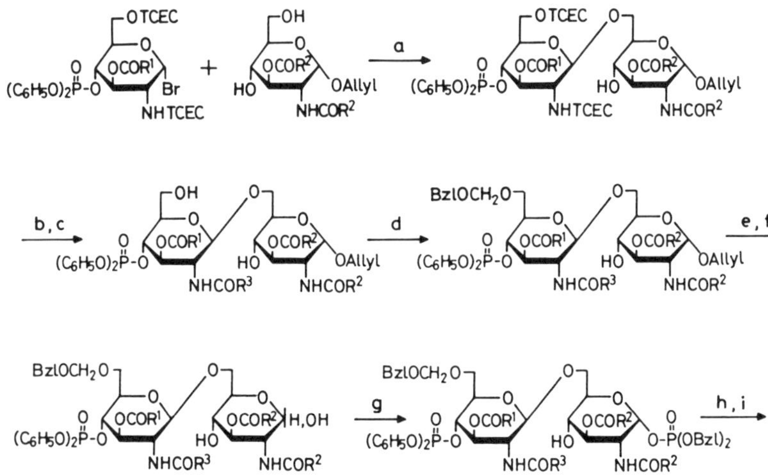

2

TCEC : CCl_3CH_2OCO, Bzl : $C_6H_5CH_2$, Allyl : $CH_2{=}CHCH_2$

R^1CO : $CH_3(CH_2)_{10}CHCH_2CO$, $CH_3(CH_2)_{12}COO$ (on CH)

R^2CO : $CH_3(CH_2)_{10}CHCH_2CO$, BzlO (on CH)

R^3CO : $CH_3(CH_2)_{10}CHCH_2CO$, $CH_3(CH_2)_{10}COO$ (on CH)

a) $Hg(CN)_2/CaSO_4$ in $CHCl_3$, reflux
b) Zn/AcOH, r.t.
c) R^3CO_2H/DCC in $CHCl_3$, r.t.
d) $BzlOCH_2Cl/(iPr)_2EtN$ in CH_2Cl_2, r.t.
e) $[Ir(COD)(PCH_3(C_6H_5)_2)_2]PF_6$ in THF
f) I_2 in aq. THF
g) $(BzlO)_2POCl$/BuLi in THF
h) H_2/Pd-black
i) H_2/PtO_2

production, antigenic activity, leukopenia inducing activity, immunoadjuvant activity, activation of human complement, macrophage stimulating activity, stimulation of murine splenocytes, and enhancement of migration of human polymorphonuclear leukocytes. We could now conclude that the endotoxin activity is expressed by the lipid A molecule which has been determined by chemical synthesis. Furthermore, the chemical synthesis can supply a pure sample of lipid A of a definite structure which is certified to be completely identical to the natural one to use as a standard.

Salmonella lipid A has been known to possess one additional palmitoyl group which was assumed to be attached to the hydroxyl group of β-hydroxymyristic acid at position 2 of *E. coli* lipid A as shown in **3**. This structure was also synthesized in our laboratory recently. Surprisingly, the biological activities exhibited by this compound were rather weaker than those of *E. coli* lipid A (**2**). Such low activity in compound **3** informed us that endotoxicity is much influenced by the delicate balance of number, size, and position of the fatty acids. In any case, such an unexpected result is clarified first by construction of the target structure by organic synthesis.

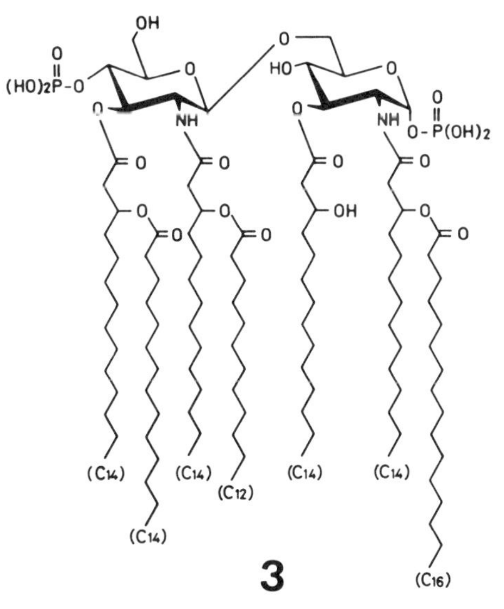

3

It has been demonstrated that monosaccharide derivatives called lipid X (**4**) and lipid Y (**5**) could be precursors in an earlier step of biosynthesis of lipid A (Takayama et al., 1983a,b). These two acylmonosaccharide phosphates became also targets of our synthetic study (Kusumoto et al., 1984). Both synthetic compounds assured the proposed structures (**4**,**5**) and verified their biological activities.

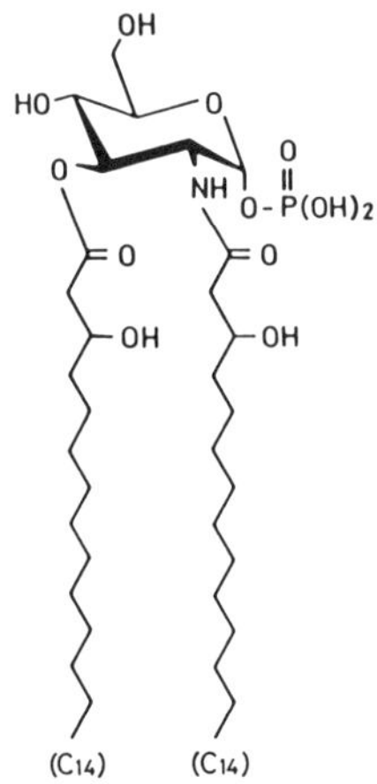

4

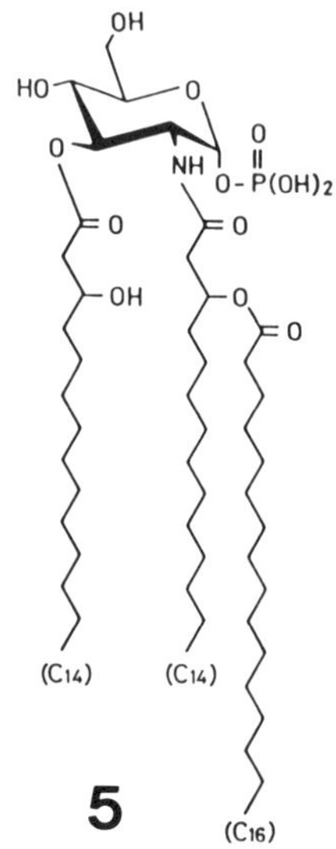

5

In addition to the success of total syntheses of natural lipid As and their precursors, the synthetic technique offered us also analogs of natural lipid A. In fact, we synthesized many structural analogs and derivatives which are somehow modified in phosphate placement or acyl groups, keeping the original β(1-6)-D-glucosamine disaccharide skeleton. From results of biological tests of these compounds, we can now discuss the role of phosphate groups or acyl functions in the exhibition of multiple endotoxic activities.

Finally, in order to clarify the significance of the presence of the 3-deoxy-D-manno-octulosonic acid (KDO) moiety in the LPS molecule, particularly in view of their effect on the antigenicity and antitumor activity of lipid A, we then investigated the structure of the oligosaccharide portion of the E. coli Re mutant F515 lipopolysaccharide by use of NMR spectroscopy and conclusively determined the linkage mode of the tetrasaccharide as α-KDO-(2-4)-α-KDO-(2-6)-β-GlcN-(1-6)-α-GlcN, as shown in **6** (Zähringer et al., 1985). A synthetic study of LPS according to the above proposed structure is now in progress.

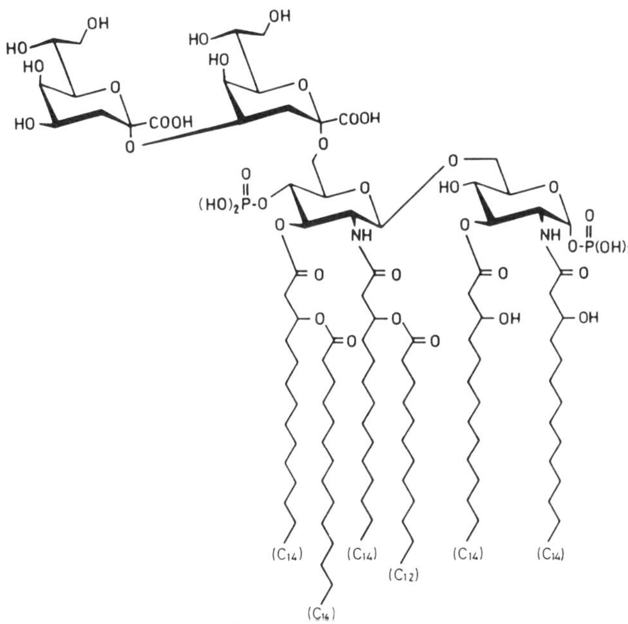

6

REFERENCES

Galanos C, Lüderitz O, Rietschel ET, Westphal O, Brade H, Brade L, Freudenberg M, Shade U, Imoto M, Yoshimura H, Kusumoto S, Shiba T (1985). Synthetic and natural Escherichia coli free lipid A express identical endotoxic activities. Eur J Biochem 148:1-5.

Galanos C, Lehmann V, Lüderitz O, Rietschel ET, Westphal O, Brade H, Brade L, Freudenberg M, Hansen-Hagge T, Lüderitz T, McKenzie G, Schade U, Strittmatter W, Tanamoto K, Zähringer U, Imoto M, Yoshimura H, Yamamoto M, Shimamoto T, Kusumoto S, Shiba T (1984). Endotoxic properties of chemically synthesized lipid A part structures. Eur J Biochem 140:221-227.

Galanos C, Lüderitz O, Rietschel, ET, Westphal O (1977).

Newer aspects of the chemistry and biology of bacterial lipopolysaccharides, with special reference to their lipid A component. In Goodwin TW (ed): "International review of biochemistry. Biochemistry of lipids." Vol 14, Baltimore: University Park Press, p 239.

Imoto M, Kusumoto, S, Shiba T, Rietschel ET, Galanos C, Lüderitz O (1985a). Chemical structure of *Escherichia coli* lipid A. Tetrahedron Lett 26:907-908.

Imoto M, Yoshimura H, Sakaguchi N, Kusumoto, S, Shiba T (1985b). Total synthesis of *Escherichia coli* lipid A. Tetrahedron Lett 26:1545-1548.

Imoto M, Yoshimura H, Yamamoto T, Shimamoto S, Kusumoto S, Shiba T (1984). Chemical synthesis of phosphorylated tetraacyl disaccharide corresponding to a biosynthetic precursor of lipid A. Tetrahedron Lett 25:2667-2670.

Imoto M, Kusumoto S, Shiba T, Naoki H, Iwashita T, Rietschel ET, Wollenweber HW, Galanos C, Lüderitz O (1983). Chemical structure of *E. coli* lipid A: Linkage site of acyl groups in the disaccharide backbone. Tetrahedron Lett 24:4017-4020.

Kanegasaki S, Tanamoto K, Yasuda T, Homma JY, Matsuura M, Nakatsuka M, Kumazawa Y, Yamamoto A, Shiba T, Kusumoto, S, Imoto M, Yoshimura H, Shimamoto T (1986). Structure-activity relationship of lipid A: Comparison of biological activities of natural and synthetic lipid A's with different fatty acid compositions. J Biochem 99:1203-1210.

Kasai N, Arata S, Mashimo J, Okuda K, Aihara Y, Kotani S, Takada H, Shiba T, Kusumoto S (1985). In vitro antigenic reactivity of synthetic lipid A analogues as determined by monoclonal and conventional antibodies. Biochem Biophys Res Commun 128:607-612.

Kusumoto S, Yamamoto M, Shiba T (1984). Chemical syntheses of lipid X and lipid Y, acyl glucosamine 1-phosphate isolated from *Escherichia coli* mutants. Tetrahedron Lett 25:3727-3730.

Kotani S, Takada H, Tsujimoto M, Ogawa T, Takahashi I, Ikeda T, Otsuka K, Shimauchi H, Kasai N, Mashimo J, Nago S, Tanaka A, Tanaka S, Harada K, Nagaki K, Kitamura H, Shiba T, Kusumoto S, Imoto M, Yoshimura H (1985). Synthetic lipid A with endotoxic and related biological activities comparable to those of a natural lipid A from an *Escherichia coli* Re-mutant. Infect Immun 49:225-237.

Kotani S, Takada H, Tsujimoto M, Ogawa T, Harada K, Mori Y, Kawasaki A, Tanaka A, Nagao S, Tanaka S, Shiba T, Kusumoto S, Imoto M, Yoshimura H, Yamamoto M, Shimamoto T (1984). Immunobiologically active lipid A analogs synthesized according to a revised structural model of natural lipid A. Infect Immun 45:293-296.

Rosner MR, Tang JY, Barzilay I, Khorana HG (1979). Structure of the lipopolysaccharide from an *Escherichia coli* heptose-less mutant.I. Chemical degradations and identification of products. J Biol Chem 254:5906-5917.

Shiba T, Kusumoto, S (1984). Chemical synthesis and biological activity of lipid A analogs. In Rietschel ET (ed): "Handbook of endotoxin, Vol 1, Chemistry of endotoxin." Amsterdam: Elsevier Science Publishers, p 284.

Takayama K, Qureshi N, Mascagni P, Nashed MA, Anderson L, Raetz CRH (1983a). Fatty acyl derivatives of glucosamine 1-phosphate in *Escherichia coli* and their relation to lipid A. J Biol Chem 258:7379-7385.

Takayama K, Qureshi N, Mascagni P, Anderson L, Raetz CRH (1983b). Glucosamine-derived phospholipids in *Escherichia coli*. J Biol Chem 258:14245-14252.

Zähringer U, Lindner B, Seydel U, Rietschel ET, Naoki H, Unger FM, Imoto M, Kusumoto S, Shiba T (1985). Structure of de-O-acylated lipopolysaccharide from the *Escherichia coli* Re mutant strain F515. Tetrahedron Lett 26:6321-6324.

Immunopharmacology of Infectious Diseases: Vaccine Adjuvants and Modulators of Non-Specific Resistance, pages 101–112

IMMUNOPOTENTIATING ACTIVITIES OF MONOPHOSPHORYL LIPID A

Edgar Ribi, J. Terry Ulrich and K. Noel Masihi

Ribi ImmunoChem Research, Inc., (E.R., J.T.U.), Hamilton, Montana 59840, and Robert Koch Institute, Federal Health Office, (K.N.M.), West Berlin, F.R.G.

INTRODUCTION

Although Gram-negative bacterial endotoxins and their active moiety, lipid A, are toxic, they also possess potentially beneficial immunopotentiating characteristics. Because of the extremely high susceptibility of humans to the toxic nature of endotoxins however, it has not been possible to utilize this biological agent in clinical applications. Attenuating the endotoxin's toxic and pyrogenic nature without eliminating its ability to stimulate beneficial immune responses was found to be possible by removal of the phosphate moiety at the C-1 position of the toxic diphosphoryl lipid A (DPL) molecule (Takayama et al., 1984b). The resulting monophosphoryl lipid A (MPL), when purified to remove traces of DPL, is at least 1,000 times less lethal and pyrogenic for rabbits than DPL or the parent endotoxin (Takayama et al., 1984a). This has made it possible to consider using MPL in humans. For example, a Phase I clinical trial has shown that MPL can be safely administered in doses of 100 $\mu g/m^2$ (Vosika et al., 1984).

In this presentation, we summarize current research results comparing various biological activities of MPL to those of DPL and endotoxin in a variety of murine models.

IMMUNOLOGICAL PROPERTIES OF MONOPHOSPHORYL LIPID A

Stimulation of the Activities of Phagocytic Cells.

The addition of MPL to mouse peritoneal macrophage cultures was shown to stimulate the phagocytosis of fluorescent beads as efficiently as did toxic DPL and reference standard endotoxin (Masihi et al., 1986b). Furthermore, as the data in Figure 1 show, MPL significantly enhanced the zymosan-induced chemiluminescence activity of mouse spleen cell cultures to levels which were comparable to those induced by DPL (Masihi et al., 1986b). Interestingly, at the dose level of 100 μg tested, the response obtained with parent endotoxin was considerably lower than that of MPL. The capacity of MPL to increase the phagocytic activities of cells in the monocyte/macrophage series suggests that it can be used to stimulate nonspecific antimicrobial and antitumor activity (see below).

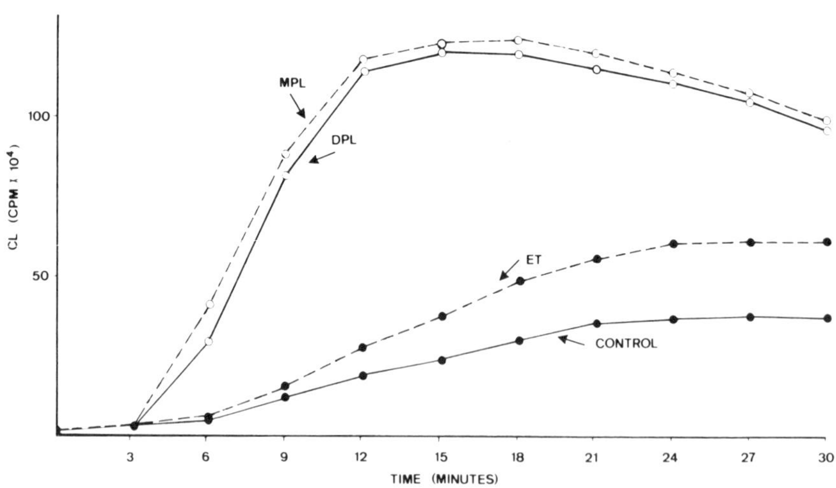

Figure 1. Stimulation of zymosan-induced chemiluminescence (CL) in BALB/c spleen cells following *in vitro* addition of 100 μg endotoxin (ET), diphosphoryl lipid A (DPL), or monophosphoryl lipid A (MPL). Methodology is described in Masihi et al. (1983).

Stimulation of Production of Macrophage Derived Mediators.

Madonna et al. (1986) recently reported that the levels of colony stimulating activity in sera of mice 6 hours after iv injection with 50 ug MPL were comparable to that obtained with 25 ug of endotoxin (Table 1, line A), confirming previous findings (Urbaschek et al., 1985). Madonna et al. (1986) also found that the interferon levels in sera collected 2 hours after iv injection with MPL (50 ug) or endotoxin (25 ug), were comparable (Table 1, line B). It has also been shown that MPL can efficiently stimulate the production of interleukin-1 by human monocytes (Table 1, line C).

TABLE 1. Stimulation of the Production of Macrophage Derived Mediators

Mediator	ET	DPL	MPL
A. Colony stimulating activity Activity of serum: CFU/ml Control: saline 0 CFU/ml	4,010±346	-	3,500±174
B. Interferon (IFN)* Antiviral activity of serum: 2 units/ml Control: saline 2 units/ml	350±50	-	200±0
C. Interleukin (IL-1)** Stimulation by human monocytes (CPM in lysates of monocytes) Control: 15,173 CPM	43,833	39,000	50,625

* Madonna et al., 1986
** Ribi, 1985

Induction of Early Endotoxin Tolerance by MPL.

MPL was shown by Madonna et al. (1986) to increase the 50% lethal dose of endotoxin by a factor of 4 when administered 3 days prior to challenge (Table 2). It was also effective in reducing the overt symptoms of endotoxicity in the challenged mice. These data demonstrate that MPL was effective in inducing a state of early tolerance to a fully toxic endotoxin.

TABLE 2. Effect of Initial MPL Exposure on LPS-Induced LD_{50} and Symptoms of Endotoxicity

	Experimental Group		
	Saline/LPS	MPL/LPS*	LPS/LPS*
LD_{50}	258 μg	1156 μg	972 μg
Symptoms			
Ruffled fur	10/12**	0/15	1/12
Conjunctivitis	5/12	2/15	0/12
Diarrhea	6/12	1/15	1/12

* Mice were injected on day 0 with saline, MPL (100 μg/mouse) or *E. coli* K235 LPS (25 μg/mouse). Three days later, the mice were challenged with *E. coli* LPS for LD_{50} and symptomatology determination.

** The proportion of mice clearly exhibiting the indicated symptom 6 hours after ip injection of *E. coli* K235 LPS (25 μg/mouse) on day 3. Injection of MPL (1-100 μg/mouse) induced none of the indicated symptoms.

Madonna et al., 1986.

Enhancement of Nonspecific Resistance Against Lethal X-irradiation.

Figure 2 shows that 100 μg of MPL given iv to mice 24 hours prior to exposure to 600 R whole body X-irradiation protected 70% of the animals (Urbaschek et al., 1985). While a dose of 10 μg of parent endotoxin was lethal for irradiated mice (10% survivors), however, it was found that a dose of 1 μg of endotoxin was not lethal and protected 75% of the animals. This protective effect is probably related to the capacity of endotoxin and MPL to induce elevated levels of colony stimulating factor and therefore to stimulate granulopoiesis (Urbaschek et al., 1980).

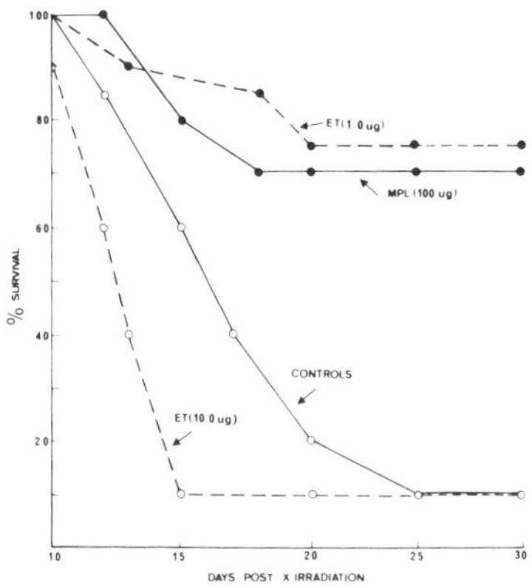

Figure 2. Survival of C_3HeB/FeJ mice receiving 600 R whole body X-irradiation 24 hours following an iv injection of endotoxin (S. minnesota R595) or MPL. Control mice were injected with saline (Urbaschek et al., 1985).

Enhancement of Nonspecific Host Resistance Against Infectious Disease.

We initially examined the effect of MPL administered in saline in protecting mice against a lethal challenge of Escherichia coli 055B5. As is seen in Figure 3, 100 µg MPL given ip in saline 1 day prior to challenge with E. coli 055B5 (5 LD_{50}) provided 100% protection. However, if the MPL treatment was given 14 days prior to challenge, no protection was achieved, indicating that the protective effect of MPL in saline was short-lived. As can also be seen in Figure 3, the protective effect is much more long-lived when the MPL is administered as an oil-in-water emulsion with trehalose dimycolate (TDM). Thus, ip pretreatment of mice with oil-in-water emulsions (1% squalane) of TDM plus MPL, or of TDM alone provided significant protection of mice even when they were challenged 14 days later.

To assess whether treatment of mice with TDM and MPL emulsions exert a protective influence through an enhanced bactericidal activity of the inflammatory cell population, we next evaluated these materials in two models using facultative intracellular parasites, namely Salmonella enteritidis (S795) and Listeria monocytogenes (EGD). The data from experiments using a S. enteritidis challenge in BALB/c mice are summarized in Table 3. These data indicate that the survivorship of mice following a lethal ip challenge (4 LD_{50}) was dependent on the dose, time of administration relative to challenge and composition of the injected material. Mice receiving 100 µg each of TDM and MPL in an oil-in-water emulsion fared consistently better than when MPL or TDM were used alone in the emulsion. MPL injected as a saline solution offered no protection even when given only 2 days prior to challenge.

TABLE 3. Survival of BALB/c Mice Injected ip with 4 LD_{50} Doses of Salmonella enteritidis (S795) Following ip Treatment with MPL or MPL + TDM

		% survivors, 14 days after challenge				
	Dose	Days post-treatment				
Treatment	(µg)	2	9	10	12	24
MPL (saline)	100	0	-	0	0	-
MPL (o/w)	100	-	55	-	-	-
MPL+TDM (o/w)	100+100	-	100	75	62	45
TDM (o/w)	100	-	25	-	25	-

Controls: For each experiment (groups of 12-20 mice) control mice were injected with saline. All mice in control group were dead within 4 days after challenge.
o/w: Oil-in-water emulsion containing 2% squalane in 0.2% tween-80 saline.

The results of our initial experiments with L. monocytogenes are shown in Figure 4. Again, it is apparent that pretreatment of mice with oil-in-water emulsion containing MPL and TDM or MPL alone or TDM alone results in significant protection of mice challenged with 5 LD_{50} of L. monocytogenes (EGD). In similar experiments (data not shown) pretreatment of mice with MPL in saline 1 or 2 days prior to infection provided no protection.

The capacity of oil-in-water emulsions containing MPL and TDM to provide a long-term protective effect is further demonstrated by the work of Masihi et al. (1986a). In these studies, iv injection of MPL and TDM in an oil-in-water emulsion (1% squalane) was able to confer protection of mice against a lethal aerogenic challenge of influenza virus administered 3 weeks later (Table 4). In addition, there was a marked reduction of the viral titer in the lungs of the treated mice.

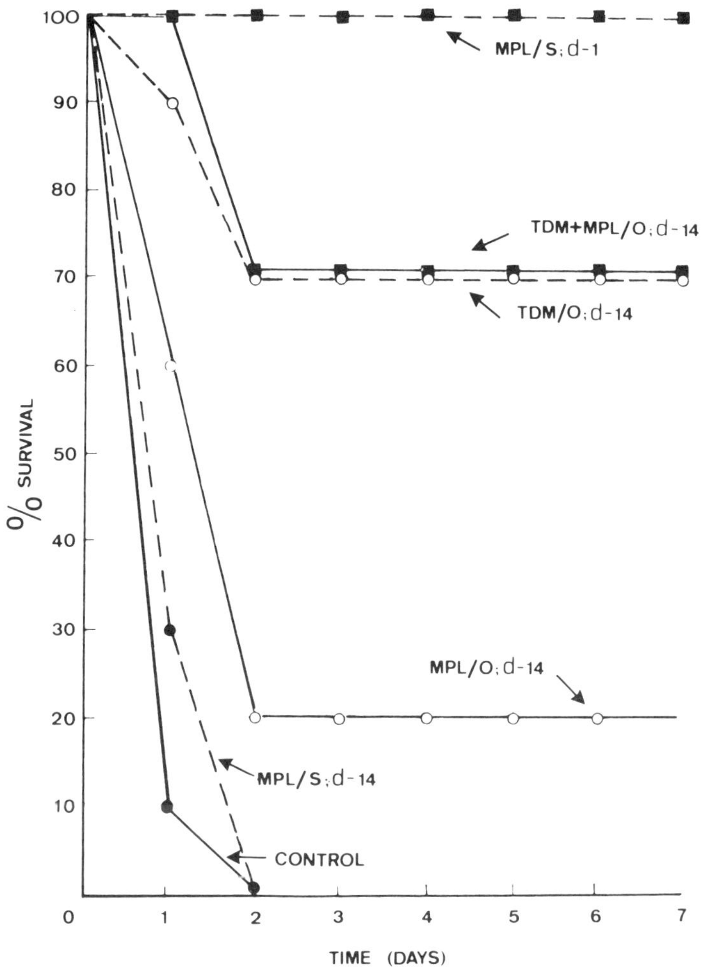

Figure 3. Survival of BALB/c mice following challenge with 5 LD_{50} Escherichia coli (055B5). Groups of 15 mice were injected ip 14 days (d-14) prior to challenge with: TDM plus MPL oil-in-water emulsion (TDM + MPL/o); TDM oil-in-water emulsion (TDM/o); MPL oil-in-water emulsion (MPL/o); or MPL in saline (MPL/s). An additional group of 15 mice was injected ip one day prior to challenge with MPL in saline (MPL/s; d-1). The dose of each component used was 100 µg per mouse.

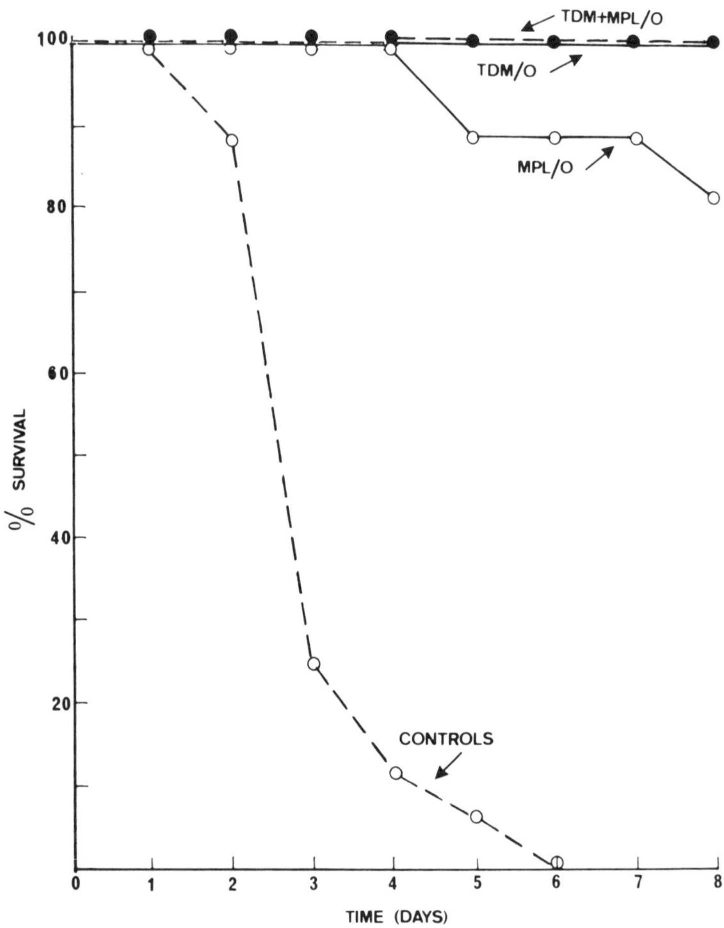

Figure 4. Survival of BALB/c mice following intraperitoneal challenge with 5 LD_{50} Listeria monocytogenes (EGD). Groups of 15 mice were injected ip 10 days prior to challenge with: TDM + MPL/o, TDM/o, or MPL/o. The dose of each component used was 100 µg per mouse. Control mice were injected with saline. For abbreviations, see legend for Figure 3.

TABLE 4. Protection Against Influenza Virus Infection by Combination of MPL and TDM*

Treatment	Dose (μg)	Survivors/ total (%)	p	Virus titer $\log_{10}$ $TCID_{50}$	p
MPL	50	0/10 (0)	-	-	-
TDM	50	0/10 (0)	-	-	-
MPL+TDM	50+50	10/10 (100)	<0.001	3.3	<0.05
Vehicle	-	0/21 (0)	-	5.0	-

* Mice in groups of 15 were treated iv with oil-in-water emulsion (1% squalane) and infected 3 weeks later with an aerosol containing A/PR/834 virus. Seventy-two hours after infection lungs of 5 mice per group were processed for viral titers on MDCK cells, and the 50% tissue culture infective dose ($TCID_{50}$) determined.

Masihi et al., 1986 (in press).

Enhancement of Antibody Formation.

We reported elsewhere that MPL markedly enhanced the adjuvant activity of TDM with weakly immunogenic antigens (Ribi, 1986). These materials are typically administered as an oil-in-water emulsion (1-2% oil). It has been found that the emulsion may be lyophilized prior to addition of the antigen. In this case the lyophilized emulsion is simply reconstituted with a saline or PBS solution containing the antigen. This new adjuvant system reproducibly elicited a greater immune response than did Freund's complete adjuvant (Ribi et al., 1986) or alum. This adjuvant system will have useful application in the development of efficacious new generation vaccines for animal and human use. These may include subunit vaccines as exemplified by a Brucella abortus extract (Ribi, 1986) or influenza A and B antigen containing bivalent vaccine (Masihi et al., 1986a), synthetic vaccines such as hepatitis B peptide (Feldner et al., 1986, Ribi, 1986) or genetically engineered antigens.

Enhancement of Antibody Formation in Immunodeficient Mice.

It is known that mice, as well as other species, become immunodeficient as they age. Tomai et al. (unpublished observation) observed a marked restoration of antibody formation when aged mice were injected with saline solutions of antigen plus MPL or DPL. These mice exhibited antibody levels which were comparable to those of young adult mice. We are currently in the process of determining whether MPL is also capable of overcoming the deficiencies in cell-mediated immune responses associated with aging. A curious observation was that, in contrast to MPL, endotoxin from smooth strains of bacteria was not effective in enhancement of the antibody production in aged mice.

Since cancer is a disease associated with immunodeficiency, this and other observations reviewed here are consistent with the observed effectiveness of MPL containing preparations in the intralesional treatment of older and larger established spontaneous sarcoid tumors in horses (Ribi and Ward, unpublished data). Clinical trials are currently underway to assess the utility of these preparations in treating several types of human cancers. Preliminary results with malignant melanoma and Kaposi's sarcoma have been very encouraging (Pinsky et al., unpublished data).

DISCUSSION

The results summarized in the preceding paragraphs lend strong support to the notion that a major site of action of MPL is the phagocytic cell system, namely the monocyte/macrophage series and possibly also the polymorphonuclear leukocytes. As a result of interaction with MPL, the phagocytic cells become activated and appear to be characterized by increased phagocytic and microbicidal activities. In the case of macrophages, activation by MPL also results in release of several mediators (colony stimulating factor, α-interferon, and interleukin-1). Activation of the phagocytic cell system is probably an important mechanism by which MPL is able to stimulate nonspecific resistance against microbial challenge.

It is important to recall from the foregoing that the activity of MPL is enhanced if it is presented in an oil-in-water emulsion containing TDM. This is consistent with the long-known observation that the activation of macrophages by bacterial endotoxins is potentiated by BCG cell walls or whole cells. We have shown that MPL possesses many of the beneficial properties and none of the harmful attributes of the endotoxic molecule (Ribi, 1986). With regards to BCG, it is well-known that TDM is one of the major adjuvant-active constituents of BCG cell walls. Thus, MPL plus TDM represents a chemically-defined version of endotoxin plus BCG, which is free of the unfavorable properties of endotoxin (Takayama et al., 1984a; Takayama et al., 1984b) and of BCG (Ribi et al., 1981).

It should also be emphasized that both TDM and MPL are amphiphilic molecules which undergo spontaneous aggregation in water to form micellar or membranous structures. Their amphiphilic nature also causes them to associate with the microscopic oil droplets present in an oil-in-water emulsion. It is interesting to speculate what role this tendency to form aggregates in water plays in the mechanism of action of these adjuvant-active compounds. We have proposed elsewhere that this is probably a key factor in at least the initial interactions between these compounds and the relevant sites in the immune system (Ribi et al., 1986).

Finally, it is very significant that MPL retains the ability of the parent endotoxin to synergistically enhance the tumor regression potency of mycobacterial cell wall adjuvants, including TDM (Ribi et al., 1986). Indeed, in our laboratory we have resorted to certain cancers rather than microbial infections as models to determine the prophylactic and therapeutic potency of chemically-defined immunostimulants of microbial origin. The low toxicity and broad spectrum of activities of MPL used alone and MPL used in combination with TDM in the laboratory models reported here indicates their potential utility as antitumor agents as well as for prevention and treatment of infectious diseases.

REFERENCES

Feldner TJ, Cantrell JL, Altman A, Dixon FJ (1986). Development of an adjuvant system with application for subunit and synthetic peptide vaccines. First Annual ASM Conference on Biotechnology, Washington DC, 20-23 March, Abstract No. 105.

Madonna GS, Peterson JE, Ribi EE, Vogel SN (1986). Early phase endotoxin tolerance: Induction by a detoxified lipid A derivative, monophosphoryl lipid A. Infect Immun 51:6-11.

Masihi KN, Azuma I, Brehmer W, Lange W (1983). Stimulation of chemiluminescence by synthetic muramyl dipeptide and analogs. Infect Immun 40: 16-21.

Masihi KN, Lange W, Brehmer W, Ribi E (1986a). Immunobiological activities of nontoxic lipid A: Enhancement of nonspecific resistance in combination with trehalose dimycolate against viral infection and adjuvant effects. Int J Immunopharmacol, in press.

Masihi KN, Lange W, Johnson AG, Ribi E (1986b). Enhancement of chemiluminescence and phagocytic activities by nontoxic and toxic forms of lipid A. J Biol Resp Mod, in press.

Ribi E (1986). Structure-function relationship of bacterial adjuvants. In Nervig RM, Gough PM, Kaeberle ML, Whetstone CA (eds): "Advances in Carriers and Adjuvants for Veterinary Biologics," Ames: Iowa State University Press, p 35.

Ribi E, Cantrell J, Feldner T, Myers K, Peterson J (1986). Biological activities of monophosphoryl lipid A. In Leive L (ed): "Microbiology-1986," Washington DC: American Society for Microbiology, p 9.

Ribi E, Cantrell J, Schwartzman S, Parker R (1981). BCG cell wall skeleton, P3, MDP and other microbial components - structure activity studies in animal models. In Hersh EM, Chirigos MA and Mastrangelo MJ (eds): "Augmenting Agents in Cancer Therapy," New York. Raven Press, p. 15.

Takayama K, Qureshi N, Raetz CRH, Ribi E, Peterson J, Cantrell JL, Pearson FC, Wiggins J, Johnson AG (1984a). Influence of fine structure of lipid A on Limulus amebocyte lysate clotting and toxic activities. Infect Immun 45: 350-355.

Takayama K, Qureshi N, Ribi E, Cantrell JL (1984b). Separation and characterization of toxic and nontoxic forms of lipid A. Rev Infect Dis 6: 439-443.

Urbaschek RM, Shadduck RK, Bona C, Mergenhagen SE (1980). Colony-stimulating factor in nonspecific resistance and in increased susceptibility to endotoxin. Microbiology 80: 115-119.

Urbaschek R, Urbaschek B, Ribi E (1985). Induction of nonspecific resistance, endotoxin tolerance and colony-stimulating activity (CSA) by nontoxic LPS components. Fed Proc 44: 1490.

Vosika GJ, Barr C, Gilberton D (1984). Phase I study of intravenous modified lipid A. Cancer Immunol Immunother 18: 107-112.

Immunopharmacology of Infectious Diseases: Vaccine Adjuvants and Modulators of Non-Specific Resistance, pages 113–123

IMMUNOMODULATION BY OUTER MEMBRANE PROTEINS ASSOCIATED WITH THE ENDOTOXIN OF GRAM-NEGATIVE BACTERIA

Barnet M. Sultzer, John P. Craig and Raymond Castagna
Department of Microbiology and Immunology, SUNY, Health Science Center at Brooklyn, Brooklyn, New York 11203

INTRODUCTION

Certain outer membrane proteins, which can be extracted in complex form associated with the lipopolysaccharide (LPS) endotoxin of Gram-negative bacteria, have been found to be potent activators of lymphocytes and macrophages (Sultzer, 1983). These proteins, which we have referred to as endotoxin protein (EP), are separable from the LPS by hot phenol-water extraction and have the property of collectively and individually activating the proliferation of B-cells from LPS hyporesponsive C3H/HeJ mice (Sultzer and Goodman, 1976). In addition, EP stimulates polyclonal antibody synthesis, activates macrophages to be cytotoxic for tumor cells, and induces interferon activity in mice (Sultzer, 1983). More recently, we have also found that EP from *Salmonella typhi* and *Bordetella pertussis* can act as adjuvants (Sultzer et al., 1985). This report will serve to amplify the evidence of the immunoregulatory activities of EP and, furthermore, describe the activation of C3H/HeJ lymphocytes and macrophages by pertussis LPS endotoxin.

MATERIAL AND METHODS

Animals. CF-1 mice were obtained from Charles River Breeding Laboratories (Wilmington, MA). CBA/J, C3H/HeJ and C3H/OuJ mice were obtained from Jackson Laboratories (Bar Harbor, Maine). Mice of both sexes were used at two to four months of age and maintained on water and Purina mouse chow *ad lib*.

Antigens and Adjuvants. Purified cholera enterotoxin was obtained from List Biological Laboratories, Inc. (Campbell, CA). Procholeragenoid (Pcg) was prepared by heating the purified toxin for 30 min. at 65°C. Cholera toxin concentrated filtrate from V. cholerae 569B was used for coating sheep erythrocytes (Kateley et al., 1974). EP was prepared from S. typhi 0-901 and B. pertussis 3779B-114 cells as previously described (Sultzer et al., 1985). Stock solutions of each EP at 1 mg/ml were prepared as pyrogen-free solutions in water and stored at -20°C. Protein-free LPS was recovered from the aqueous phase of the phenol-water fraction of the trichloracetic acid extracted endotoxin of each organism. In addition, protein-free LPS was extracted directly from acetone dried cells of B. pertussis by the phenol-chloroform-petroleum ether method (Galanos et al., 1969). Highly purified S3 pneumococcal polysaccharide was generously provided by Dr. G. Schiffman. Polymyxin B sulfate was obtained from Sigma Chemical Co. (St. Louis, MO).

Lymphocyte Cultures. Single cell suspensions were prepared from spleens, and the cells cultured in RPMI-1640 medium supplemented with fetal calf serum (Gibco Laboratories, Grand Island, N.Y.), 100 U of penicillin per ml and 100 μg of streptomycin as previously described (Sultzer and Goodman, 1976). For cultures depleted of macrophages, the spleen cells were treated with carbonyl iron (Sultzer and Goodman, 1976). In those cultures depleted of T-cells, monoclonal anti-thy 1.2 antibody and Low Tox rabbit complement from Accurate Chemical and Scientific Corp. (Westbury, N.Y.) were used. DNA synthesis was measured by incorporation of [^{3}H]-thymidine. Interleukin-1 (IL-1) activity from peritoneal macrophage cultures stimulated with EP or LPS was assayed by using C3H/HeJ thymocytes (Mizel, 1980).

Plaque-forming Cell Assay. Direct (IgM) and indirect (IgG) plaque-forming cells were measured in a modified Jerne system using erythrocytes (SRBC) or SRBC coated with cholera enterotoxin. Spleen cells were cultured at various concentrations in 35 mm plastic petri dishes or 16 mm well plates at 37°C in an atmosphere of 83% N_2, 10% CO_2 and 7% O_2 in the presence or absence of antigen and/or adjuvant added at the initiation of the culture. All cultures were done in triplicate and fed daily with 0.1 ml of culture medium. For determining IgM plaques against S3 pneumococcal polysaccharide, SRBC were coated with S3 by the chromium chloride method (Baker et al., 1969). For polyclonal antibody experiments, the spleen cell cultures were incubated with or without EP or LPS alone. The plaque assay was done after 72 hrs of culture using trinitrophenylated (TNP) coated SRBC as the substrate (Rittenberg and Pratt, 1969).

Gel Electrophoresis. Analytical polyacrylamide gel electrophoresis (PAGE) was performed with the discontinuous sodium dodecyl sulfate (SDS) buffer system (Laemmli, 1970) using slab gels as previously described (Sultzer, et al., 1985). The stacking gel was 14% acrylamide with 4M Urea. The samples were dissolved in an SDS and 2-mercaptoethanol buffer. The gel was run 3 hrs against a voltage of 200-240 V and stained by the silver method (Tsai and Frasch, 1982).

RESULTS AND DISCUSSION

The results of previous experiments have clearly shown that the EP from both *S. typhi* and *B. pertussis* enhanced the immune response to cholera enterotoxin in mice after immunization with cholera toxoid (Sultzer et al., 1985). The degree of protection in mice challenged with lethal toxin 6 weeks after immunization with antigen and adjuvant was increased 5 to 27 times over that obtained when cholera toxoid was given alone. Furthermore, serum from these mice prior to challenge showed higher antitoxin levels which correlated with the enhanced degree of protection.

In more recent experiments, we have used the T-dependent antigen SRBC and the so-called T-independent antigen S3 pneumococcal polysaccharide. Splenic lymphocytes from mice which were immunized with SRBC and given *S. typhi* EP (TEP) or *B. pertussis* EP (PEP) simultaneously produced 5 to 7 times more IgG plaque forming cells (PFC) than mice which received the antigen alone (Table 1). In the case of the S3 pneumococcal polysaccharide, the enhancement of IgM-PFCs by both TEP and PEP was detected at high and low dose of antigen. Of additional interest is the fact that when *S. typhi* LPS is given under the same regimen, a significant depression of 70-88% in IgM plaques is obtained (data not shown).

Next we turned to lymphocyte cultures to dissect, if possible, how EP could adjuvant antibody production. Both TEP and PEP are potent polyclonal activators of antibody synthesis. As shown in Table 3, both TEP and LPS stimulate

TABLE 1.

ADJUVANT EFFECT OF ENDOTOXIN PROTEIN
ON IGG RESPONSE TO SHEEP ERYTHROCYTES IN CBA/J MICE

	MEAN NO. INDIRECT PFC/10^6 SPLEEN CELLS[1]			
	EXP. 1		EXP. 2	
ANTIGEN/ADJUVANT[2]	7 DAYS	14 DAYS	7 DAYS	14 DAYS
SRBC	89	22	56	35
SRBC + TEP	439 (4.9)[3]	157 (7.1)	315 (5.6)	109 (3.1)
SRBC + PEP	590 (6.6)	163 (7.4)	297 (5.3)	140 (4.0)

1. 4-5 MICE PER GROUP.
2. SRBC (0.5%) GIVEN I.V. WITH ADJUVANT (10 µG).
3. ( ) STIMULATION INDEX.

TABLE 2.

ENHANCEMENT OF IGM ANTIBODY TO S3
PNEUMOCOCCAL POLYSACCHARIDE IN MICE
BY ENDOTOXIN PROTEIN

ANTIGEN/ADJUVANT (µG)[1]	TOTAL MEAN PFC/SPLEEN[2] AT 5 DAYS	% INCREASE
S3 (0.1)	3,178	-
+ TEP (10)	5,106	60.7
+ PEP (10)	5,459	71.8
S3 (1.0)	5,898	-
+ TEP (10)	10,903	84.9
+ PEP (10)	8,761	48.5

1. ANTIGEN AND ADJUVANT GIVEN SIMULTANEOUSLY BY I.P. ROUTE.
2. DIRECT PLAQUES, MEAN OF 4 MICE PER GROUP. (CF-1).

large numbers of PFC to TNP-SRBC; however, the response to TEP is not inhibited by polymyxin B as is the case with LPS, indicating that TEP is not contaminated with any residual LPS. In previous studies, the stimulation in culture by EP of antibody synthesis to cholera toxoid and SRBC has been demonstrated to equal or surpass the adjuvant effect of LPS (Sultzer et al., 1985). When splenic lymphocytes derived from SRBC primed mice are used in culture, the secondary PFC response can be enhanced as well (Table 4). The optimal response is obtained when both the antigen and adjuvant are cultured with cells primed with both SRBC and TEP. Enhancement of Ig-PFC to SRBC using the same protocol also has been obtained (data not shown).

The requirement for accessory cells for the adjuvant effect of EP was also examined. Depletion of T-cells or macrophages significantly reduced the direct PFC to cholera toxoid as shown in Tables 5 and 6: however, it is important to note that a substantial portion of the overall enhancement is due to polyclonal activation which is not decreased and in some cases enhanced by removal of macrophages or T-cells.

TABLE 3.

EFFECT OF POLYMYXIN B ON POLYCLONAL ACTIVATION STIMULATED BY ENDOTOXIN AND ENDOTOXIN PROTEIN

	MEAN NO. OF PFC/10^6 SPLEEN CELLS[a]			
PB (μG)	LPS (10)[b]	EP (10)[b]	LPS (1)	EP (1)
0	548	486	646	430
5	103 (81%)[c]	523 (-)	82 (87%)	440 (-)
10	74 (86%)	445 (8%)	48 (93%)	561 (-)

a. ALL CULTURES WERE HARVESTED AFTER 72 HRS OF INCUBATION AND PLAQUED AGAINST TNP-SRBC. CBA/J MOUSE SPLEEN CELLS.

b. LPS AND EP DERIVED FROM *SALMONELLA TYPHI* 0-901 AND USED AT 10 AND 1 MICROGRAM PER CULTURE.

c. (%) INHIBITION.

TABLE 4.

ADJUVANT EFFECT OF ENDOTOXIN PROTEIN ON CULTURES OF ANTIGEN PRIMED LYMPHOCYTES[a]

	PRIMED WITH			
	SRBC		SRBC + TEP	
CULTURED WITH	CBA/J	CF-1	CBA/J	CF-1
0	7[b]	246	5	228
SRBC	22	1367	49	440
SRBC + TEP	963 (43.8)[c]	3261 (2.4)	2708 (55.3)	2626 (5.9)

a. SPLENIC LYMPHOCYTES CULTURED 5 DAYS AFTER PRIMING INJECTION.

b. MEAN NO. OF DIRECT PFC/10^6 SPLEEN CELLS AFTER 5 DAYS OF CULTURE.

c. ( ) FOLD-INCREASE OVER MICE PRIMED WITH SRBC OR SRBC+TEP.

In view of the role of macrophages as accessory cells for the adjuvant effect of EP and since EP has been shown to activate mouse macrophages to be cytotoxic for tumor cells, we investigated the possibility that macrophage Interleukin-1 (IL-1) activity could be stimulated by EP. For this purpose, resident peritoneal macrophages from normal mice were collected, plated and cultured in the presence of each stimulant at 100 μg per culture. After twenty-four hours, the culture supernatants were harvested and assayed for IL-1 activity by the C3H/HeJ thymocyte assay. The results (Fig. 1) clearly show that supernatants synergize with Concanavalin A to stimulate thymocyte proliferation. We conclude, therefore, that EP like LPS can stimulate IL-1 activity from mouse macrophages which may very well contribute to the adjuvanticity of EP.

TABLE 5. EFFECT OF T-CELLS ON THE ADJUVANTICITY OF EP IN MURINE LYMPHOCYTE CULTURES[1]

	Mean No. PFC/10^6 Spleen Cells					
	CBA/J			C3H/OuJ		
Antigen/Adjuvant	S.C.	S.C.-T[4]	% (change)	S.C.	S.C.-T[4]	% (change)
None	15	2		0	9	
PCG[2]	6	0		60	9	(- 85)
TEP[3]	415	615	(+ 48)	380	395	(+ 4)
PCG + TEP	1590	620	(- 61)	520	250	(- 52)

1. 6 days of culture, direct PFCs measured against cholera toxin coated SRBC.
2. Procholeragenoid antigen at 1 µg/ml of culture.
3. TEP at 10 µg/ml of culture.
4. Depletion by monoclonal anti-Thy 1.2 plus C' varied from 86% to 100% as measured by Con A response assay.

TABLE 6. EFFECT OF MACROPHAGES ON THE ADJUVANTICITY OF EP IN MURINE LYMPHOCYTE CULTURES[1]

	Mean No. PFC/10^6 Spleen Cells		
Antigen/Adjuvant	Undepleted	Depleted[2]	(% change)
None	0	0	
PCG[3]	0	0	
TEP[4]	177	292	(+ 65)
PCG + TEP	569	85	(- 85)
PEP[4]	272	238	(- 13)
PCG + PEP	1450	417	(- 71)

1. 6 days of culture, direct PFCs measured against cholera toxin coated SRBC.
2. Macrophage depletion by carbonyl iron method.
3. Procholeragenoid antigen at 1µg/ml of culture.
4. TEP and PEP at 10µg/ml of culture.

As a by-product of the extraction of PEP, we recovered LPS using the phenol-water method (PW) for purifying LPS from the Boivin endotoxin. The LPS recovered contained less than 1% protein and was mitogenically inactive on C3H/HeJ splenic lymphocytes (Sultzer et al., 1985). However the yields were relatively small and since pertussis LPS is similar to rough (R) enteric LPS, we adopted the phenol-chloroform-petroleum ether (PCE) method (Galanos et al., 1969) which efficiently extracts R-LPS. By this procedure, we obtained essentially protein-free pertussis LPS which, surprisingly, was active as a mitogen for C3H/HeJ spleen cells (Table 7). In fact the activity of PLPS is amplified when C3H/HeJ B-cells are used (Table 8), whereas the typical enteric LPS or the PW-PLPS is essentially inactive. As expected, all of the LPS preparations are active on the LPS responsive CBA/J and C3H/OuJ

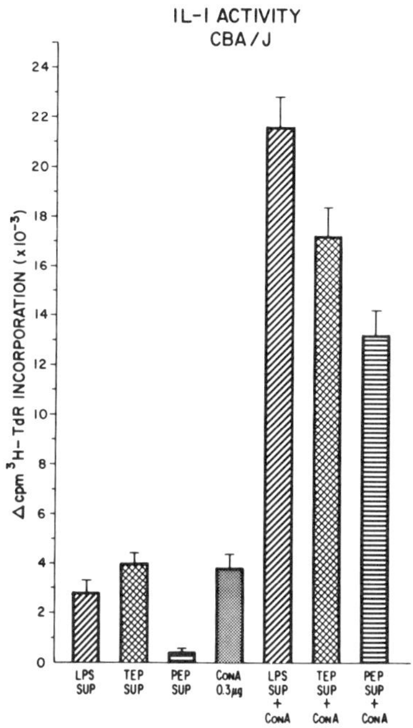

Figure 1. Interleukin-1 activity in the supernatants of EP stimulated CBA/J macrophages.

strains, regardless of the source or extraction method used.

When these pertussis LPS preparations were analyzed by SDS-PAGE, a clear difference was obtained (Fig. 2). The PW-LPS demonstrated one major band, whereas the PCE-LPS produced 2 major bands (1,2), a diffuse area of staining between the major bands (3), and the suggestion of a faster-migrating minor band (4). From these results, it appears that the major species (2) is inactive on C3H/HeJ B-cells and the slowest migrating species (1) is most likely responsible for the mitogen effect observed with C3H/HeJ cells. Indeed, in a preliminary experiment wherein we have separated the two major molecular species of the PCE-PLPS by hydroxylapatite chromatography, (1) is mitogenic for C3H/HeJ spleen cells whereas (2) is not, although both components activate C3H/OuJ cells.

TABLE 7. STIMULATION OF DNA SYNTHESIS IN C3H/HEJ SPLENIC LYMPHOCYTES BY PERTUSSIS LIPOPOLYSACCHARIDE[1]

LPS, μG/CULTURE		MEAN NET CPM OF ^{3}H-TDR INCORPORATION	
EXP. 1		C3H/HEJ	CBA/J
PLPS (PW)[1]	1	98	42,433
	10	767	43,350
	100	1,086	9,927
EXP. 2		C3H/HEJ	C3H/OUJ
PLPS (PCE)[2]	0.1	3,683	36,920
	1.0	10,966	23,294
	10.0	16,199	10,622

1. PERTUSSIS LPS (PW) EXTRACTED BY PHENOL-WATER METHOD.
2. PERTUSSIS LPS (PCE) EXTRACTED BY PHENOL-CHLOROFORM-PETROLEUM ETHER METHOD.

TABLE 8. STIMULATION OF DNA SYNTHESIS IN C3H/HEJ B-ENRICHED SPLENIC LYMPHOCYTES BY PERTUSSIS LIPOPOLYSACCHARIDE ENDOTOXIN

LPS, μG/CULTURE		MEAN NET CPM OF ^{3}H-TDR INCORPORATION			
SPLEEN CELLS		C3H/HEJ	(SI)	C3H/OUJ	(SI)
PLPS[1]	0.1	11,666	(7.0)	49,688	(5.3)
"	1.0	8,636	(5.5)	41,583	(4.6)
"	10.0	5,847	(4.0)	37,781	(4.2)
TLPS[2]	0.1	439	(1.2)	35,581	(4.1)
"	1.0	541	(1.3)	35,736	(3.9)
"	10.0	607	(1.3)	23,990	(3.1)
B-CELLS[3]					
PLPS	0.1	6,900	(3.9)	50,798	(9.5)
"	1.0	13,680	(6.8)	58,155	(10.9)
"	10.0	30,230	(13.8)	53,729	(10.0)
TLPS	0.1	459	(1.2)	42,716	(8.2)
"	1.0	830	(1.4)	49,549	(9.3)
"	10.0	650	(1.3)	22,860	(4.8)

1. PERTUSSIS LPS EXTRACTED BY PHENOL-CHLOROFORM-PETROLEUM ETHER. NO PROTEIN DETECTED (LOWRY).
2. LPS FROM *S. TYPHI* 0-901 BY PHENOL WATER METHOD. LESS THAN 1.0% PROTEIN (LOWRY).
3. SPLEEN CELLS DEPLETED OF T-CELLS BY MONOCLONAL ANTI-THY 1.2 AND C' (96% DEPLETION BY CON A ASSAY).

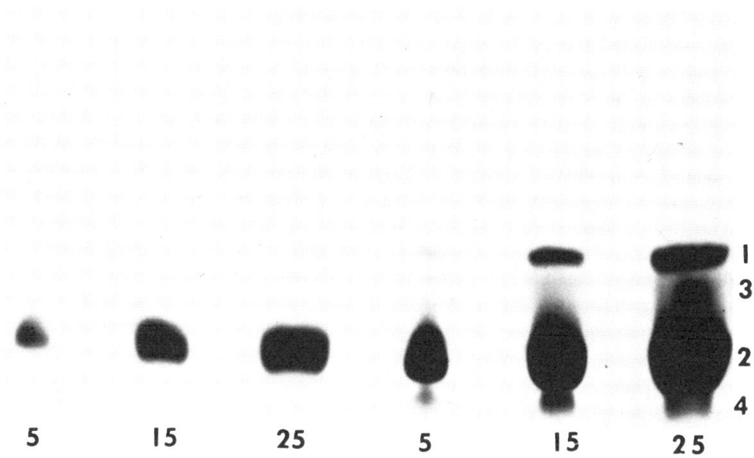

Figure 2. SDS-PAGE slab gel of pertussis LPS. The left three lanes are PW-LPS. The right three lanes are PCE-LPS at the concentrations shown in micrograms.

Polymyxin B inhibition experiments using lipid-enriched fractions of LPS produced by acetic acid hydrolysis revealed that the mitogenic activity of the pertussis glycolipid fraction could be significantly reduced. As shown in Table 9, a comparable reduction in activity is evident in the cultures from both C3H/OuJ and C3H/HeJ mice in the presence of PB suggesting that the lipid of pertussis LPS, at least in part, is responsible for the mitogenic activity on C3H/HeJ cells in contrast to the results of previous experiments (Girard et al., and Le Dur et al., 1980).

TABLE 9. EFFECT OF POLYMYXIN B ON THE STIMULATION OF DNA SYNTHESIS IN SPLENIC LYMPHOCYTES BY PERTUSSIS LPS

	Mean Net cpm of ^{3}H-TdR-Incorporation	
Mitogen (μg)	C3H/OuJ	C3H/HeJ
PL[1], 0.1	36,429	8,661
" , 1.0	57,016	14,542
PL, 0.1 + PB[2]	10,828 (70%)[3]	1,611 (78%)
", 0.1 + PB	37,607 (34%)	9,018 (38%)

1. PL = pertussis glycolipid from acetic acid hydrolyzed pertussis LPS according to the method of Le Dur, et al. 1980.

2. PB = polymyxin B at 10 μg per culture.

Taken together, these data provide evidence to suggest that a specific molecular species of pertussis LPS has the property of activating C3H/HeJ B-cells, which are ordinarily unresponsive to the lipid-A from enteric LPS. Further studies on the chemistry of PLPS may provide an insight into the nature of the deficiency of C3H/HeJ B-cells in terms of their response to various lipids derived from lipopolysaccharide endotoxins.

SUMMARY

From the results presented, we conclude that the outer membrane proteins we have separated from the endotoxin complex of S. typhi and B. pertussis are potent adjuvants. The antibody response to both T-dependent and T-independent antigens can be enhanced. Lymphocyte culture experiments indicate that both T-cells and macrophages are important accessory cells in the adjuvant process, although clearly polyclonal activation independent of accessory cell participation, also supports the enhanced response to any one antigen selected. In addition, we have found that a particular molecular species of pertussis LPS can act as a polyclonal activator of C3H/HeJ LPS hyporesponsive lymphocytes and that the lipid of this species of LPS contributes to its mitogenicity for C3H/HeJ B-cells

ACKNOWLEDGEMENTS

We thank Lynne Torpie and Eileen Meaney for their excellent technical assistance and Janice Howard for the preparation of this manuscript. This work was supported in part by the Office of Naval Research, Contract N00014-84-K-0693.

REFERENCES

Baker PJ, Stashak PW, Prescott B (1969). Use of erythrocytes sensitized with purified pneumococcal polysaccharides for the assay of antibody and antibody-producing cells. Appl. Microbiol. 17: 422-426.

Galanos C, Luderitz O, Westphal O (1969). A new method for the extraction of R lipopolysaccharides. Eur. J. Biochem. 9: 245-249.

Girard R, Chaby R, Bordenava G (1981). Mitogenic response of C3H/HeJ mouse lymphocytes to polyanionic polysaccharides obtained from Bordetella pertussis endotoxin and from other bacterial species. Infect. Immun. 31: 122-128.

Le Dur A, Chaby R, Szabó L (1980). Isolation of two protein-free and chemically different lipopolysaccharides from Bordetella pertussis phenol-extracted endotoxin. J. Bacteriol. 143: 78-88.

Mizel SB (1980). Studies on the purification and structure-function relationships of murine lymphocyte activating factor (Interleukin 1). Mol. Immunol. 17: 571-577.

Rittenberg MB, Pratt KL (1969). Antitrinitrophenyl (TNP) plaque assay: Primary response of BALB/c mice to soluble and particulate immunogen. Proc. Soc. Exp. Biol. Med. 132: 575-581.

Sultzer BM (1983). Lymphocyte activation by endotoxin and endotoxin protein: The role of the C3H/HeJ mouse. In: Nowotny, A. ed, Beneficial Effects of Endotoxin. Plenum Press, N.Y., 227-248.

Sultzer BM, Craig JP, Castagna R (1985). The adjuvant effect of pertussis endotoxin protein in modulating the immune response to cholera toxoid in mice. Develop. biol. Standard. 61: 225-232.

Immunopharmacology of Infectious Diseases: Vaccine Adjuvants and Modulators of Non-Specific Resistance, pages 125–137

CHEMICAL CHARACTERIZATION AND IMMUNOENHANCING ACTIVITIES OF PURIFIED CYTOPHAGA EXOPOLYMER

William R. Usinger
Robert I. Mishell

Department of Microbiology and Immunology
University of California, Berkeley
Berkeley, CA 94720

OVERVIEW

A recently described species of Cytophaga sheds into its growth medium macromolecules that potentiate murine immune responses (Usinger et al. 1985). We observed that these molecules augmented the generation of antigen-specific, primary humoral immune responses by cultured murine spleen cells; therefore we designated them as in vitro adjuvants (Shiigi et al. 1977, Mishell et al. 1981). Prior to identifying the genus of this gliding bacteria, we designated the adjuvant "GBA", for gliding bacteria adjuvant. We have subsequently investigated several biochemical and immunoregulatory properties of GBA and developed protocols for purifying the active material.

The biologically-active adjuvant appears to consist of basic amino-sugar polymers ranging in size from 5 - 500 x 10^6 daltons. These contain an average of 1 nitrogen atom per monosaccharide; none of the amines are in the primary configuration. The biological activities of the polymers are stable to treatment with detergent, mild acid and base, and boiling. Purified polymers contain <1% non-polysaccharide contaminants and retain the immunoregulatory activities displayed by the crude material. In picomolar quantities, the polymers cause B lymphocytes to proliferate and to secrete immunoglobulin. They also stimulate macrophages to synthesize and/or secrete Interleukin 1 (IL-1) and colony stimulating factors (CSF).

Recent preliminary experiments indicate that GBA augments

in vivo humoral immune responses and may cause significant increases in the level of natural killer cell activity. Because of the adjuvant's broad biological activities and unusual composition, combined with its high specific activity and possible limited side-effects, we believe GBA has promise as a potentially beneficial immunoenhancing compound for use in human and veterinary medicine. We are therefore attempting to determine the exact chemical nature of the biologically active polymer and are investigating the mechanisms by which the adjuvant mediates its various biological effects.

RESULTS

We performed an extensive series of experiments with the crude Cytophaga adjuvant to determine the charge, size, and stability to various chemical and enzymatic treatments of its biologically active components. Fractions resulting from these procedures were assayed for their mitogenic activity on murine spleen cells. The results of these experiments were used to devise a purification protocol as shown (Figure 1).

PROTOCOL FOR THE PRODUCTION AND PURIFICATION OF GBA

CYTOPHAGA GROWN TO LATE LOG PHASE
|
BACTERIA REMOVED BY CENTRIFUGATION
|
CONCENTRATION OF SUPERNATANT BY ULTRAFILTRATION
|
ORGANIC PRECIPITATION
|
DIALYSIS
|
DNASE/RNASE TREATMENT
|
PROTEOLYTIC DIGESTION
|
BOIL IN DETERGENT
|
GEL FILTRATION (SEPHAROSE 4B)
|
DESALTING
|
POLYMYXIN B ADSORPTION
|
LYOPHILIZATION

The protein contaminants of the Cytophaga adjuvant purified by this protocol were reduced from 5% to 0.5% and a yellow pigment, flexirubin, was reduced to undetectable levels.

The specific activity of the polymer purified by this means was increased 25 - 100 fold, while the overall yield was approximately 10%. This suggests that some of the contaminants removed during purification may be inhibitors of the bioassays that were employed to measure activity, since at most a 10 fold increase in activity would result from removing 90% neutral contaminants.

The biochemical properties of the purified adjuvant are summarized below (Figure 2).

Physical and Chemical Properties of GBA

Protein	<0.5%
Nucleic Acid	$A^{1\%}_{260} = 0$
Endotoxin	0.01 - 0.05%
Pigment	$A^{1\%}_{455}$ <0.05%
Size	Runs in void of A150
Electron Microscopy	Spherical particles; $2 \times 10^6 - 4 \times 10^8$ daltons
Sedimentation	Biologically active particles pellet at 100,000 x g in 1 hr
Elemental Analysis	C 47.08; H 7.11; N 5.83; O 39.99
1° Amines	<0.02%
Charge	pI >8.6
Biologically stable to:	Boiling, denaturants, detergent, mixed glycosidases

The result of several experiments suggests that GBA is a large polymer of amino sugars. Estimates of the exopolymer's size ($5 - 500 \times 10^6$ daltons) obtained from gel filtration in dissociating buffers are consistent with those calculated from the particle diameters observed in electron micrographs (Figure 3). Quantitative analysis of carbon, nitrogen, oxygen and hydrogen indicates that the elemental composition of GBA is similar to amino sugar polymers. Chitin (poly N-acetyl glucosamine) for example is 47.3% C, 39.4% O, 6.4% H, and 6.9% N compared to 47.1% C, 40.0% O, 7.1% H, and 5.9% N for GBA. The basic charge (pI >8.6) of GBA is in the range of amino sugar polymers. Its reactivity in the phenol-sulfuric hexose assay (Figure 4) is also similar to that of amino sugar polymers and is substantially less than the reactivity of unsubstituted sugar polymers such as dextran. We are now attempting to identify the individual monosaccharide components of GBA. We plan to analyze hydrolyzed subunits by gas-liquid chromatography and mass spectrometry once appropriate hydrolytic conditions have been determined.

Electron Micrograph of Purified GBA

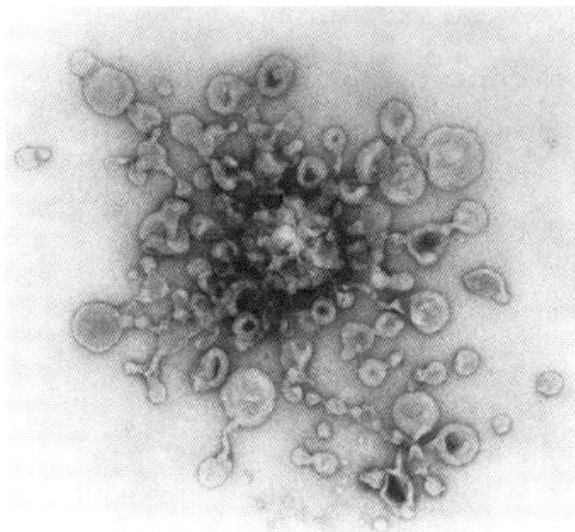

Figure 3: A droplet of purified GBA, diluted in H_2O, was applied to glow-discharged grids and stained with uranyl acetate. After washing, grids were examined by electron microscopy (80,000 fold magnification).

Phenol Sulfuric Hexose Assay

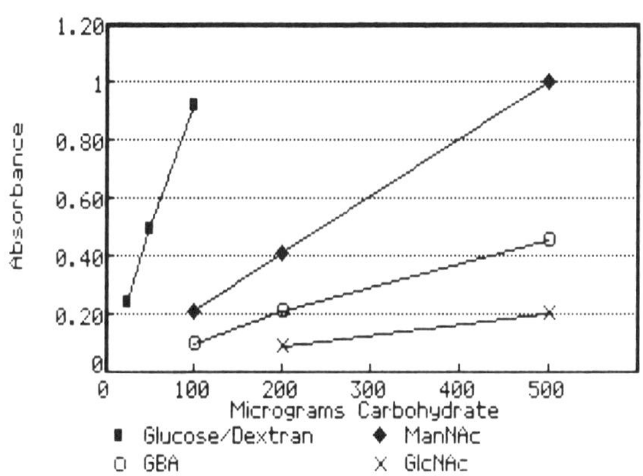

Figure 4: See text for details.

The adjuvant is active in several biological assays. To measure adjuvanticity in vitro, murine spleen cell cultures were established under conditions that are unfavorable for the induction of primary humoral immune responses to sheep red cells (Mishell and Dutton 1967, Shiigi et al. 1977). As shown in Figure 5, mouse spleen cells cultured under such conditions generate few antibody forming cells; but cultures supplemented with adjuvant generate strong antigen-specific responses. The minimum dose required to induce significant responses is approximately 100 ng.

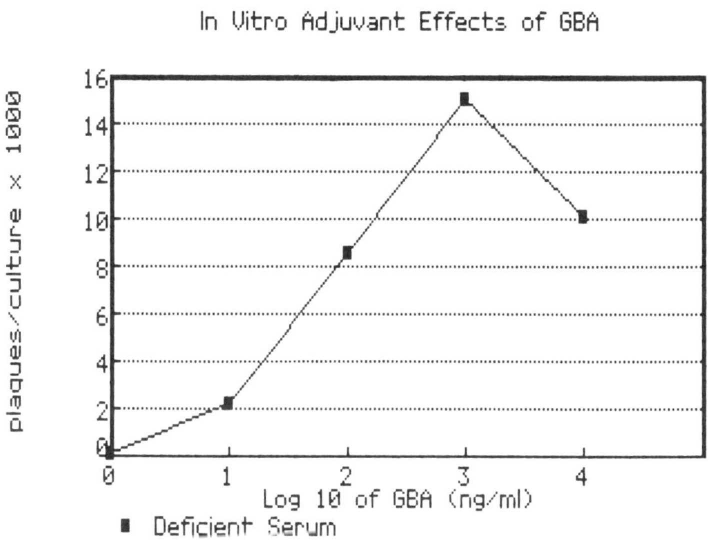

Figure 5: BDF_1 mouse spleen cells (4×10^6 cells/culture in 1 ml volumes) were cultured with sheep erythrocytes (antigen) in medium containing "nonsupportive" fetal calf serum and the indicated quantities of GBA. After 5 days, cells were harvested and assayed for the number of antibody-forming cells in a direct plaque assay.

GBA is mitogenic and activates murine B cells polyclonally to secrete immunoglobulin (Figures 6 and 7). These experiments indicate that GBA is active over a broad dose range and is only minimally inhibitory at very high doses.

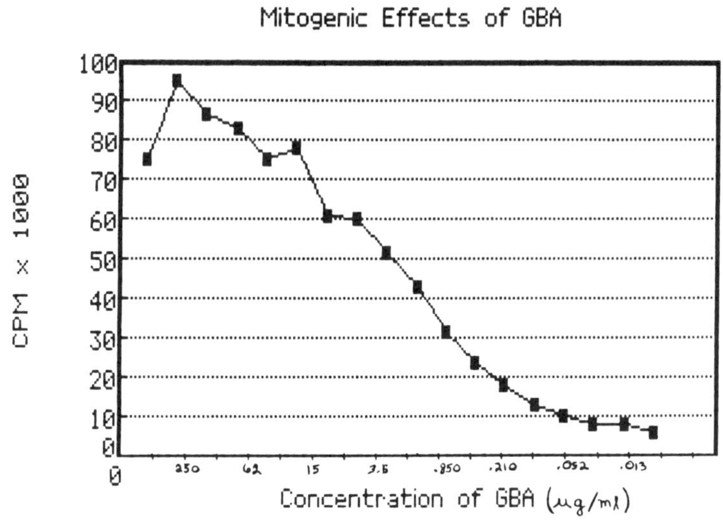

Figure 6: BDF_1 mouse spleen cells (2×10^6 cells/ml) were cultured with the indicated doubling dilutions of GBA, pulsed with ^{3}H-thymidine after 48 hours, and harvested and assayed 24 hours later for incorporation of radioactivity.

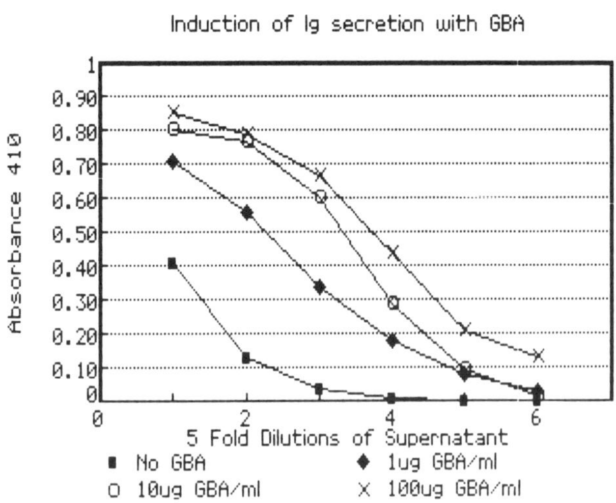

Figure 7: BDF_1 mouse spleen cells (1×10^6 cells/ml) were incubated for 5 days with 0, 1, 10 or 100 ug of GBA. Supernatants were analyzed for total Ig by a sandwich EIA assay.

In a collaborative study with Dr. Gayle D. Wetzel, Department of Biology, University of California, San Diego, we found that GBA directly stimulates B cells to proliferate. Individual B cells were placed in Terisaki wells and their responses to dextran sulfate, lipopolysaccharide (LPS) and GBA alone and in various combinations were determined visually. The results of such an experiment are shown in Table 1. This experiment indicates that GBA can deliver a proliferative signal to individual B cells by itself, in contrast to LPS, which requires dextran sulfate as a cofactor.

INDIVIDUAL B CELLS RESPOND TO GBA

INDUCERS	% INPUT CELLS YIELDING CLONES
LPS (25) + DXS (40)	21.2 ± 4.0
DXS (40)	<0.3
GBA 10 μG/ML	10.1 ± 2.6
" 1 μG/ML	0.5 ± 0.7
" 0.1 μG/ML	<0.3
GBA 10 μG/ML + DXS (20)	41.6 ± 6.4
" 1 μG/ML + DXS (20)	2.7 ± 1.3
" 0.1 μG/ML + DXS (20)	0.8 ± 0.9

Table 1: Murine spleen cells, depleted of T cells, were placed in Terisaki wells (10 ul/culture) at several cell concentrations. After plating, wells were examined microscopically to identify those wells containing a single cell. Six days later, the wells containing single cells were reexamined for colony formation.

GBA also induces the synthesis and/or secretion of IL-1 by human and IL-1 and CSF by murine macrophages. The effects of GBA on the secretion of IL-1 by the murine myelomonocytic cell line, WEHI 265, are shown in Figure 8. These findings together with those of the studies with B cells indicate that the polymers may exert their adjuvant effects by multiple pathways involving separately B cells and macrophages as direct targets.

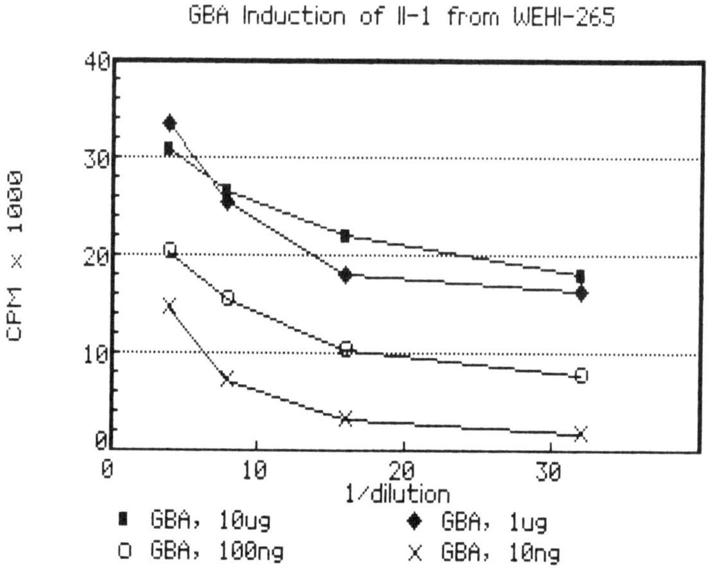

Figure 8: WEHI 265 myelomonocytes were cultured with the indicated quantities of GBA. After 3 days, supernatants were collected; dilutions of these supernatants were tested for IL-1 activity by the thymocyte comitogen assay. Uninduced control supernatants were similarly tested and found to contain less than 2000 cpm of activity at the highest concentration (results not shown).

Recently we have begun to investigate the in vivo effects of GBA. To study the immunoenhancing properties of GBA in vivo, we immunized mice intraperitoneally with suboptimal amounts of antigen. The antigen was emulsified in an oil-in-water vehicle with and without GBA. Primary antibody titers were determined 9 days later by solid phase ELISA. A representative experiment using cytochrome C as the immunogen is shown in Figure 9. This study showed that the inclusion of GBA resulted in primary humoral responses 25-50 fold greater than those of controls using antigen alone. Similar results have been obtained with lysozyme and ovalbumin.

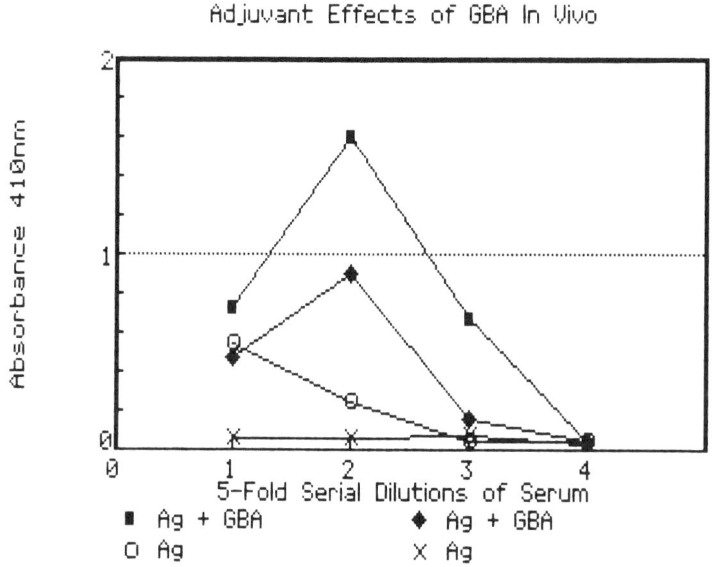

Figure 9: Two pairs of BALB/c mice (4 total) were injected with 10 ug of cytochrome C ± 50 ug GBA emulsified in a mixture of L121 pluronic polyol, Tween 80 and squalane. Nine days later, mice were bled and the sera were tested for antibody by solid-phase ELISA.

Preliminary experiments to determine the effects of GBA on natural killer cell activity were performed in collaboration with Dr. Phyllis B. Blair, Department of Microbiology and Immunology, University of California, Berkeley. Sets of mice were injected intraperitoneally with GBA, poly(IC) or saline. Eighteen hours later, spleens were removed and assayed for their NK activity against standard ^{51}Cr-labelled YAC targets. As shown in Table 2, GBA induced increases in NK activity of 300-400% over saline controls, responses that were similar to those that occurred in mice injected with poly(IC). Whether GBA increases NK activity by inducing gamma interferon, as does poly(IC), (Zarling 1980), or activates NK cells by inducing IL-2 (Kuribayashi et al. 1981) or employs yet another pathway remains to be investigated.

Induction of Natural Killer Cells, *In Vivo*

E/T Ratio	Inducers of NK		
	None	GBA	Poly(IC)
25	0.9	3.4	12.1
50	8.5	15.9	25.2
100	9.6	24.5	33.9

Table 2: Numbers are the averages of percent lysis directed against ^{51}Cr-labelled YAC target cells mediated by C57BL/CRL spleen cells 18 hours after intraperitoneal injection of the indicated inducers.

DISCUSSION/SUMMARY

We have isolated and purified a set of large and basic aminosugar polymers that display a broad range of immunological activities *in vitro* and *in vivo*. The purified exopolymer is active in picomolar quantities. At high concentrations it results in minimal inhibition of several *in vitro* assays. Moreover, it is well-tolerated by mice at doses that induce substantial responses *in vivo*. These studies suggest that GBA may have a favorable therapeutic index and exhibit fewer deleterious side-effects than have been reported with other adjuvants.

Biological studies show that GBA potentiates humoral immune responses *in vitro* and *in vivo* and that it directly activates macrophages and B lymphocytes. Similar properties have been described for other natural substances with strong immunoenhancing activity such as LPS (Morrison and Ryan 1979), peptidoglycan (Heymer and Reitschel 1977), and outer membrane proteins of gram negative bacteria (Chen et al. 1980). The induction of IL-1 provides a clear example of the importance of macrophages in mediating the effects of GBA and other adjuvants. Many adjuvants including GBA induce macrophages to synthesize and/or secrete IL-1. Recently, Hoffmann et al. (1984) reported that purified IL-1 itself potentiates *in vitro* humoral immune responses. Thus induction of IL-1 is very likely a major pathway of exogenous adjuvant action.

GBA may also exert some of its adjuvant activities through direct effects on B cells. According to one model of B cell activation, proposed by Goodman and Weigle (1985), two distinct signals are required for antigen-specific B cell responses. One is an "early" inductive signal to B cells that initiates nonspecific activation, marked by proliferation and polyclonal Ig secretion. The second mimics the T_H second signal to B cells; it can bypass the need for T cells. Clearly, GBA delivers the first signal to B cells, as shown in Figures 6 and 7. Whether GBA also delivers the T_H-like signal proposed by Goodman and Weigle for the guanosine ribonucleoside adjuvant remains to be demonstrated.

A similar adjuvant effect may result from enhancement of T_H cell activity - a pathway of adjuvant actions suggested as one utilized by LPS (Bismuth et al. 1985). The possible individual pathways of adjuvant activity, described above, are not mutually exclusive nor exhaustive. We believe that the mechanisms of adjuvant action probably involve multiple cellular and hormonal interactions and that some of the hormones may not as yet have been identified.

A potentially important area for further investigation is to determine whether exogenous adjuvants induce regulatory hormones that act selectively on B and T subsets to alter the quality as well as quantity of immune responses. Studies to investigate the existence of such regulatory hormones will be facilitated by the availability of several chemically diverse, well-characterized, purified adjuvants such as GBA. These adjuvants may be especially suitable reagents for investigating the hypothesis that the induction of cellular or humoral responses or of specific isotypes by environmental antigens are mediated by regulatory hormones produced by macrophages and other antigen-nonspecific target cells as a result of adjuvant stimulation. Accordingly, isotype selection may depend more on adjuvant-specific reactions than reactions that are specific for antigen.

The potency of GBA on mammalian immune reactions is somewhat paradoxical since the Cytophaga species from which it is obtained is killed by temperatures of greater than 30°C and therefore is not pathogenic for mammals. One hypothesis that may explain the potent immunoreguatory activity of the Cytophaga exopolymer is that the carbohydrate structures of the adjuvant are recognized by mammalian cell-surface lectins that were evolutionarily selected and conserved because of their capacities to bind similar sugars present on the surfaces of pathogenic microbes. These putative mammalian receptors may be a means by which host defense systems can respond efficiently to classes of structurally-similar substances. Lectins that recognize microbial carbohydrates are thought to be important components of the host defense systems of invertebrates. Such lectins have been found on the surfaces of hemocytes and as soluble constituents of the hemolymph of many invertebrate species (Sharon and Lis 1972; Pistole 1978). Consistent with this hypothesis is our preliminary finding that GBA binds to the surface of WEHI 265 cells, as detected by indirect fluorescence. Possibly the same lectins that promote phagocytosis by invertebrates are present on mammalian macrophages where they bind appropriate polysaccharides and initiate the pathways of adjuvant action. Greater understanding of the chemistry and biology of GBA and other adjuvants will help determine the validity of these hypotheses.

REFERENCES

Bismuth G, Duphot M, Theze J (1985). LPS and specific T cell responses: Interleukin 1 (IL-1)-independent amplification of antigen-specific T helper (T_H) cell proliferation. J Immunol 134:415.

Chen YU, Hancock REW, Mishell RI (1980). Mitogenic effects of purified outer membrane proteins from Pseudomonas aeruginosa. Infect Immun 28:178.

Goodman MG, Weigle WO (1985). Dissociation of inductive from differentiative signals transmitted by C8-substituted guanine ribonucleosides to B cells from SJL mice. J Immunol 134:91.

Heymer B, Reitschel ET (1977). Biological properties of peptidoglycans. In Schlessinger D (ed): "Microbiology 1977," Washington DC: Am Soc Microbiol, p 344.

Hoffmann MK, Mizel SB, Hirst JA (1984). IL-1 requirement for B cell activation revealed by use of adult serum. J Immunol 133:2566.

Kuribayashi K, Gillis S, Kern DE, Henney CS (1981). Murine NK cell cultures: Effects of interleukin-2 and interferon on cell growth and cytotoxic reactivity. J Immunol 126:2321.

Mishell RI, Chen YU, Clark GC, Gold MR, Hill JL, Kwan E, Lee DA (1981). Induction of murine lymphocytes and macrophages by components of bacterial cell walls and membranes. In Shockman GD, Wicken AJ (eds): "Chemistry and biological activities of bacterial surface amphiphiles," New York: Academic Press, p 327.

Mishell RI, Dutton RW (1967). Immunization of dissociated spleen cell cultures from normal mice. J Exp Med 126:423.

Morrison DC, Ryan JL (1979). Bacterial endotoxins and host immune responses. Adv Immunol 28:293.

Pistole TG (1978). Broad-spectrum bacterial agglutination activity in the serum of the horse shoe crab, Limulus polyphemus. Devel Comp Immunol 2:65.

Sharon N, Lis H (1972). Lectins: Cell agglutinations and sugar-specific proteins. Science 177:949.

Shiigi SM, Capwell RR, Grabstein KH, Mishell RI (1977). Sera and the in vitro induction of immune responses. III. Adjuvant obtained from gliding bacteria with properties distinct from enteric bacterial lipopolysaccharide. J Immunol 119:679.

Usinger WR, Clark GC, Gottschalk E, Holt S, Mishell RI (1985). Characteristics of bacterium GB-2, a presumptive Cytophaga species with novel immunoregulatory properties. Current Microbiology 12:203.

Zarling, J. M. 1980. Augmentation of human natural killer cell activity by purified interferon and polyribonucleotides. In Herberman RB (ed): "Natural Cell-Mediated Immunity against Tumors," New York: Academic Press, p 698.

ACKNOWLEDGMENTS

The authors gratefully acknowledge the fine technical assistance of Ms. Laurie Bost, Mr. Zollie A. Griffin, and Mr. Jon Karpilow; Dr. Phyllis B. Blair and Dr. Gayle D. Wetzel for their collaborative experimental work; and Dr. Charles Harden and Dr. Alexander Glazer for helpful discussions. This work was supported by funds from the Office of Naval Research (N14-84-K0626) and a grant from the Gustavus and Louise Pfeiffer Research Foundation.

Immunopharmacology of Infectious Diseases: Vaccine Adjuvants and
Modulators of Non-Specific Resistance, pages 139–154

IMMUNOLOGICAL PROTECTION AGAINST MUCOSAL PATHOGENS BY DIRECT STIMULATION OF ANTIBODY-FORMING CELLS IN THE GUT-ASSOCIATED LYMPHOID TISSUES

John D. Clements, Frank L. Lyon, and
Robert F. Garry
Department of Microbiology and Immunology,
Tulane University School of Medicine, New
Orleans, Louisiana 70112

INTRODUCTION

Microbial pathogens can infect a host by one of several mechanisms. They may enter through breaks in the integument induced by trauma, they may be introduced by vector transmission, or they may interact with a mucosal surface. After colonization, the pathogen may elaborate one or more toxins or invade to cause systemic disease. The majority of human pathogens initiate disease following infection of mucosal surfaces and represent the single largest cause of morbidity and mortality among the world's populations. Diarrheal and respiratory illness together account for more than 15 million deaths annually and are among the most common debilitating infectious diseases afflicting people of all ages around the globe. While extensive research has been conducted to determine the role cell mediated immunity and serum antibody play in protection against infectious agents, little is known about the role of mucosal immunity. A major limitation to the development of effective immunoprophylaxis against mucosal pathogens is the inability to stimulate significant levels of mucosal antibody directed against specific virulence determinants.

The results of much recent research have indicated the potential of developing new vaccines for bacteria, viruses and parasites that are important human pathogens. Surface proteins, which play a role in the pathogenesis of these agents, are being identified and the immunodominant peptides of these proteins are being characterized and synthesized or produced by recombinant DNA methods for use as vaccines. While some of these peptides are natively immunogenic and protective as vaccines, available evidence indicates that many peptides considered as vaccine candidates will not, in their native state, produce significant levels of antibody or antibody that protects the host. Of the several approaches to enhance the immunogenicity of such peptides, one of the more attractive is linkage of the peptide (hapten) to an immunogenic protein (carrier). Vaccines composed of a carrier protein with linked haptens can generate functional anti-hapten antibody, even if the hapten is not immunogenic, and may also generate antibody to the carrier. Furthermore, the antibody response to such antigens can be class specific (depending upon the route of delivery), long-lived, and capable of being boosted (Klipstein et al., 1982a; Klipstein et al., 1982b). While this approach to vaccines is extremely attractive, important theoretical and technical questions need to be answered. These include the importance of charge and configuration of the carrier to vaccine efficacy; the length, density, and mechanism of linkage of the hapten; potential toxicity of the linking reagents or linker molecules; and the problem of predicting protection in humans from studies in the laboratory or in animal models.

We have isolated and extensively characterized a protein from *E. coli* which should be useful as a carrier in a variety of conjugate vaccines. This protein, designated LT-B, binds to the G_{M1} ganglioside on the surface of cells where it remains localized for antigen processing by components of the immune system. If administered parenterally, LT-B induces a serum response to itself and to haptens covalently linked to the molecule even in the absence of an adjuvant. Likewise, LT-B administered orally has been shown in both animal models and in human volunteers, to induce a serum IgG and mucosal IgA response to itself and to appropriately linked haptens.

We have utilized recombinant DNA technology to construct a plasmid containing the genes for the production of LT-B and have developed a simple method for purifying LT-B free of contaminating endotoxin and other proteins (Clements et al., 1983; Clements and El-Morshidy, 1984). Preliminary studies with two different haptens have given evidence of the potential usefulness of this molecule as a carrier.

ABROGATION OF ORALLY INDUCED TOLERANCE

As a part of the preceding investigation, we began studying the phenomenon of immune tolerance following oral administration of antigen. It is well known that oral immunization can lead to the production of systemic tolerance in response to subsequent parenteral injection of the specific antigen (Challacombe and

Tomasi, 1980). It has also recently been demonstrated that administration of cholera toxin (CT) can abrogate oral tolerance to an unrelated antigen (Elson and Ealding, 1984a). Although the mechanism for this abrogation is unknown, it is presumed to result from an alteration of the regulatory environment in the gut associated lymphoid tissue, shifting it toward responsiveness. Both subunits of CT (and also of the heat-labile enterotoxin of *E. coli* [LT]) have immunoregulatory potential. The binding subunit can mediate thymocyte proliferation (Spiegel et al., 1985) and act as an efficient carrier for stimulation of anti-hapten IgA responses to unrelated antigens (Elson and Ealding, 1984b; McKenzie and Halsey, 1984). The A subunit, on the other hand, stimulates adenylate cyclase by ADP-ribosylation of the GTP binding component in the regulatory center of the adenylate cyclase complex (Finkelstein, 1973).

In the course of these investigations, we discovered that simultaneous administration of LT with an orally administered antigen can also abrogate the development of tolerance to that antigen. We were interested in determining the parameters of this effect and in determining the relative contributions of the two subunits. Three groups of BALB/c mice were immunized in this experiment. On day 0, each group was immunized orally as follows: Group A received 0.5 ml of PBS, Group B received 0.5 ml of PBS containing 5 mg of Ovalbumin, and Group C received 0.5 ml of PBS containing 5 mg of Ovalbumin and 25 µg of LT. This regimen was repeated twice again on days 7 and 14. On day 21, all animals were immunized i.p. with 1 µg of Ovalbumin in 20% Maalox. On day 28, all animals were sacrificed and assayed for serum IgG antibodies directed against Ovalbumin by ELISA. As seen in Figure 1, animals primed orally with Ovalbumin developed a significantly lower ($p \leq 0.005$) serum IgG anti-Ovalbumin response following subsequent parenteral immunization with Ovalbumin than those receiving PBS alone (35 µg/ml vs 95 µg/ml). On the other hand, animals primed orally with Ovalbumin <u>and</u> LT developed a significantly higher ($p \leq 0.0005$) serum IgG anti-Ovalbumin response than those in either of the other two groups (3,194 µg/ml). Interestingly, the simultaneous administration of LT with Ovalbumin not only overcame tolerance to Ovalbumin caused by oral feeding, but also acted as an adjuvant for the antigen.

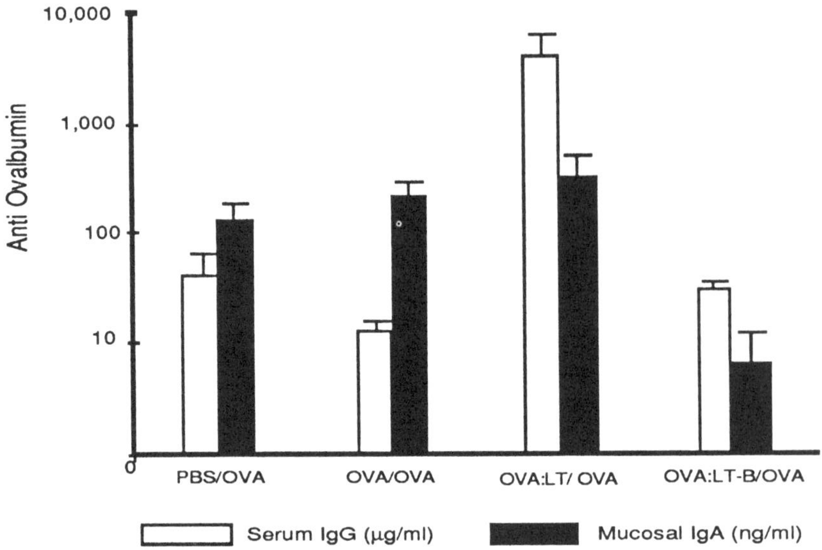

Figure 1. Abrogation of oral tolerance to Ovalbumin by LT. Groups of mice were fed on days 0, 7, and 14 with 5 mg Ovalbumin, 5 mg Ovalbumin plus 25 μg LT, 5 mg Ovalbumin plus 17 μg LT-B, or PBS. All animals were boosted i.p. on day 21 with 1 μg Ovalbumin then assayed on day 28 for the presence of serum antibodies to Ovalbumin.

We next wanted to determine if the observed response was a function of the binding component of the molecule (LT-B) or of the enzymatically active subunit A. We were in a unique position to make this determination since LT-B derived from the holotoxin by dissociation chromatography is invariably contaminated with residual traces of LT, and since our LT-B recombinant clones produce LT-B free of any contaminating subunit A. We therefore repeated the above experiment except that, in place of LT we substituted an equimolar amount of LT-B (17 μg vs 25 μg). Also seen in Figure 1, there were no significant differences between groups primed orally with Ovalbumin and LT-B and those primed with Ovalbumin alone or PBS alone.

These experiments clearly demonstrated that the ability to abrogate the induction of tolerance is a function of the A subunit of LT. Presumably, the B subunit is also required to facilitate penetration of the A subunit into the cell. We next initiated a series of experiments designed to determine the effect of varying the timing and route of delivery of the LT in concert with the orally administered antigen. For this experiment, three groups of BALB/c mice were immunized as above. On day 0, each group was immunized orally as follows: Group A received 0.5 ml of PBS, Group B received 0.5 ml of PBS containing 5 mg of Ovalbumin, and Group C received 0.5 ml of PBS containing 5 mg of Ovalbumin and 25 µg of LT. This regimen was repeated twice again on days 7 and 14. Group D received 0.5 ml of PBS containing 5 mg of Ovalbumin on day 0 and 0.5 ml of PBS containing 5 mg of Ovalbumin and 25 µg of LT on days 7 and 14. Group E received 0.5 ml of PBS containing 5 mg of Ovalbumin on days 0 and 7 and 0.5 ml of PBS containing 5 mg of Ovalbumin and 25 µg of LT on day 14. On day 21, all animals were immunized i.p. with 1 µg of Ovalbumin in 20% Maalox. On day 28, all animals were sacrificed and assayed for serum IgG and mucosal IgA antibodies directed against Ovalbumin by ELISA.

As seen in Figure 2, animals receiving LT with Ovalbumin subsequent to the initial Ovalbumin prime (Groups D and E) developed a significantly lower ($p \leq 0.005$) serum IgG anti-Ovalbumin response than those in the group receiving LT with Ovalbumin in the initial immunization (Group C). This may reflect either a timing-to-event phenomenon reflecting the shorter timing of LT administration prior to i.p. administration of the antigen or, conversely, may represent a decreased effectiveness resulting from prior immunologic experience with the antigen. The effect of LT administration on the development of mucosal IgA was also determined (Fig. 3). There was a significant ($p \leq 0.025$) increase in mucosal IgA anti-Ovalbumin (70 ng/ml) when LT was administered with the Ovalbumin during each of the three oral priming events (Group C). However, if the animals were immunized with Ovalbumin first, subsequent administration of LT with Ovalbumin failed to produce a detectable mucosal IgA anti-Ovalbumin response.

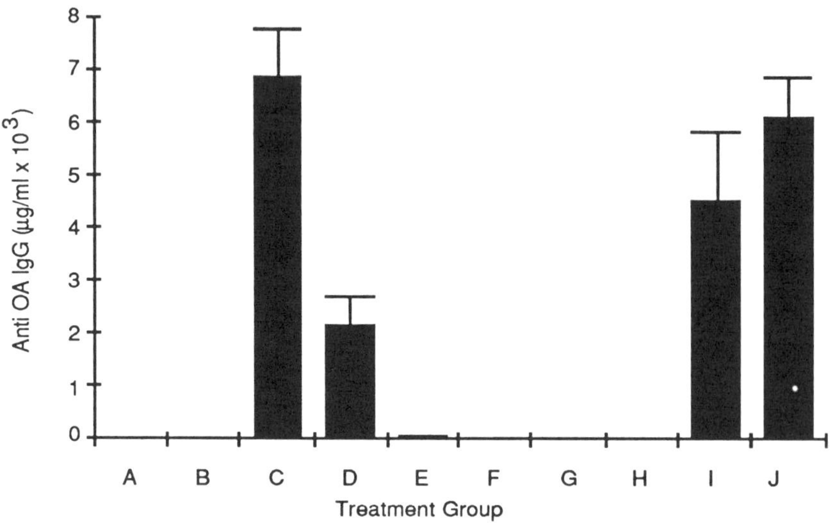

Figure 2. Serum IgG anti-Ovalbumin responses following immunization with Ovalbumin or with Ovalbumin and LT. (See text for details).

The effect of timing of the LT administration was also examined. Two groups of BALB/c mice were immunized for this study. Group G received 0.5 ml of PBS containing 5 mg of Ovalbumin on days 0, 7, and 14, and received 0.5 ml of PBS containing 25 µg of LT and days 1, 8, and 15. Group H received 0.5 ml of PBS containing 25 µg of LT and days 0, 7, and 14, and received 0.5 ml of PBS containing 5 mg of Ovalbumin on days 1, 8, and 15. As above, all animals were immunized i.p. with 1 µg of Ovalbumin in 20% Maalox on day 21. On day 28, all animals were sacrificed and assayed for serum IgG and mucosal IgA antibodies directed against Ovalbumin by ELISA. Animals receiving LT before each administration of Ovalbumin had a slight but significantly higher ($p \leq 0.05$) level of serum IgG (Fig. 2H) and mucosal IgA (Fig. 3H) anti-Ovalbumin than those orally primed with PBS alone (Figs. 2A and 3A), those orally primed with PBS containing Ovalbumin (Figs. 2B and 3B), or those orally primed with Ovalbumin the day before each administration of LT (Figs. 2G and 3G).

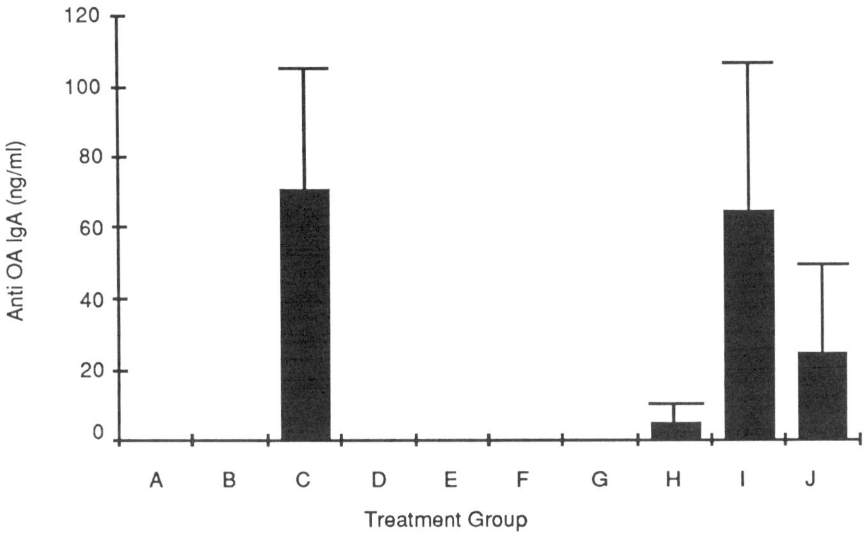

Figure 3. Mucosal IgA anti-Ovalbumin responses following immunization with Ovalbumin or with Ovalbumin and LT. (See text for details).

Three additional groups of mice were also immunized. Group F received 0.5 ml of PBS containing 5 mg of Ovalbumin on days 0, 7, and 14. Group J received 0.5 ml of PBS containing 5 mg of Ovalbumin and 25 µg of LT an days 0, 7, and 14. On day 21, both groups of animals were immunized i.p. with 1 µg of Ovalbumin and 25 µg of LT in 20% Maalox. On day 28, all animals were sacrificed and assayed for serum IgG and mucosal IgA antibodies directed against Ovalbumin as above. The parenteral administration of LT did not effect the abrogation of tolerance by orally administered LT. Thus, the serum IgG (Fig. 2F) and mucosal IgA (Fig. 3F) anti-Ovalbumin responses in animals boosted parenterally with with LT were not significantly different than control values. Moreover, parenteral boosting with LT neither enhanced nor diminished the serum IgG (Fig. 2J) and mucosal IgA (Fig. 3J) anti-Ovalbumin response when compared to animals receiving oral priming with LT (Figs. 2C and 3C).

The last group of animals in this study received 0.5 ml of PBS containing 5 mg of Ovalbumin and 25 µg of LT on day 0, and 0.5 ml of PBS containing 5 mg of Ovalbumin on days 7 and 14. On day 21, all animals were immunized i.p. with 1 µg of Ovalbumin in 20% Maalox. On day 28, all animals were sacrificed and assayed for serum IgG and mucosal IgA antibodies directed against Ovalbumin. Interestingly, serum IgG (Fig. 2I) and mucosal IgA (Fig. 3I) anti-Ovalbumin responses in animals receiving LT on only a single occasion, that being upon first exposure to the antigen, were not significantly different from those observed in animals receiving three oral priming doses with LT, thereby indicating that the alteration of the regulatory environment in the gut associated lymphoid tissue which shifts it toward responsiveness occurs early upon first exposure to the antigen and demonstrates memory in favor of responsiveness.

Clearly, LT has significant immunoregulatory potential, both as a means of abrogation of tolerance to specific antigens and as an adjuvant. We have begun a series of experiments to further examine these effects. The questions addressed include (i) the effect of varying the i.p. challenge dose after oral priming is complete, (ii) the effect of varying the dosage of LT, (iii) the ability of LT to abrogate tolerance once it is firmly established, rather than prevent the induction of tolerance, (iv) the effect of administration of LT with multiple antigens, and (v) the effects on the different cell types involved.

STUDIES ON MUCOSAL IMMUNITY TO HERPESVIRUS

The herpesvirus group includes two important human pathogens which can initiate infection at mucosal surfaces (Allen and Rapp, 1982). Herpes simplex virus type 1 (HSV-1) is the etiological agent of cold sores, ulcerative lesions of the labial mucosa (herpetic gingivostomatitis). HSV-1 is also capable of infecting the conjunctiva, the mucosal surface surrounding the eye. The virus may spread from the conjunctiva to other tissues in the eye thereby posing a serious hazard to sight. In fact, herpes keratitis is the leading infectious cause of blindness in this country. HSV-1 is also capable of infecting the mucosal surfaces of the genitalia and is becoming of increasing importance as a venereal pathogen (CDC, 1982). Herpes simplex virus type 2 (HSV-2), a related virus, infects primarily mucosal surfaces of the male and female genital tract and is a common sexually transmitted pathogen. HSV-2 is also the causative agent of herpetic meningoencephalitis which is acquired by a neonate during passage through an infected birth canal and is associated with a high fatality rate (circa 50%). By all accounts the incidence of HSV-1 and HSV-2 induced venereal disease is approaching epidemic proportions, especially among those in their late teens to early thirties (CDC, 1982). There are currently no protective vaccines against HSV-1 or HSV-2 liscensed for human use, nor are there any chemotherapeutic agents which are efficacious in the cure of genital herpes (Allen and Rapp, 1982; Babuik and Rouse, 1979).

The genomes of HSV-1 and HSV-2 encode several distinct envelope glycoproteins (Balachandran et al., 1982). The HSV-1 glycoproteins designated gB, gC, gD and gE have been shown by immunological and biochemical criteria to be structurally similar to corresponding glycoproteins of HSV-2 (Allen and Rapp, 1982; Babuik and Rouse, 1979). Analyses of the DNA sequences of the genes encoding these pairs of HSV-1 and HSV-2 glycoproteins confirms the relatedness (Bzik et al., 1984). The herpesvirus envelope glycoproteins represent the major viral antigens recognized by immunoprecipitating antibodies and are important in a protective humoral immune response (Allen and Rapp, 1982). The herpesvirus-specified glycoproteins are also the major viral antigens which are found on the surface of infected cells rendering them potentially important targets for immune effector mechanisms which control the spread of virus by the destruction of infected cells (Allen and Rapp, 1982; Babuik and Rouse, 1979). Indeed, recovery from primary infection with herpesviruses appears to be mediated by a combination of humoral and cellular immune mechanisms. Not surprisingly, considering the extensive homology of the envelope glycoproteins, recovery from HSV-1 or HSV-2 infection offers significant protection against systemic infection by the other virus (Allen and Rapp, 1982). However, systemic immunization with nonviable, attenuated or subunit vaccines has proven uniformly inefficient in generating protective immunity to infection by HSV-1 or HSV-2 at mucosal surfaces (Babuik and Rouse, 1979; Breinig et al., 1978; Oakes and Lausch, 1984). Antibodies specific for HSV-2 have been found in the cervicovaginal (mucosal) secretions of HSV-2 infected women or mice (McDermott et al., 1984; Mendis et al., 1981; Morahan et al., 1977). It has been established that mice surviving intravaginal challenge with HSV-2 were resistant to a subsequent intravaginal challenge with HSV-2, but susceptible to a systemic infection (Nahmias et al., 1967). These results suggest that mucosal immunity may confer resistance to herpesvirus infection.

Recent studies in our laboratory have demonstrated the efficacy of direct stimulation of antibody forming cells in the lymphoid tissues with toxoid antigens as a means of stimulating significant levels of specific antitoxic immunoglobulin A with neutralizing activity, as well as production of specific antitoxic serum immunoglobulin G (Clements et al., 1986). These studies employed an auxotrophic mutant of *Salmonella enteritidis* as a vehicle for delivery of cloned antigenic determinants directly to the antibody forming cells of the gut-associated lymphoid tissues (GALT). The present study was designed to determine whether a herpesvirus antigen so delivered would be presented in such a manner as to stimulate production of an immune response with a significant mucosal component. As a model, we chose glycoprotein B of Herpes simplex virus type 1, although we feel that any information we obtain will be broadly applicable to a variety of antigens for which secretory immunity may be important.

The gene coding for glycoprotein B of HSV-1 has been cloned and the nucleotide sequence determined (Bzik et al., 1984). We have obtained a copy of that clone (kindly provided by S. Person, Pennsylvania State University) which consists of HSV-1 DNA representing 0.345 to 0.376 map units inserted into the M13 derived cloning vector plasmid pUC9 (Fig.4). Translation of these sequences would yield a 100.3 kilodalton polypeptide constituting the backbone of gB. This is not, however, an expressing clone of HSV-1 gB. In order to convert this to an expressing clone, it was necessary to insert the gB gene into an expression vector.

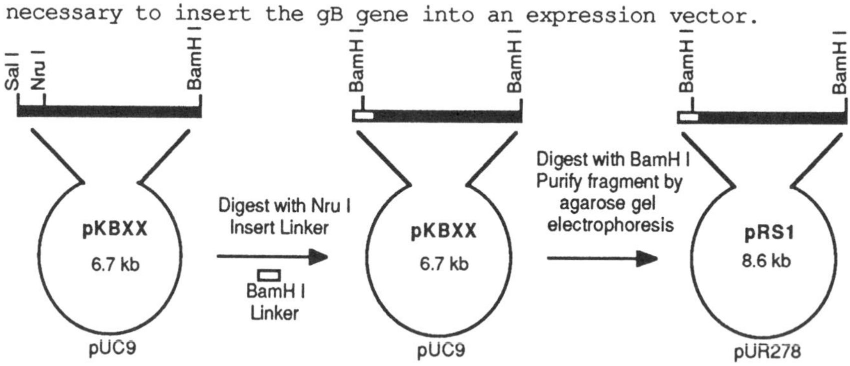

Figure 4. Construction of plasmid pRS1.

Construction of an expressing clone of HSV glycoprotein b

Our initial attempt at construction of an expressing clone was based upon a computer generated analysis showing a translation start codon at position 790 in the pKBXX nucleotide sequence. Upstream from that site at position 484 is a unique restriction site for the restriction endonuclease *Nru*I. This enzyme creates a blunt cut which, when ligated into a *Sma*I cut pUC8 should have created an in-frame construct. A series of recombinant plasmids was created by this method but none could be confirmed to express an immunologically relevant recombinant protein. A series of new constructs was made using the set of cloning vectors pUR 278, 288, 289 (Rüther and Müller-Hill, 1983). These plasmids have four unique cloning sites, *Bam*HI, *Sal*I, *Xba*I, and *Hind*III, at the 3' end of the *lac* Z gene in all frames. Because in these vectors all cloning sites exist in all frames, any inserted sequence should be expressed in one of the plasmids.

First, synthetic *Bam*HI linkers were phosphorylated using polynucleotide kinase essentially as described by Maniatis, et al. (1982). Plasmid pKBXX, purified by the procedure of Birnboim and Doly (1979), was then digested with *Nru*I, and an additional *Bam*HI linker was inserted at that site (Fig. 4). Following phenol/chloroform extraction and ethanol precipitation, the recovered DNA was used to transform *E. coli* K-12 derivative JM83 (*ara* Δ*lac-pro str*A *thi* f80*dlac*Z ΔM15) (Vieira and Messing, 1982). A series of transformants was selected on the basis of insertional inactivation of the *lac* function on the plasmid (white colonies on X-gal) and ampicillin resistance. Isolates were then screened using agarose gel electrophoresis of plasmid preparations purified by cesium chloride density centrifugation. One transformant contained a plasmid yielding two distinct bands of appropriate size upon digestion with *Bam*HI was selected for further study. The derivative plasmid yielded two fragments of 3.4 kb and 3.2 kb when digested with *Bam*HI, and electrophoresed through 0.65% agarose. The larger of these represented then HSV-1 sequence. This fragment was eluted from the gel and inserted into the *Bam*HI site of each of the pUR series plasmids as indicated above. Prior to the ligation reaction, each plasmid was digested with *Bam*HI then dephosphorylated with calf intestinal alkaline phosphatase. The recovered DNA was used to transform *E. coli* strain JM83. Transformants were screened for insertional inactivation of the *lac* function on the plasmid and ampicillin resistance. Isolates from each transformation were then analyzed by agarose gel electrophoresis of plasmid DNA purified by cesium chloride density centrifugation. Transformants that contained plasmids yielding two distinct bands of appropriate size upon digestion with *Bam*HI were selected for further study.

A minicell producing strain of *E. coli*, DS410 (Dougan and Sherrat, 1977), was subsequently transformed with plasmids isolated from each of the recombinant series. Transformants were processed for minicell production (Achtman et al., 1979), labeled with ^{35}S-Methionine, and electrophoresed through a 10-13% gradient SDS-PAGE gel which was subsequently autoradiographed to detect proteins coded for by the plasmids. Companion gels were run and stained for total protein. The autoradiograms and stained gels (Fig. 5) demonstrated the presence of a single unique high molecular weight protein band at approximately 105,000 daltons in the DS410 transformant receiving plasmid DNA from a recombinant plasmid derived from the *Bam*HI gB fragment and plasmid pUR 278. No corresponding band was seen in transformants receiving recombinant plasmids derived from either of the other two pUR plasmids, nor was it present in minicell lysates from cells containing plasmid pUR 278 alone. The recombinant plasmid coding for expression of this protein band was designated pRS1.

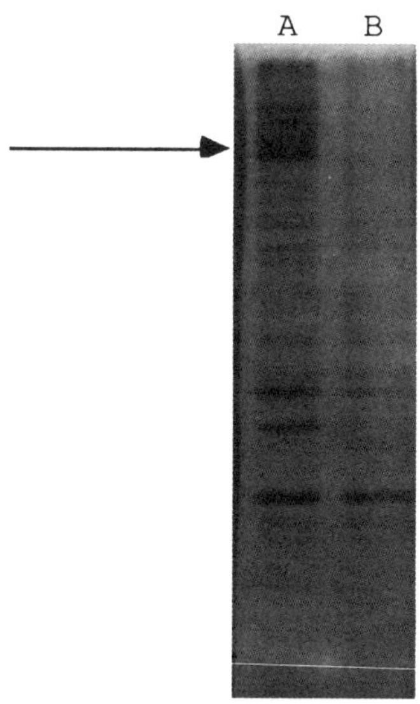

Figure 5. Analysis of minicells. *E. coli* strain DS410 was transformed with plasmids isolated from each of the recombinant series. Transformants were processed for minicell production, labeled with ^{35}S-Methionine, and electrophoresed through a 10-13% gradient SDS-PAGE gel. Shown is a coomassie blue stained gel of (A) *E. coli* strain DS410 containing plasmid pUR 278 with HSV DNA inserted in the *Bam*HI site and (B) *E. coli* strain DS410 containing plasmid pUR 278.

Characterization of recombinant gB (rgB)

In order to examine the immunologic characteristics of the recombinant protein, the minicell preparations were repeated and the recombinant protein extracted from the SDS-PAGE. The recombinant gB was identified in a stained section of the gel and the corresponding region from the unstained portion of the gel was excised, emulsified in TEAN buffer (Clements and Finkelstein, 1979), and dialysed against TEAN containing 0.1% SDS. BALB/c mice were immunized with approximately 50 μg of the extracted protein given i.p. in Freund's complete adjuvant. Following a boost at 10 days with an additional 50 μg in Freund's incomplete adjuvant, mice were bled and the serum separated.

Virus neutralization assay

African Green Monkey Kidney Cells (AGMK) cells were maintained and passaged in Eagle's minimal essential medium (MEM) supplemented with 10% fetal bovine serum. A thymidine kinaseless (tk^-) mutant of Herpes simplex virus type 1 (HSV-1) was propogated on AGMK cells. For the neutralization assay, AGMK cells were seeded in 96-well tissue culture dishes at 5 X 10^4 cells per well. Sera from mice which had been immunized with recombinant gB or an irrelevant antigen (control serum) were added to aliquots of HSV-1. The mixtures were then used to infect the monolayers of AGMK cells. Cells were challenged with HSV-1 at a multiplicity of infection of 10 pfu per cell or mock infected in the presence of the mouse serum. After 18 hr, the ability of the mouse serum to neutralize HSV-1 infectivity was quantitated by counting the number of cells in each well which were rounded or spindle-shaped, the typical cytopathic effect (CPE) induced by HSV-1. As seen in Figure 6, the antiserum raised in mice against recombinant gB was able to protect AGMK cells against the cytopathic effects of HSV-1 (50% protection was provided at a 1/64 dilution of the serum). These results established that recombinant gB produced in bacteria was capable of eliciting production of potent neutralizing antibodies. We are currently extending these studies to determine if these antibodies are cross-neutralizing between different species of herpesvirus and the potential for use of recombinant gB as an effective immunoprophylactic.

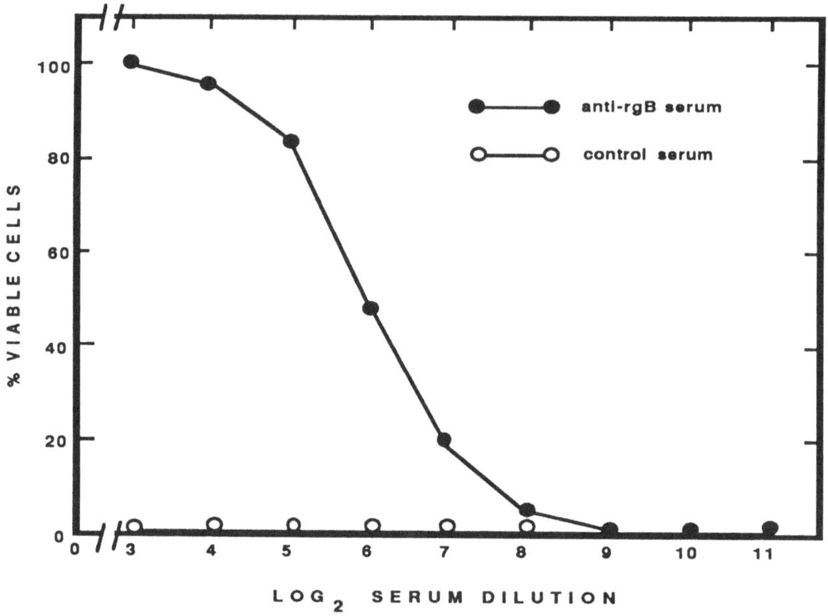

Figure 6. Neutralization of HSV-1 by antisera to recombinant gB. Aliquots of HSV-1 were incubated for 1 hr at 4°C with serial dilutions of an antiserum against gB raised in mice, or with control mouse serum. Preparations were then used to infect monolayers of AGMK cells growing in culture.

REFERENCES

Achtman M, Manning PA, Edelbluth C, Herrlich P (1979). Export without proteolytic processing of inner and outer membrane proteins encoded by F sex factor tra cistrons in *Escherichia coli* minicells. Proc Natl Acad Sci 76:4837.

Allen WP, Rapp F (1982). Concept review of genital herpes vaccines. J Infect Dis 145:413-421.

Babuik LA, Rouse BT (1979). Immune control of herpes virus latency. Can J Microbiol 25:267-274.

Balachandran ND, Harnish WE, Rawls WE, Bacchetti S (1982). Glycoproteins of Herpes simplex virus type 2 as defined by monoclonal antibodies. J Virol 44:344-355.

Birnboim HC, Doly J (1979). A rapid alkaline extraction procedure for screening recombinant plasmid DNA. Nucleic Acids Res 7:1513.

Breinig MC, Wright LC, McGeorge MB, Morahan PS (1978). Resistance to vaginal or systemic infection with Herpes simplex virus type 2. Arch Virol 57:25-34.

Bzik DJ, Fox BA, DeLuca NA, Person S (1984). Nucleotide sequence specifying the glycoprotein gene, gB, of Herpes simplex virus type 1. Virol 133:301-314.

CDC (1982). Genital Herpes Infection- United States, 1966-1979. MMWR 31:138-139.

Challacombe SJ, Tomasi TB, Jr (1980). Systemic tolerance and secretory immunity after oral immunization. J Exp Med 152: 1459-1472.

Clements JD, Finkelstein RA (1979). Isolation and characterization of homogeneous heat-labile enterotoxins with high specific activity from *Escherichia coli* cultures. Infect Immun 24:760-769.

Clements JD, Flint DC, Engert RF, Klipstein FA (1983). Cloning and molecular characterization of the B subunit of *Escherichia coli* heat-labile enterotoxin. Infect Immun 40:653-658.

Clements JD, El-Morshidy S (1984). Construction of a potential live oral bivalent vaccine for typhoid fever and cholera-*Escherichia coli*- related diarrheas. Infect Immun 46:564-569.

Clements JD, Lyon F, Lowe KL, Farrand AL, El-Morshidy S (1986). Oral immunization of mice with an attenuated strain of *Salmonella enteritidis* containing a recombinant plasmid which codes for production of the B subunit of the heat-labile enterotoxin of *Escherichia coli*. Infect Immun (In Press).

Dougan G, Sherratt D (1977). The transposon Tn1 as a probe for studying ColE1 structure and function. Molec Gen Genet 151: 151.

Elson CO, and Ealding W (1984a). Generalized systemic and mucosal immunity in mice after mucosal stimulation with cholera toxin. J Immunol 132:2736-2741.

Elson CO, and Ealding W (1984b). Cholera toxin feeding did not induce oral tolerance in mice and abrogated oral tolerance to an unrelated protein antigen. J Immunol 133:2892-2897.

Finkelstein, RA (1973). Cholera. CRC Critical Reviews in Microbiology 2:553-623.

Klipstein FA, Engert RF, and Clements JD (1982a). Development of a vaccine of cross-linked heat-stable and heat-labile enterotoxins that protects against *Escherichia coli* producing either enterotoxin. Infect Immun 37:550-557.

Klipstein FA, Engert RF, and Clements JD (1982b). Arousal of mucosal secretory immunoglobulin A antitoxin in rats immunized with *Escherichia coli* heat-labile enterotoxin. Infect Immun 37:1086-1092.

Maniatis T, Fritsch EF, Sambrook J (1982). "Molecular Cloning: A Laboratory Manual." New York: Cold Spring Harbor, p 396.

McDermott MR, Smiley JR, Leslie P, Brais J, Rudzroga HE, Bienenstock J (1984). Immunity in the female genital tract after intravaginal vaccination of mice with an attenuated strain of Herpes simplex virus type 2. J Virol 51:747-753.

McKenzie SJ, Halsey JF (1984). Cholera toxin B subunit as a carrier protein to stimulate a mucosal immune response. J Immunol 133:1818-1824.

Mendis LN, Best JM, Banatvala JG (1981). Class-specific antibodies (IgG and IgA) to membrane antigens of Herpes simplex virus type-2 infected cells in patients with cervical dysplasia and neoplasia. Int J Cancer 27:669-677.

Morahan PS, Breing MC, McGeorge MB (1977). Immune responses to vaginal or systemic infection of BALB/cJ mice with Herpes simplex virus type 2. J Immunol 119:2030-2036.

Nahmias AJ, Naib ZM, Highsmith AK, Josey WE (1967). Experimental genital Herpes simplex virus infection in the mouse. Pediatric Res 1:209-210.

Oakes JE, Lausch RN (1984). Monoclonal antibodies suppress replication of virus type 1 in trigeminal ganglia. J Virol 51:656-661.

Rüther U, Müller-Hill B (1983). Easy identification of cDNA clones. EMBO J 2:1791-1794.

Spiegel S, Fishman PH, Weber RJ (1985). Direct evidence that endogenous G_{M1} ganglioside can mediate thymocyte proliferation. Science 230:1285-1287.

Vieira J, Messing J (1982). The pUC plasmids, an M13mp7- derived system for insertion mutagenesis and sequencing with synthetic universal primers. Gene 19:259-268.

Immunopharmacology of Infectious Diseases: Vaccine Adjuvants and Modulators of Non-Specific Resistance, pages 155–164

NATURAL AND SYNTHETIC TREHALOSE DIESTERS AS IMMUNOMODULATORS.

E. LEDERER, G. LEMAIRE, J.P. TENU and J.F. PETIT

Institut de Biochimie, Université Paris-Sud, 91405 Orsay, France.

Many of the immunoactive bacterial compounds, such as lipopolysaccharides, peptidoglycans and their derivatives will be discussed in detail by others in this symposium. We shall restrict ourselves to trehalose diesters ("cord factors"), which are characteristic for the CMN group of bacteria (Corynebacteria, Mycobacteria, Nocardiae) (for reviews see Asselineau and Asselineau, 1978; Goren, 1982; Lederer, 1979, 1984; Lemaire et al., 1985, 1986).

The mycolic acids esterifying trehalose in 6,6' position are different in each of the genera; mycolic acids are α-branched β-hydroxy acids of the general formula:

$$R\text{-}CH(OH)\underset{\substack{|\\R'}}{CH}\ CO_2H$$

The R' in α is a straight saturated alkyl chain from C_{14} to C_{24}; the hydroxylated chain can have double bonds, methyl or methylene substituents.

Three types of natural mycolic acids are known:

1- Corynomycolic acids (C_{28} to C_{36}), in Corynebacteria, for instance: $CH_3(CH_2)_{14}\text{-}CH(OH)\text{-}\underset{\substack{|\\C_{14}H_{29}}}{CH}\text{-}CO_2H$

2- Nocardomycolic (or nocardic) acids (C_{40} to C_{60}), for instance:

$$CH_3(CH_2)_aCH{=}CH(CH_2)_bCH{=}CH\text{-}(CH_2)_cCH{=}CH(CH_2)_dCH(OH)\text{-}\underset{\substack{|\\C_{14}H_{29}}}{CH}\text{-}CO_2H$$

(a + b + c + d = 32, 34, 36.)

3- Mycobacterial mycolic acids (C_{60} to C_{90}) produced by mycobacteria, for instance: $C_{84}H_{164}O_3$:

$$CH_3(CH_2)_{19}\underbrace{CH\text{-}CH}_{CH_2}(CH_2)_{14}\underbrace{CH\text{-}CH}_{CH_2}\text{-}(CH_2)_{17}CH(OH)\text{-}\underset{\substack{|\\C_{24}H_{49}}}{CH}\text{-}CO_2H$$

The nomenclature of trehalose diesters is variable. The term "cord factor" should be restricted to natural 6,6'-diesters of trehalose. P_3 is a mycobacterial lipid identical with cord factor. The term TDM (for trehalose dimycolate) has been generally accepted.

I- BIOLOGICAL PROPERTIES OF TDM.

Bekierkunst (1968) was the first to show that TDM was an efficient immunomodulator.

Due to their insolubility in aqueous solvents, trehalose diesters have usually been dissolved in mineral or vegetable oil and then emulsified in saline: the properties of these oil in water emulsions (TDM/o) vary according to the nature and proportion of oil .

TDM can also be prepared as autoliposomes of approximately 1 μm in diameter where the lamellae consist of TDM, the interlamellar fluid being water; these autoliposomes, (TDM/w) are injected in saline (Kato, 1970; Lepoivre et al., 1982).

While most of the mycobacterial trehalose dimycolates have analogous biological properties, TDM from *M. avium* is inactive (Masihi et al., 1985).

A- Toxicity.

TDM/w is apyrogenic and after i.p. injection in mice, is devoid of gross long term toxicity (Orbach et al., 1983). Intratracheal administration of TDM/w in rats induces small granulomas in the lung which regress within a few weeks (Masse and Nolibé, to be published). I.v. injections of TDM/o causes lung granulomas the importance of which depends on the % of oil and the size of the oil droplets. Under very severe conditions (i.p. injection in mineral oil) TDM causes interstitial and hemorrhagic pneumonitis (Seggev et al., 1984). Synthetic lower analogs, discussed later, are devoid of toxicity (Yarkoni et al., 1978; Numata et al., 1985). Anticancer phase I and II clinical trials of *M.smegmatis* cell wall skeleton + TDM showed no significant hematopoietic, renal, hepatic or pulmonary toxicity (Vosika et al., 1983). I.v injection of TDM/o or TDM/w sensitizes to endotoxins, but far less than a comparable weight of BCG (Parant et al., 1977).

B- Adjuvant activity.

TDM increases the ability of killed microbes or

purified antigens to vaccinate against a variety of microorganisms: Listeria monocytogenes, (Le Garrec et al.,1981), Brucella abortus (Woodard et al.,1980) and Entamoeba histolytica (Sharma et al.,1985). Protection is accompanied by an increased DTH and in most cases by enhanced antibody titers.

C- Stimulation of non-specific resistance

a) - Protection against bacteria.

TDM/o protects mice against intracellular bacteria such as L. monocytogenes (Parant et al., 1977, 1978), Salmonella typhi and S. typhimurium (Yarkoni and Bekierkunst, 1976), as well as against the extracellular Klebsiella pneumoniae (Parant et al., 1977, 1978). TDM/w protects mice against K. pneumoniae and L. monocytogenes (Parant et al., 1977). In these experiments trehalose dicorynomycolate from C. diphtheriae and its synthetic racemic isomer ("C76") were equally active.

b- Protection against parasites.

TDM in FIA protects mice against Trypanosoma cruzi (Leon et al. 1983); TDM/w is active against T. musculi (Vincendeau et al., 1986) and against parasites growing within erythrocytes, such as Babesia microti (Clark, 1979) and Plasmodium berghei (Kumar et al., 1984). I.p. injection of TDM in 1% squalane protects mice against infection by Toxoplasma gondii (Masihi et al., 1985). TDM/w protects also mice against the trematode Schistosoma mansoni (Olds et al., 1980).

Even injected 14 days after infection of mice with tetrathyridia of Mesocestoides corti, TDM/w reduces parasite burden (White, Thompson and Penhale, submitted).

The absence of correlation between the mode of administration of TDM and the route of the challenge is interesting. Furthermore, the immunostimulation by TDM increases gradually over weeks: mice were better protected against B. microti 7 weeks after an i.v. injection of 200 µg of TDM/w than after 3 or 5 weeks (Clark, 1979). Mice were protected against P. berghei 6 weeks after a second i.p. injection of 250 µg of TDM/w (Kumar et al. 1984). In both cases, the mice surviving the first challenge were protected against a second challenge several months later.

c- Protection against viruses.

TDM emulsified with MDP (in 1% oil + 0.02% Tween) and injected i.v. protects mice against an aerosol challenge with influenza virus (Masihi et al., 1984,

1985). Intranasal administration of TDM/w protects mice against a lethal challenge with Sendai virus (Numata et al., 1985).

d- Antitumor activity.

Antitumor properties of TDM will not be described here. Briefly, TDM/o can prevent tumor growth or even induce tumor regression. The presence in the emulsion of a second immunostimulant (cell wall skeleton, endotoxin, muramylpeptides) strongly increases the effect. TDM/w, injected i.p., protects mice against the growth of syngeneic tumor cells (P815, L1210). Intratracheal administration of TDM/w to rats protects 30% of the animals against syngeneic P77 fibrohistiocytoma.(See Lederer and Chedid, 1982; Lemaire et al., 1985, 1986).

II- BIOLOGICAL PROPERTIES OF SYNTHETIC TREHALOSE DIESTERS

Synthetic 6,6'-trehalose diesters are non toxic and much less granulomagenic, but are usually less active (Yarkoni et al, 1978). "C100", a trehalose diester with a synthetic C_{44} mycolic acid and "C76", a synthetic racemic isomer of the dicorynomycolate of trehalose have qualitatively the same biological activities as TDM. Even trehalose dipalmitate, (C_{44}), was active in oil against infection of mice by S. mansoni (Olds et al.,1980). Some synthetic analogs have also antitumor properties in rats (Pimm et al., 1979). A recent paper (Numata et al., 1985) describes the synthesis of a series of trehalose 6,6'-diesters of fatty acids (linear, or α-branched or α-branched, β-hydroxylated). No lethal toxicity was observed in mice injected with 400 µg of the analogs in 9% oil. The cytolytic activity of mouse peritoneal macrophages was potentiated by TDM/o, TDM/w and some synthetic analogs. TD(BH48), a diester with a C_{48} synthetic mycolic acid was even slightly more active than TDM for activation of macrophages. TD(BH32), (="C76") also stimulates non-specific resistance against Sendai virus infection, as well as TDM, after intranasal application.

III- SYNERGISM OF TDM WITH OTHER IMMUNOMODULATORS.

TDM and MDP, both emulsified together in oil (or squalane) with Tween or Arlacel, injected intralesionally, cause regression of the line 10 hepatocarcinoma in strain 2 guinea pigs (McLaughlin et al., 1980; Yarkoni et al.,1981). Such an effect has also been described for mice infected by M.tuberculosis or influenza virus (Masihi et al., 1984). Oil emulsions of TDM, MDP and killed B. abortus are more effective as vaccines than bacteria in FCA (Woodard et al., 1980).

Quite recently Ribi Immunochem (Hamilton, Montana) has proposed a new adjuvant: "RAS" (Ribi adjuvant system) containing a monophophoryl lipid A (MPL) and TDM; RAS is said to be more active than FCA. An antiinfective synergistic activity of MPL+TDM in mice to aerogenic influenza virus infection is reported in this meeting by E. Ribi.

IV- MECHANISM OF ACTION OF TDM.

A- Cellular targets of TDM.

The primary target cell of TDM has not been unambiguously identified. *In vitro*, TDM can stimulate macrophage interaction with T. cruzi (Kierszenbaum et al.,1984) and produces proliferation of T cells (Kierszenbaum et al., 1981). Anyhow, several arguments point to the macrophage as the main effector cell of TDM *in vivo* : 1)TDM is active especially against intracellular microbes; 2) protection of mice against influenza virus is abrogated by silica, dextran sulfate and carrageenan (Masihi et al., 1984); 3) a few days after i.p. injection of TDM, macrophages in peritoneal exudates are modified as described below.

B- Properties of macrophages elicited by TDM/w.

Murine macrophages obtained 7 days after an i.p. injection of TDM/w are different from both resident and inflammatory macrophages. They have a decreased level of alkaline phosphodiesterase and β-galactosidase. They do not secrete or contain plasminogen activator. They produce large quantities of H_2O_2 (1 nmole/min/10^6 macrophages) after triggering by phorbol myristate acetate (Lepoivre et al., 1982). Upon zymosan triggering, they release as much arachidonate metabolites as resident cells but produce PGE_2 and thromboxane A_2 rather than PGI_2. The conversion of leukotriene C to leukotriene D is efficient but biosynthesis of Platelet Activating Factor is low (Drapier et al., 1983).

TDM/w elicited macrophages are in the same functional state as pyran-elicited macrophages : they are not fully activated for tumor cytotoxicity but only primed. To become cytotoxic for tumor cells, primed macrophages have to receive a second signal delivered *in vitro* by a short pulse with 10 ng/ml LPS or 1 μg/ml MDP. Such a mild in vitro treatment is inefficient on resident or inflammatory macrophages. The final activation of TDM/w primed macrophages by LPS or MDP is accompanied by a 3-fold increase in their glucose consumption and secretion of new polypeptides (Grand-Perret et al., 1986).

Reisser et al. (1984) obtained rat peritoneal macrophages cytotoxic for tumor cells 7 days after i.p. injection of 200 ug TDM/w.

Alveolar macrophages from rats, 3 days after intratracheal administration of 200 μg TDM/w, are primed and become cytotoxic for tumor cells after culture in vitro with 40 ng/ml LPS (Nolibé et al., 1985).

C- Mechanism of action of TDM on macrophages.

Since in vitro addition of TDM/w to resident or inflammatory macrophages does not modify their degree of activation, as judged by their cytotoxic activity against tumor cells, the action of TDM/w on macrophage activation is probably indirect. T-cells do not seem involved as macrophages recovered from thymectomized, irradiated mice treated with TDM are cytotoxic by culture in vitro in LPS containing media (Orbach-Arbouys et al., 1983).

TDM could exert its action through host factors. Indeed, Ramanathan et al., (1980), have demonstrated that TDM/w activates the alternative pathway of complement in guinea-pigs and man. Retzinger et al., (1981,1982), have shown that TDM-coated hydrophobic beads, which are comparable to TDM/w, bind proteins, especially plasma fibrinogen, which might give rise to activating molecules such as the fibrino-peptide B. The immunomodulating properties of TDM may thus be due to its capacity to form a particular type of interface favoring adsorption of proteins.

CONCLUSIONS

TDM, especially as suspension in water, is devoid of pyrogenicity and long term toxicity. Injected i.v. or i.p. or given intranasally, it protects experimental animals against a vast array of infectious agents: viruses, intracellular microbes, or extracellular organisms, or parasites growing within erythrocytes. In some cases, the ability of TDM-activated macrophages to produce activated oxygen species might be involved, but in other cases, such as parasites growing within erythrocytes, cytotoxic proteins produced by activated macrophages (TNF or others) might be implicated.

The fact that TDM acts in synergy with MDP or LPS indicates that trehalose diesters have specific targets. This synergism should find applications in veterinary and clinical medicine.

Asselineau C. and Asselineau J. (1978). Trehalose-containing glycolipids. Prog. Chem. Fats other Lipids, 16, 59-99 Pergamon Press.

Bekierkunst A. (1968). Acute granulomatous response produced in mice by trehalose-6,6'dimycolate. J.Bact, 96, 958-961.

Clark I.A. (1979). Protection of mice against Babesia microti with cord factor COAM, zymosan, glucan, Salmonella and Listeria. Parasite Immunol., 1, 179-186.

Drapier J.C., Roubin R., Petit J.F. and Benveniste J. (1983). Lipid mediator synthesis in peritoneal macrophages from mice injected with immunostimulants. Biochim. Biophys. Acta 751, 90-98.

Goren M.B. (1982). Immunoreactive substances of Mycobacteria. Amer.Rev.Resp.Dis., 125, 50-69.

Grand-Perret T., Lepoivre M., Petit J.F. and Lemaire G. (1986). Macrophage activation by trehalose dimycolate. Requirement for an expression signal in vitro for antitumoral activity. Biochemical markers distinguishing primed and fully activated macrophages. Europ. J. Immunol., 16, 332-338.

Kato M. (1970). Site II specific inhibition of mitochondrial oxidative phosphorylation by trehalose-6-6'-dimycolate (cord factor) of Mycobacterium tuberculosis Arch. Biochem. Biophys. 140, 379-390.

Kierszenbaum F. and Walz D.R. (1981). Proliferative responses of central and peripheral rat lymphocytes elicited by cord factor (trehalose 6,6'-dimycolate) Infect. Immun., 33, 115-119.

Kierszenbaum F., Zenian A. and Wirth J.J. (1984). Macrophage activation by cord factor (trehalose 6,6' dimycolate). Enhanced association with and intracellular killing of Trypanosoma cruzi. Infect.Immun., 43, 531-535.

Kumar P., Ahmad S. and Lederer E. (1984). Protection de souris contre Plasmodium berghei par le tréhalose dimycolate (TDM) en suspension aqueuse. C.R.Acad.Sc. Paris, T.298, Série III p.453-456.

Lederer E. (1979). Cord factor and related synthetic trehalose diesters. Springer Semin.Immunopathol., 2, 133-148.

Lederer E. (1984). Chemistry of mycobacterial cord factor and related natural and synthetic trehalose esters. In:"The Mycobacteria a source book". Eds. J.Wayne and G.P. Kubica. Marcel Dekker Inc., New York; Part A p.361-378.

Lederer E. and Chedid L. (1982). Immunomodulation by sysnthetic muramylpeptides and trehalose diesters in "Immunological approaches to cancer therapeutics". Ed. E. Mihich, J. Wiley and Son, New York, 107-135.

Le Garrec Y. Galleli A. and Audibert F. (1981). Induction of resistance to Listeria monocytogenes in mice treated with a combination of inactivated bacteria potentiated by trehalose dimycolate. Ann. Immunol. (Inst. Pasteur) 132D, 271-280.

Lemaire G., Tenu J.P., Petit J.F. and Lederer E. (1985). Effects of microbially derived products on mononuclear phagocytes. In: The Reticuloendothelial System. A comprehensive treatise. Vol.8, Pharmacology. ed. J.W. Hadden & A. Szentivanyi. Plenum Press New-York & London, 183-245.

Lemaire G., Tenu J.P., Petit J.F. and Lederer E. (1986). Natural and synthetic trehalose diesters as immunomodulators. Medicinal Res.Revs, in press.

Leon L.L., Queiroz-Cruz M., Galvao-Castro B., Soares G.H., Lima A.O. et Lederer E. (1983). Protection de souris par le dimycolate de tréhalose (TDM) contre une infection létale par Trypanosoma cruzi. C.R.Acad.Sc. Paris, T.297, Série III, 335-337.

Lepoivre M., Tenu J.P., Lemaire G. and Petit J.F. (1982). Antitumor activity and hydrogen peroxide release by macrophages elicited by trehalose diesters. J. Immunol., 129, 860-866.

McLaughlin C.A., Schwartzman S.M., Horner B.L., Jones G.H., Moffatt J.G., Nestor J.J. Jr and Tegg D. (1980). Regression of tumors in guinea pigs after treatment with synthetic muramyl dipeptides and trehalose dimycolate. Science, 208, 415-416.

Masihi K.N., Brehmer W., Lange W., Ribi E. and Schwartzman S. (1984). Protective effect of muramyl dipeptide analogs in combination with trehalose dimycolate against aerogenic influenza virus and Mycobacterium tuberculosis infections in mice. J.Biol.Resp.Modif., 3, 663-666.

Masihi K.N., Brehmer W., Lange W. Werner H. and Ribi E. (1985). Trehalose dimycolate from various Mycobacterial species induces differing anti-infectious activities in combination with Muramyl dipeptide. Infect.Immun., 50, 938-940.

Nolibé D., Tenu J.P., Lepoivre M. and Petit J.F. (1985) Activation of rat alveolar macrophages by intratracheal administration of trehalose dimycolate (TDM). Int. J. Immunopharmac. 7, 279.

Numata F., Nishimura K., Ishida H., Ukei S., Tone Y., Ishihara C., Saiki, I., Sekikawa I. and Azuma I. (1985). Lethal and adjuvant activities of cord factor (trehalose 6,6' dimycolate) and synthetic analogs in mice. Chem. Pharm. Bull., 33, 4544-4555.

Olds G.R., Chedid L., Lederer E. and Mahmoud A.A.F. (1980). Induction of resistance to Schistosoma mansoni by natural cord factor and synthetic lower homologs. J. Infect. Dis., 141, 473-478.

Orbach-Arbouys S., Tenu J.P. and Petit J.F. (1983). Enhancement of in vitro and in vivo antitumor activity by cord factor (6,6'-dimycolate of trehalose) administered suspended in saline. Int.Arch.Allergy & Applied Immunol., 71, 67-73.

Parant M., Audibert F., Parant F., Chedid L., Soler E., Polonsky J. and Lederer E. (1978). Non-specific immunostimulant activities of synthetic trehalose 6,6'-diesters (lower homologues of cord factor). Infect.Immun., 20, 12-19.

Parant M., Parant F., Chedid L., Drapier J.C., Petit J.F., Wietzerbin J. and Lederer E. (1977). Enhancement of nonspecific immunity to bacterial infection by cord factor (6,6'-Trehalose Dimycolate). J.Infect. Dis., 135, 771-777.

Pimm R., Baldwin W., Polonsky J. and Lederer E. (1979) Immunotherapy of an ascitic rat hepatoma with Cord Factor (Trehalose-6,6'-dimycolate) and synthetic analogues. Int. J. Cancer 24, 780-785.

Ramanathan V.D., Curtis J. and Turk J.L. (1980). Activation of the alternative pathway of complement by Mycobacteria and cord factor. Infect.Immun., 29, 30-35.

Reisser D., Jeannin J.F. et Martin F. (1984), Effet in vivo et in vitro du dimycolate de trehalose (TDM) sur l'activité tumoricide des macrophages péritonéaux de rats. C.R.Acad.Sc.Paris, t.298 -Série III, 181-184.

Retzinger G.S., Meredith S.C., Hunter, R.L., Takayama K. and Kezdy F.J. (1982). Identification of the physiologically active state of the mycobacterial glycolipid trehalose 6,6'-dimycolate and the role of fibrinogen in the biologic activities of trehalose 6,6'-dimycolate monolayers. J.Immunol., 129, 735-744.

Retzinger G.S., Meredith S.C., Takayama K., Hunter R.L. and Kezdy F.J. (1981). The role of surface in the biological activities of trehalose 6,6'-dimycolate. Surface properties and development of a model system. J. Biol. Chem., 256, 8208-8216.

Seggev J.S., Goren M.B. and Kirpatrick C.H. (1984). The pathogenesis of trehalose dimycolate induced interstitial pneumonitis. Cell.Immunol., 85, 428-435.

Sharma A., Haq A., Ahmad S. and Lederer E. (1985). Vaccinationof rabbits against Entamoeba histolytica with aqueous suspension of trehalose dimycolate as the adjuvant. Infect.Immun., 48, 634-637.

Vincendeau P., Daulouède S. et Ripert C. (1986). Effet protecteur du dimycolate de tréhalose lors de l'infestation de la souris par Trypanosoma musculi. C.R. Acad. Sc. Paris, T. 302, Série III, n°14, 529-532.

Vosika G. and Gray R. (1983). Phase I study of i.v. mycobacterial cell wall skeleton and cell wall skeleton combined with trehalose dimycolate. Cancer Treatment Reports 67, 785-790.

Woodard L., Toone N. and McLaughlin C. (1980) Comparison of muramyl dipeptide, trehalose dimycolate and dimethyl dioctadecyl ammonium bromide as adjuvants in Brucella abortus 45/20 vaccine. Infect. Immun. 30,409-412.

Yarkoni E. and Bekierkunst A. (1976) Non-specific resistance against infection with Salmonella typhi and Salmonella typhimurium induced in mice by Cord Factor (trehalose-6,6'-dimycolate) and its analogues. Infect. Immun. 14,1125-1129.

Yarkoni E., Lederer E. and Rapp H.J. (1981). Immunotherapy of experimental cancer with a mixture of synthetic muramyl dipeptide and trehalose dimycolate. Infect. Immun., 32, 273-276.

Yarkoni E., Rapp H.J., Polonsky J. and Lederer E. (1978), Immunotherapy with an intralesionally administered synthetic cord factor analogue. Int.J.Cancer, 22, 564-569.

Immunopharmacology of Infectious Diseases: Vaccine Adjuvants and Modulators of Non-Specific Resistance, pages 165–170

THE DIFFERENTIAL ADJUVANT ACTIVITY OF $Al(OH)_3$ AND SAPONIN

Robert H. R. Bomford

Department of Experimental Immunobiology, The Wellcome Research Laboratories, Beckenham, Kent BR3 3BS, U.K.

INTRODUCTION

Saponin is a mixture of water-soluble triterpene glycosides extracted from the bark of the South American tree Quillaia saponaria (Dalsgaard, 1978). It is highly surface-active on account of the hydrophobic triterpene and hydrophilic sugar moieties, and is exploited as a foaming agent in the soft drinks industry.

The adjuvant action of saponin was discovered half a century ago (Thibault et Richou, 1936) and it has been used in a variety of veterinary vaccines ever since, particularly those against foot-and-mouth disease virus (Dalsgaard, 1978).

Most recently, saponin has attracted attention on account of its powerful adjuvant activity for experimental vaccines against parasitic protozoa (Scott et al., 1984), and also its ability to form stable and highly-immunogenic complexes with the surface proteins of enveloped viruses (Morein and Simons, 1985). There is also evidence that its adjuvant activity differs from that of $Al(OH)_3$ in both the types of antigen with which it is effective (Bomford, 1984; Bomford et al., 1985), and the components of the immune response which are stimulated (Scott et al., 1984).

SAPONIN AS AN ADJUVANT FOR ANTI-PARASITE VACCINES

The potential of saponin as an adjuvant for anti-parasite vaccines was first recognized with Trypanosoma *cruzi* in mice (Johnson et al., 1963) and later with *Plasmodium berghei* in rats (Desowitz, 1975), *P. yoelii* in the mouse (McColm et al., 1982) and *P. knowlesi* in monkeys (Mitchell et al., 1979).

The basis for the selective efficacy of saponin relative to $Al(OH)_3$ and a variety of other adjuvants for the potentiation of protective immunity against *T. cruzi* in the mouse has been investigated in some detail (Scott et al., 1984). It was found that the immune response to *T. cruzi* stimulated by saponin differed from that with $Al(OH)_3$ in two respects. Firstly, saponin but not $Al(OH)_3$ elicited IgG2a and IgG2b anti-*T. cruzi* antibodies; and secondly, saponin also provoked a delayed-type hypersensitivity (DTH) response, whereas $Al(OH)_3$ did not. However, protection against *T. cruzi* infection was correlated with DTH rather than IgG2 antibody since another adjuvant, squalane, stimulated IgG2 without DTH, and failed to confer protection.

THE COMPLEXING OF SAPONIN WITH ANTIGENS

Saponin is a potent haemolysin, probably on account of its ability to complex with cholesterol in cell membranes producing lesions which, in the electron microscope, resemble those caused by the lytic components of complement (Dourmashkin et al., 1962). This may in part explain why saponin is a strong adjuvant for whole-cell parasite vaccines, and also for sheep erythrocytes (SRBC) (Bomford, 1980a,b).

After SRBC have been lysed by saponin, the immunogenic fraction is found in the particulate material sedimented by centrifugation rather than in the soluble supernatant, indicating that saponin complexed with membrane fragments retains its adjuvanticity (Bomford, 1982).

Saponin forms morphologically-defined, stable and highly immunogenic complexes with proteins released from the envelopes of viruses such as parainfluenza, influenza, measles and rabies (Morein et al., 1984; Morein and Simons, 1985). These particles, named ISCOMS ('immunostimulating complexes') appear in the electron microscope as pitted spheres about 30nm in diameter, and presumably consist of a mixed micelle of saponin and envelope protein, although the orientation of the components within the complex has not yet been determined. ISCOMS are more immunogenic than free or micellar viral subunits, and permit a considerable economy in the dose of both antigen and saponin relative to that needed without complex formation (Morein and Simons, 1985). This is important, expecially in view of the necessity to avoid the irritant and inflammatory effects of saponin. The potential of ISCOMS for veterinary viral subunit vaccines has recently been demonstrated by inducing protective immunity against feline leukemia with ISCOMS prepared from the feline leukemia virus (Osterhaus et al., 1985).

One reason for the strong immunogenicity of ISCOMS may be the fact that the particles contain many molecules of antigen and adjuvant which simultaneously interact with the target cell in the immune system, whether this be antigen-presenting cell or lymphocyte, which is presently unknown. This form of local targeting of antigen and adjuvant would ensure that a supra-threshold dose of both components is received by the responding cells, leading to a single-hit kinetics of activation. In this respect, ISCOMS could provide an important guide to the formulation of other adjuvants in micro-particulate form.

DIFFERENTIAL EFFICACY OF SAPONIN AND $Al(OH)_3$ FOR STRONG AND WEAK ANTIGENS

The first indication that the relative adjuvant efficacy of saponin and $Al(OH)_3$ can depend on the nature of the antigen came from studies using SRBC and bovine serum albumin (BSA), where it was found that saponin was more effective with the former antigen, and the opposite was the case with the latter (Bomford, 1980a). Saponin may be a good adjuvant for SRBC because, as mentioned above, it can form complexes with cholesterol in the membrane. However in further studies using DNP conjugates of BSA, fowl gamma globulin (FGG) and keyhole limpet haemocyanin (KLH) as antigens, saponin was superior for the strong antigen DNP-KLH, whereas the response to the weaker antigens DNP-BSA and DNP-FGG was best potentiated by $Al(OH)_3$ (Bomford, 1984). This result could still be explained by factors such as the molecular weight of the antigen (KLH being much larger than BSA or FGG) or on the ability of saponin to form complexes with KLH and not with the other antigens. However, these possibilities were excluded in experiments using human growth hormone in genetically high and low responder mice (Bomford et al., 1985). Here, using the same antigen, $Al(OH)_3$ but not saponin elicited a humoral response in the low-responder mice, whereas saponin was the better adjuvant in the high responding strain.

The reasons for this differential adjuvant efficacy are as yet unknown, although the results are compatible with the hypothesis that $Al(OH)_3$ is better than saponin at preventing the triggering of T suppressor cells down-regulating the response to intrinsically weak antigens.

CONCLUSIONS

Considerable progress has been made in delineating the characteristics of saponin as an adjuvant. Given an antigen of a suitable type, which means one that is an intrinsically strong antigen in the species in question and which preferably has the correct amphiphilic nature to interact with saponin to form ISCOMS, saponin is capable of stimulating a humoral response which includes IgG2 isotypes and also cell-mediated immunity. This is of importance in providing protective immunity to parasitic protozoa and retroviruses such as FeLV. It is worth pointing out that there is another category of compounds, the polyene antibiotics such as nystatin and amphotericin B, which share with saponin the property of binding to cholesterol in cell membranes, and which show similar adjuvant properties (Blanke et al., 1977; Bomford, 1980b; Little et al., 1983).

The fundemental mechanism of the adjuvant action of saponin remains unknown. It is possible that it does no more than cause cell destruction leading to the release of inflammatory mediators which mediate adjuvant activity. There is some evidence against this simple hypothesis. The local inflammatory effect of saponin at the site of injection can be blocked by injecting it together with liposomes containing cholesterol, and this does not abolish to adjuvant activity (Scott et al., 1985). There is some information on the cellular site of saponin action. The potentiation of the response to SRBC by saponin does not take place in athymic mice (Bomford, 1982) showing that for the response to T-dependent antigens saponin cannot substitute for T cells. It has recently been shown that saponin is an effective adjuvant for T-independent antigens (Flebbe and Braley-Mullen, 1986) suggesting that it may act on B cells.

Finally, it is not yet clear whether saponin will be acceptable for human vaccines, in view of its haemolytic and inflammatory activity. It remains to be determined whether, by the application of ISCOM technology, sufficiently small doses of saponin can be used to avoid any deleterious side-effects.

REFERENCES

Blanke TJ, Little JR, Shirley SF, Lynch RG (1977). Augmentation of murine immune responses by amphotericin B. Cell Immunol 33:180.

Bomford R (1980a). The comparative selectivity of adjuvants for humoral and cell-mediated immunity I. Effect on the antibody response to bovine serum albumin and sheep red blood cells of Freund's incomplete and complete adjuvants, alhydrogel, Corynebacterium parvum, Bordetella pertussis, muramyl dipeptide and saponin. Clin exp Immunol 39:426.

Bomford R (1980b). Saponin and other haemolysins (vitamin A aliphatic amines, polyene antibiotics) as adjuvants for SRBC in the mouse. Evidence for a role for cholesterol-binding in saponin adjuvanticity. Int Archs Allergy appl Immun 63:170.

Bomford R (1982). Studies on the cellular site of action of the adjuvant activity of saponin for sheep erythrocytes. Int Archs Allergy appl Immun 67:127.

Bomford R (1984). Relative adjuvant efficacy of $Al(OH)_3$ and saponin is related to the immunogenicity of the antigen. Int Archs Allergy appl Immun 75:280.

Bomford R, Aston R, Ivanyi J (1985). Reversal of Il-2-restricted hyporesponsiveness to human growth hormone by the use of aluminium hydroxide as adjuvant. Immunogenetics 21:505.

Dalsgaard K (1978). A study of the isolation and characterization of the saponin Quil A. Evaluation of its adjuvant activity, with a special reference to the application in the vaccination of cattle against foot-and-mouth disease. Act Vetinaria Scand Suppl 69:1.

Desowitz RS (1975). Plasmodium berghei: Immunogenic enhancement of antigen by adjuvant addition. Exp Parasitol 38:6.

Dourmashkin RR, Dougherty RM, Harris RJC (1962). Electron microscope observations on Rous sarcoma virus and cell membranes. Nature 194:1116.

Flebbe LM, Braley-Mullen H (1986). Immunopotentiation by SGP and Quil A II. Identification of responding cell popu-

lations. Cell Immunol 99:128.
Johnson P, Neal RA, Gall D (1963). Protective effect of killed trypanosome vaccines with incorporated adjuvants. Nature 200:83.
Little JR, Abegg A, Plut E (1983). The relationship between adjuvant and mitogenic effects of amphotericin methyl ester. Cell Immunol 78:224.
McColm AA, Bomford R, Dalton L (1982). A comparison of saponin with other adjuvants for the potentiation of protective immunity by a killed Plasmodium yoelii vaccine in the mouse. Parasite Immunology 4:337.
Mitchell GH, Richards WHG, Coller A, Kietrich FM, Dukor P (1979). Nor-MDP, saponin, corynebacteria and pertussis organisms as immunological adjuvants in experimental malaria vaccination of macaques. Bull WHO 57 (Suppl 1): 189.
Morein B, Sundquist B, Hoglund S, Dalsgaard K, Osterhaus A (1984). Iscom, a novel structure for antigenic presentation of membrane proteins from enveloped viruses. Nature 308:457.
Morein B, Simons K (1985). Subunit vaccines against enveloped viruses: virosomes, micelles and other protein complexes. Vaccine 3:83.
Osterhaus A, Weiger K, Uytdehaag F, Jarrett O, Sundquist B, Morein B (1985). Induction of protective immune response in cats by vaccination with feline leukemia virus ISCOM. J Immunol 135:591.
Scott MT, Bahr G, Moddaber F, Afchain D, Chedid L (1984). Adjuvant requirements for protective immunization of mice using a Trypanosoma cruzi 90K cell surface glycoprotein. Int Archs Allergy appl Immun 74:373.
Scott MT, Goss-Sampson M, Bomford R (1985). Adjuvant activity of saponin: Antigen localisation studies. Int Archs Allergy appl Immun 77:409.
Thibault P, Richou R (1936). Sur l'accroissement de l'ammunite antitoxique sous influence de l'addition de diverses substances a l'antigene (anatoxins diptherique et tetanique). C R Soc Biol 121:718.

Immunopharmacology of Infectious Diseases: Vaccine Adjuvants and Modulators of Non-Specific Resistance, pages 171–180
Published 1987 by Alan R. Liss, Inc.

LIPOSOMES AS CARRIERS FOR A MALARIA PEPTIDE VACCINE: DEVELOPMENTAL ASPECTS

Roberta L. Richards, Robert A. Wirtz, Wayne T. Hockmeyer and Carl R. Alving

Departments of Membrane Biochemistry (R.L.R., C.R.A.), Entomology (R.A.W.) and Immunology (W.T.H.), Walter Reed Army Institute of Research, Washington, DC 20307-5100

INTRODUCTION

There is a great need for a vaccine against malaria. Malaria is one of the most prevalent diseases in the world, and afflicts between 150 million and 300 million people each year. The infection is initiated by infected anopheline mosquitoes injecting sporozoites into the bloodstream of humans. The sporozoites pass through the bloodstream directly to the liver. In the liver, they are transformed into merozoites and then are released back into the bloodstream. The merozoites invade erythrocytes, undergo asexual reproduction and then are released back into the bloodstream, where they invade more erythrocytes. Thus, both the sporozoite and the merozoite are stages in the life cycle of the malaria parasite that are prospective targets for a vaccine.

The major advantage of a vaccine against the sporozoite stage is that the parasites would be stopped before they reach the bloodstream. After entering the bloodstream a substantial fraction of the parasites always are inside erythrocytes and not available to antibody. It is already known that immunization with irradiated sporozoites protects both animals and humans against sporozoite-induced malaria (Nussenzweig et al., 1969; Clyde et al., 1975). This protection is mediated in part by antibodies which recognize a protein, the circumsporozoite (CS) protein, on the surface of the sporozoite.

A region in the middle of the CS protein composed of 37 asn-ala-asn-pro tetrapeptide repeats interspersed with 4 asn-val-asp-pro tetrapeptides appears to be important in eliciting protective antibodies (Dame et al., 1984; Young et al., 1985; Ballou et al., 1985). Recently the gene encoding the CS protein of the human malaria parasite, Plasmodium falciparum, has been cloned and sequenced (Dame et al., 1984; Young et al., 1985). Peptides derived from the repeat region of the CS protein have been conjugated to proteins (e.g., albumin) and have been used in animal immunogenicity studies (Ballou et al., 1985; Enea et al., 1984; Zavala et al., 1985). Antibodies raised against the peptides recognized native CS protein, as manifested by circumsporozoite precipitation (CSP) reactions, and also blocked sporozoite invasion of human hepatoma cells (Ballou et al., 1985).

In the above studies the peptide-protein conjugates were completely nonimmunogenic when used alone. To achieve immunogenicity, conjugation of peptide to a protein, and emulsification of the peptide-protein conjugates with complete Freund's adjuvant were required in order to elicit high titer anti-CS protein antibodies. Freund's adjuvant is not acceptable for use in human vaccines and this has prompted the examination of liposomes as a potential alternative safe and effective adjuvant (Alving et al., 1986).

Liposomes are spherical phospholipid vesicles which form spontaneously when dried phospholipids are mixed vigorously with aqueous solutions. Molecules, such as drugs or peptides, that are present in the aqueous phase during liposome formation are encapsulated within the vesicles. Other lipids, including lipophilic adjuvants such as lipid A and muramyl dipeptide (MDP), can also be incorporated in the lipid bilayer (Alving et al., 1986). When liposomes are administered parenterally, the vast majority are rapidly taken up by phagocytic reticuloendothelial cells, especially in the liver, spleen, bone marrow and lung (Lopez-Berestein et al., 1984). Large doses of liposomes are now being used effectively and safely as carriers of antimicrobial agents in humans (Lopez-Berestein et al., 1985). No toxic effects of liposomes have yet been detected in humans (Lopez-Berestein et al., 1984).

Immunomodulators, including macrophage activating factor and MDP, when carried by liposomes cause efficient activation of macrophages (Fidler et al., 1982). Since macrophages, and particularly Kupffer cells, are major sites for immunological processing of certain antigens (Rosenstreich, 1981; Diamond, 1982; Unanue, 1984), and macrophages are also the principal sites for expression of the activities of certain adjuvants (Allison, 1979), encapsulation in liposomes of a nonimmunogenic peptide should result in enhanced immunogenicity of the peptide. In this report we summarize evidence that liposome-encapsulation of CS peptide conjugated to bovine serum albumin (BSA) resulted in excellent immunogenicity of the CS peptide-BSA conjugate in the absence of other adjuvants.

MATERIALS AND METHODS

The CS peptide used in these studies, 16 amino acids in length, was synthesized as described previously (Ballou et al., 1985). The 16 amino acids comprised 4 repeats of asn-ala-asn-pro. The BSA conjugate of the CS peptide (CS-peptide-BSA) was prepared with the use of succinimidyl 4(N-maleimidoethyl) cyclohexane-1-carboxylate and contained 15 to 25 CS peptides per molecule of BSA (Marglin and Merrifield, 1970). CS-peptide-BSA was used either alone or encapsulated in liposomes as an antigen to immunize rabbits.

Liposomes (multilamellar) were prepared as described previously (Alving et al., 1984 and 1986) from a mixture of dimyristoyl phosphatidylcholine, cholesterol, dicetyl phosphate, and, where indicated, lipid A prepared from Escherichia coli 0111 lipopolysaccharide in molar ratios of 1:0.75:0.11:0.02. The liposomes were washed twice in 0.15 M NaCl by centrifuging at 29,000 x g to remove unencapsulated antigen.

Rabbits (2 per group) were immunized by intravenous injection of 1 ml of either CS-peptide-BSA in 0.15 M NaCl or CS-peptide-BSA encapsulated in liposomes lacking or containing lipid A. Each rabbit received boosting injections at 4 and 29 weeks after the primary injection. For the primary injection, all 6 rabbits received 8-9 μg each of CS-peptide-BSA alone or in liposomes containing or lacking lipid A. The boosting injections were 2-5 μg of

CS-peptide-BSA in liposomes containing or lacking lipid A and 30 µg of CS-peptide-BSA in saline. Blood was drawn from the rabbits at 2-4 week intervals and the sera assayed for antibodies to CS protein.

Enzyme-linked immunosorbent assays (ELISA) were carried out in wells of polystyrene microtiter plates as described previously (Young et al., 1985; Alving et al., 1986).

Some of the immune sera were tested in the circumsporozoite precipitation (CSP) assay. CSP reactions were performed essentially as described by Vanderberg et al. (1969). Aliquots (5 µl) containing 500-1000 P. falciparum salivary gland sporozoites resuspended in medium 199 were mixed with 5 µl of serum on a microscope slide, sealed under a coverslip rimmed with petroleum jelly and incubated at 37°C for 1 hour. Reactions were evaluated under phase contrast microscopy at 400x magnification. A 2+ reaction consisted of a granular precipitate on the surface of the sporozoites while a 4+ reaction gave a long, thread-like filament at one end of the sporozoites.

Immunofluorescence antibody assays (IFA) were also performed. Sporozoites were isolated from mosquito salivary glands, diluted in saline or culture medium containing 0.1% BSA, counted using a hemocytometer, and diluted to 2000 to 5000 sporozoites per 10 µl. Aliquots (10 µl) were spread onto each well of multiwell printed IFA slides, air dried at RT, and stored at -70°C. IFAs were initiated by spreading 20 µl volumes of serum, diluted 1/50 or 1/100 with blocking buffer, onto the wells of an IFA slide. After incubation for 20 minutes at RT in a moist chamber, the serum samples were aspirated and the wells washed with 2 drops of PBS. Aliquots (20 µl) of fluorescein isothiocyanate-conjugated goat anti-rabbit antibody (Kirkegard and Perry, Gaithersburg, MD) diluted 1:40 with blocking buffer were then added to each well. After a second 20 minute incubation, the wells were washed with 3 drops of PBS, mounted in glycerol and examined by fluorescence microscopy at 500x magnification.

RESULTS

Figure 1 shows the ELISA titer at 4 weeks after

intravenous immunization with liposome-encapsulated CS-peptide-BSA. Each line represents the mean ELISA activity of serum from 2 rabbits tested against a thyroglobulin conjugate of the same CS peptide. Antibody activity was measured spectrophotometrically and the maximum measurable absorbance (A_{414}) in the assay was 2.0. When rabbits were immunized with the CS-peptide-BSA in liposomes containing lipid A, high titer antibodies were obtained. A lower titer of antibody was obtained after immunization with liposomes lacking lipid A. There was no measurable activity in the preimmunization bleedings, and also none in the serum taken at 4 weeks from rabbits immunized with CS-peptide-BSA alone (not shown).

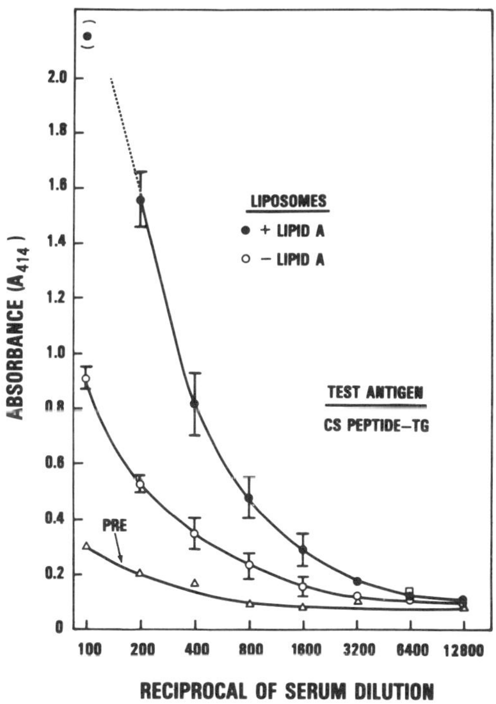

Figure 1. ELISA antibody activity in rabbit sera 4 weeks after immunization with liposome-encapsulated CS-peptide-BSA. Each line represents the mean activity of serum from 2 rabbits tested against a thyroglobulin conjugate of the same CS peptide. The maximum measurable absorbance (A_{414}) was 2.0. From Alving et al., 1986.

Table 1. Circumsporozoite Precipitation Assay[c]

Immunogen	Rabbit Number	Strength of reaction (0-4+)[a]	Number of sporozoites positive[b]
Liposomes containing CS-peptide-BSA	430	2+	8
Liposomes containing CS-peptide-BSA and lipid A	431	4+	20

[a]In each case the preimmunization bleeding showed no reactivity.
[b]A total of 25 randomly chosen sporozites was examined for each serum sample.
[c]From Alving et al., 1986.

Serum from 1 rabbit in each group immunized with liposome-encapsulated CS peptide-BSA, taken 2 weeks after the primary immunization, was tested for activity in the circumsporozoite precipitation assay. This in vitro assay correlates well with in vivo protection. As can be seen in Table 1, serum from both rabbits tested was active in the CSP assay.

Figure 2 shows a partial quantification of the results of an immunofluorescence assay on sera obtained at 2 weeks after immunization. The degree of fluorescence induced by binding of antibodies to intact sporozoites was rated from 0 to 4+ for each of the rabbits immunized with liposome-encapsulated CS-peptide-BSA. Serum from both rabbits immunized with lipid A containing liposomes was strongly positive in the IFA. The rabbits immunized with liposomes lacking lipid A gave a much weaker reaction in the IFA, but both did react.

As Figure 3 shows, antibody levels against the CS peptide, as measured by ELISA, have remained high over a long period of time. This figure shows the response with time for the most active rabbit of each group. Although the antibody levels had started dropping within 5 weeks

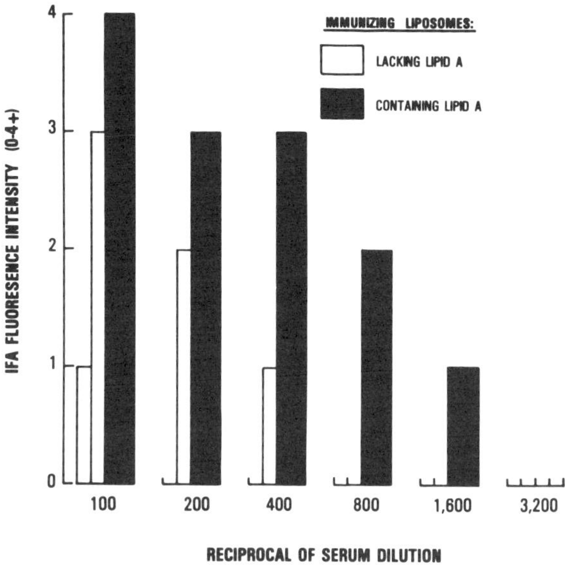

Figure 2. Partial quantification of the IFA. The degree of fluorescence induced by the antisera was rated from 0 to 4+ for each 2 rabbits immunized with liposomes containing CS peptide-BSA without lipid A and 2 rabbits with the same liposomes containing lipid A. From Alving et al., 1986.

after the first boost, a second boost at 29 weeks resulted in antibody levels which remained high for at least 25 weeks in the rabbit immunized with CS-peptide-BSA encapsulated in liposomes containing lipid A. A lesser antibody response was obtained when CS-peptide-BSA was encapsulated in liposomes lacking lipid A. No antibody response was observed after immunization with CS-peptide-BSA alone until after the second boost, and this response was always lower than that observed in rabbits immunized with antigen encapsulated in liposomes lacking or containing lipid A.

DISCUSSION

The results summarized here show that a very poorly immunogenic BSA-conjugated peptide from the repeat region of the CS protein of Plasmodium falciparum was made highly immunogenic by encapsulation in liposomes. The

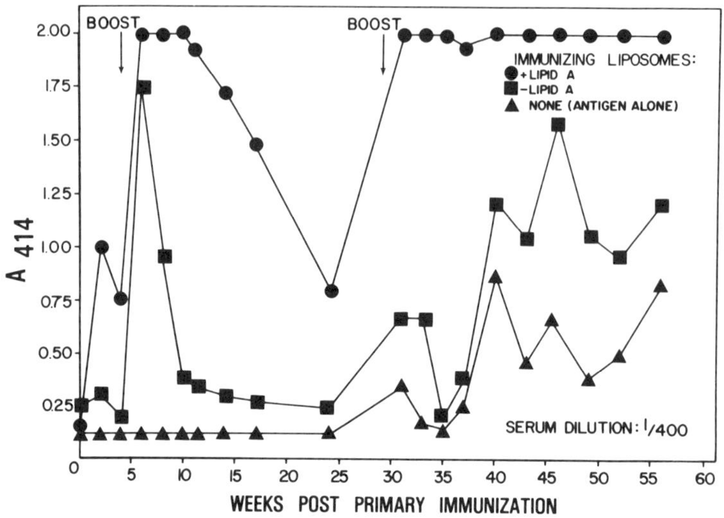

Figure 3. ELISA anti-CS-peptide antibody activity of rabbit sera with time. The most active rabbit of each group is shown. The maximum measurable response was A_{414} of 2.0. From Alving et al., 1986.

antibodies produced reacted with the peptide antigen itself and also with native CS protein and with intact living sporozoites. Previous results showed a strong correlation between protection against sporozoite-induced malaria and reactivity both with native CS protein and with intact living sporozoites (Nussenzweig et al., 1969; Vanderberg et al., 1969; Clyde et al., 1975; Rieckmann et al., 1979). In addition, studies now in progress on the use of liposomes in humans suggest that there will be few problems with toxicity (Coune et al., 1983 Lopez-Berestein et al., 1984; Lopez-Berestein et al., 1985;. Thus encapsulation in liposomes has made possible production of antibody against a virtually nonimmunogenic malaria antigen. The immune response is long-lived, of relatively high titer, and probably protective against sporozoite-induced malaria. Liposomes therefore show promise as a nontoxic carrier serving also as adjuvant for nonimmunogenic synthetic peptides as antigens in a human malaria vaccine.

REFERENCES

Allison AC (1979). Mode of action of immunological adjuvants. J Reticuloendothel Soc 26: 619.

Alving CR, Shichijo S, Mattsby-Baltzer I (1984). Preparation of liposomes in immunological studies. In Gregoriadis G (eds): "Liposome Technology, Vol 2", Boca Raton: CRC Press, p. 158.

Alving CR, Richards RL, Moss J, Alving LI, Clements JD, Shiba T, Kotani S, Wirtz RA, Hockmeyer WT (1986) Effectiveness of liposomes as potential carriers of vaccines. Applications to cholera toxin and human malaria sporozoite antigen. Vaccine (in press).

Ballou WR, Rothbard J, Wirtz RA, Gordon DM, Williams JS, Gore RW, Schneider I, Hollingdale MR, Beaudoin RL, Maloy WL, Miller LH, Hockmeyer WT (1985). Immunogenicity of synthetic peptides from circumsporozoite protein of Plasmodium falciparum. Science 228: 996.

Clyde DF, McCarthy VC, Miller RM, Woodward WE (1975). Immunization of man against falciparum and vivax malaria by use of attenuated sporozoites. Am J Trop Med Hyg 24: 397.

Coune A, Sculier J, Frühling J, Stryckmans P, Brassine C, Ghanem G, Laduron C, Atassi G, Ruysschaert JM, Hildebrand J (1983). Iv administration of a watar-insoluble antimitotic compound entrapped in liposomes. Preliminary report on infusion of large volumes of liposomes to man. Cancer Treat Rep 67: 1031.

Dame JB, Williams JL, McCutchan TF, Weber JL, Wirtz RA, Hockmeyer WT, Maloy WL, Haynes JD, Schneider I, Roberts D, Sanders GS, Reddy EP, Diggs CL, Miller LH (1984). Structure of the gene encoding the immunodominant surface antigen on the sporozoite of the human malaria parasite Plasmodium falciparum. Science 225: 593.

Diamond B (1982). Macrophages and the immune response. In Arias I, Popper H, Schachter D, Shafritz DA (eds): "The Liver: Biology and Pathobiology." New York: Raven Press, p 525.

Enea V, Ellis J, Zavala F, Arnot DE, Asavanich A, Masuda A, Quakyi I, Nussenzweig RS (1984). DNA cloning of Plasmodium falciparum circumsporozoite gene: Amino acid sequence of repetitive epitope. Science 225: 628.

Fidler IJ, Barnes Z, Fogler WE, Kirsh WE, Bugelski P, Poste G (1982).. Involvement of macrophages in the eradication of established metastases following intra-

venous injection of liposomes containing macrophage activators. Cancer Res 42: 496.
Lopez-Berestein G, Fainstein V, Hopfer R, Mehta K, Sullivan MP, Keating M, Rosenblum MG, Mehta R, Luna M, Hersh EM, Reuben J, Juliano RL, Bodey GP (1985). Liposomal amphotericin B for the treatment of systemic fungal infections in patients with cancer: a preliminary study. J Infect Dis 151: 704.
Lopez-Berestein G, Kasi L, Rosenblum MG, Mehta K, Sullivan MP, Keating M, Rosenblum MG, Mehta R, Luna M, Hersh EM, Reuben J, Juliano RL, Bodey GP (1984). Clinical pharmacology of ^{99m}Tc-labelled liposomes in patients with cancer. Cancer Res 44: 375.
Marglin A, Merrifield RB (1970). Chemical synthesis of peptides and proteins. Ann Rev Biochemistry 39: 841.
Nussenzweig R, Vanderberg J, Most H (1969). Protective immunity produced by the injection of x-irradiated sporozoites of Plasmodium berghei IV Dose response, specificity and humoral immunity. Milit Med 134: 1176.
Rosenstreich DL (1981). The macrophage. Oppenheim JJ, Rosenstreich DL, Potter M (eds): "Cellular Functions in Immunity and Inflammation," New York: Elsevier/North Holland, p 127.
Rieckmann KH, Beaudoin RL, Cassells JS, Sell KW (1979). Use of attenuated sporozoites in the immunization of human volunteers against falciparum malaria. Bull WHO 57: 261.
Unanue ER (1984). Antigen-presenting function of the macrophage. Ann Rev Immunol 2: 395.
Vanderberg J, Nussenzweig RS, Most H (1969). Protective immunity produced by injection of x-irradiated sporozoites of Plasmodium berghei. V In vitro effects of immune serum on sporozoites. Milit Med 134: 1183.
Young JF, Hockmeyer WT, Gross M, Ballou WR, Wirtz RA, Trosper JH, Beaudoin RL, Hollingdale MR, Miller LH, Diggs CL, Rosenberg M (1985). Expression of Plasmodium falciparum circumsporozoite proteins in Escherichia coli for potential use in a human malaria vaccine. Science 228: 958.
Zavala F, Tam JP, Hollingdale MR, Cochrane AH, Quakyi I, Nussenzweig RS, Nussenzweig V (1985). Rationale for development of a synthetic vaccine against Plasmodium falciparum malaria. Science 228: 1436.

Immunopharmacology of Infectious Diseases: Vaccine Adjuvants and Modulators of Non-Specific Resistance, pages 181–190

MODULATION OF ANTIGEN PRESENTATION AND HOST MEDIATORS BY BLOCK COPOLYMER ADJUVANTS.

Robert L. Hunter and Beth Bennett

Department of Pathology, Emory University, Atlanta, GA 30322
Supported by USPHS Grant ES03791.

The predominant paradigm of research on immunologic adjuvants is that each compound has a specific reactive site which interacts with receptors on cells or otherwise stimulates a specific response. However, investigators have long recognized that many adjuvants are surface active agents in that they contain both hydrophilic and hydrophobic groups. The physicochemical properties which contribute to surface activity are nonspecific but are subject to diverse subtle variations. Our studies were undertaken to identify the critical parameters of surface activity which contribute to adjuvant action. The nonionic block copolymer surfactants manufactured by BASF Wyandotte are composed of blocks or chains of hydrophilic polyoxyethylene (POE) and blocks of hydrophobic polyoxypropylene (POP) attached in one of four configurations, Figure 1. By varying the size of the blocks of POP and POE, dozens of preparations have been produced which span nearly the entire range of available nonionic surfactants. It seemed unlikely that major differences between the biologic activities of these copolymers could be due to active sites on one which were not present on many others. Consequently, they provide an ideal model for studying the physicochemical parameters which contribute to adjuvant activity.

In initial studies with triblock copolymers, one of the preparations, L121, proved to be a powerful adjuvant for stimulating antibody formation to BSA following injection in an oil-in-water emulsion (Hunter et al, 1981). L101 was less effective in stimulating antibody, but was more effective in inducing DTH and granulomas. The other triblock copolymers had little activity for either. The physical form of the emulsions was important. In most experiments, lyophilized BSA was homogenized with the hydrocarbon and surfactant before addition of PBS.

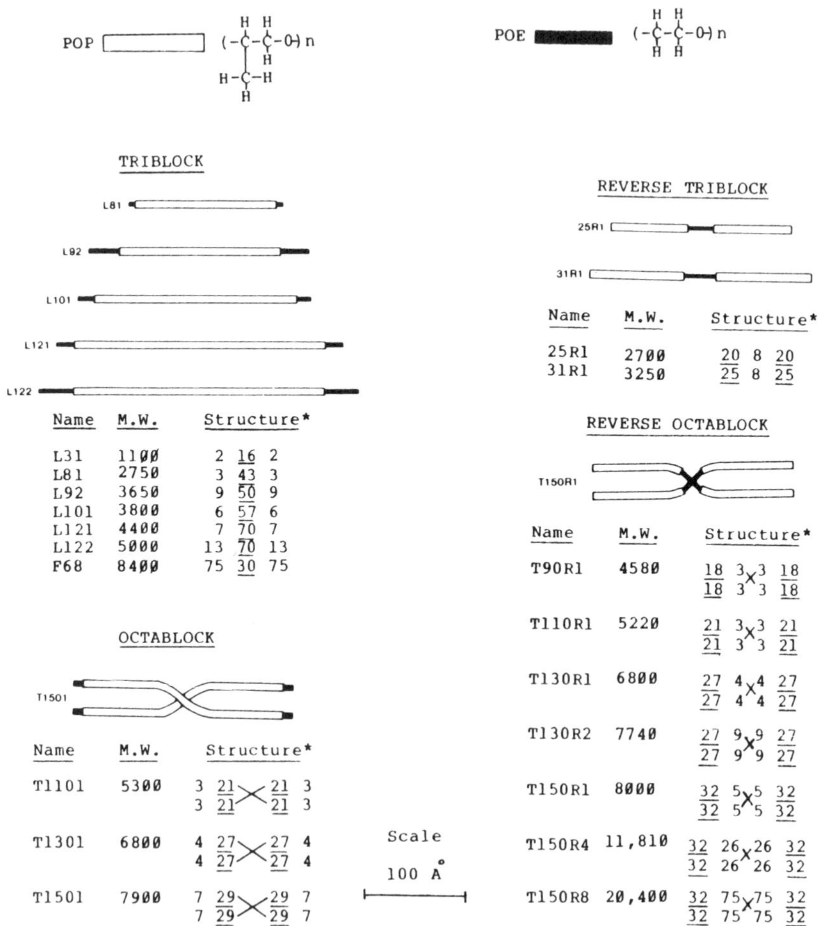

Figure 1, Structure of Block Copolymers. The copolymers were obtained from BASF Wyandotte, Wyandotte, Michigan, who sell them under the trade names of Pluronic and Tetronic polyols. They are composed of blocks of hydrophilic polyoxyethylene (POE) attached to blocks of hydrophobic polyoxypropylene (POP). The diagrams are drawn to scale for both length and thickness. *Numbers represent the units of oxyethylene and oxypropylene (underlined) in each block.

Emulsions prepared identically except that BSA was dissolved in the PBS rather than being mixed with the hydrocarbon and surfactant were ineffective. Our early experiments included immunizations with chemically modified proteins, especially lipid-conjugated BSA, which selectively stimulates DTH, and a variety of hydrocarbon vehicles in addition to the copolymers. Each component proved to have a role in determining both the intensity and class of immune response.

The copolymers and other surfactants with adjuvant activity were found to have hydrophile-lipophile balance (HLB) values less than 2 and, thus, would be classified as spreading agents. Spreading agents are insoluble in water and do not emulsify or solubilize lipids or membranes. Instead, they adhere to lipids and influence the interaction of soluble macromolecules with them. We demonstrated a correlation between the ability of copolymers to promote retention of soluble macromolecules on the surface of oil drops and their activity as adjuvants. The local concentration of antigen fixed to a surface is far higher than can be achieved by comparable amounts of material free in solution. It appeared that the copolymers which were adjuvants produced a concentrated surface matrix presentation of antigen to cells of the immune system. HLB determinations permitted the identification of surfactants which are large and hydrophobic enough to remain attached to oil drops and promote retention of proteins. We proposed that these were the minimal properties of a compound which enabled it to have this type of adjuvant activity.

The situation quickly became more complex. Continuing experiments demonstrated a greater variety and intensity of immune and inflammatory responses than anticipated. Consequently, we undertook studies using all available copolymers with low HLB values (Hunter and Bennett, 1984). Eleven of the 17 had nominally 10% POE by weight and, therefore, differed only in the size of blocks and their mode of linkage. Each was characterized by thin layer chromatography (TLC) and nuclear magnetic resonance (NMR) to determine its purity and composition. Mice were injected with 1.25 mg of each copolymer with 50.0 ug of BSA in an oil-in-water emulsion to evaluate its adjuvant and inflammatory properties.

Each of the copolymers produced a characteristic pattern of immune response and inflammation, Table 1. The most effective adjuvants were the largest polymers with 10% hydrophilic POE on the ends of the molecules (L121, L101 and T1501). The antibody titers rose progressively following a single injection to reach a peak at six weeks.

Block	Antibody Titer[a] (6 wk)	C3 Conversion[b]	Microscopic Structure[c]
Triblock			
L81	2178 ± 233	10%	oil
L92	1664 ± 201	<10%	oily ppt
L101	84,328 ± 8899	57%	fibers
L121	67,814 ± 5916	66%	fibers
L122	184 ± 45	35%	fibers and ppt
Reverse Triblock			
25R1	434 ± 107	10%	oil
31R1	264 ± 64	11%	oil
Octablock			
T1101	4799 ± 816	21%	oil and oily fibers
T1301	10,432 ± 1245	72%	oily fibers
T1501	136,245 ± 13,033	90%	fibers
Reverse Octablock			
T90R1	<100	<10%	oil
T110R1	472 ± 114	<10%	oil
T130R1	583 ± 145	<10%	oil
T130R2	518 ± 136	-	-
T150R1	268 ± 73	11%	oil
T150R4	1558 ± 245	-	-
T150R8	<100	-	-
None	<100	0%	-

Table 1, Responses to block copolymer surfactants in oil-in-water emulsions with BSA.

[a]Titer of antibody against BSA measured by an ELISA 6 wk after single injection of antigen and copolymer in an oil-in-water emulsion ± the standard error on groups of 10 animals.

[b]The percent reduction in native C3 following incubation of 25 mg/ml copolymer with 30% normal human serum for 2 hours at 37°C as measured by agarose gel electrophoresis and immunofixation.

[c]The structure assumed by the copolymer in aqueous suspension as seen with phase contrast microscopy. (ppt = fine precipitate)

Increasing the length of the POE chains caused the preparations to lose their activity as adjuvants. For example, the emulsion containing L121 stimulated a mean antibody titer to BSA greater than 67,000, while a similar emulsion containing L122 stimulated a mean titer of only 184. L121 and L122 differ only in the length of the POE chains. Shortening the length of the POP chains produced agents with lower adjuvant activity, but greater toxicity as measured by inflammation in the foot at the site of the injection. Placement of the POE at the center of the molecule flanked by chains of POP produced reverse copolymers which were weak adjuvants but stimulated granulomatous inflammation. Intensity of the inflammatory responses in the footpads did not correlate with antibody titers.

The data in Table 1 demonstrate two additional correlations of relevance to our studies. The ability of a block copolymer to function as an adjuvant for antibody formation correlated with its ability to activate complement and with the microscopic structure it formed in saline (Hunter and Bennett, 1986). Four of five block copolymers which activated complement significantly more than controls were powerful adjuvants. The fifth, L122, induced some of the manifestations of antibody formation, especially germinal center hyperplasia. Since all of the block copolymers used were poorly soluble or insoluble in water, they each formed some type of aggregate upon addition to Hank's Balanced Salt Solution (HBSS). Each of the polymers which activated complement formed fibrous structures. All of the remaining copolymers formed spherical masses with smooth surfaces which resembled oil drops.

The formation of spherical structures by some of the polymers demonstrated that the interfacial tension between them and water was sufficient to overwhelm ordering forces within the polymers. This implied that their surfaces were relatively hydrophobic. Similarly, the fineness of the fibrous structures formed by other copolymers indicated that they had hydrophilic surfaces which permitted expression of a tendency to form linear structures.

The copolymers were examined with scanning electron microscopy, Figure 2. The fibrous surfaces formed by the two best adjuvant copolymers, L121 and T1501, differed significantly from one another. L121 formed flat flakes

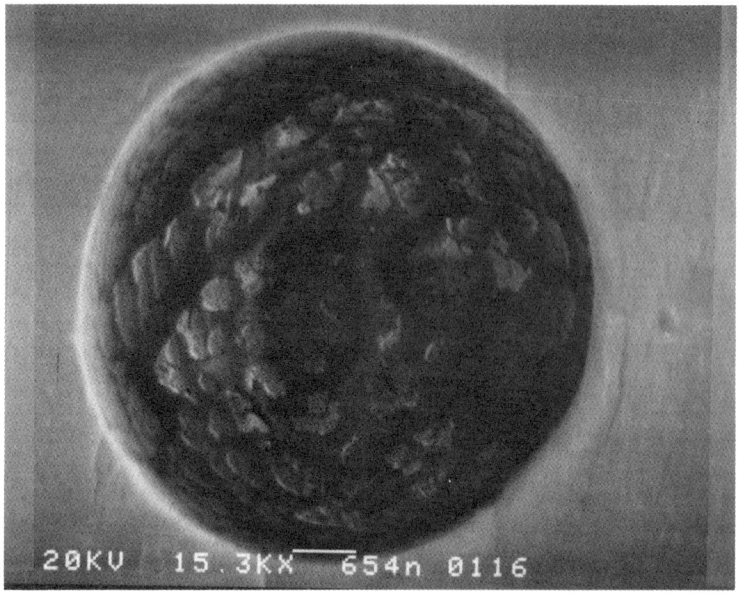

Figure 2, Scanning electron micrograph of an emulsion of L121 and T150R1 with oil and BSA. The two copolymers have separated from one another on the surface of the droplet. The light areas are a thick continuous mass of protein adherent to the surface in of copolymer L121. The dark areas are copolymer T150R1 with little adherent protein. (15300X).

which appeared to peel off the surface while T1501 formed distinct cylindrical micelles. Similarly, the structures formed by 31R1 and T150R1 both demonstrated relatively smooth surfaces, but that of T150R1 contained regular arrays of linear structures while 31R1 showed no irregularities at the highest magnification. These data demonstrate that the large octablock copolymers, T1501 and T150R1, form linear liquid crystalline surface structures. T1501, with a hydrophilic surface, forms linear micelles while T150R1 forms a surface composed of alternating arrays of hydrophilic and hydrophobic domains with a periodicity of approximately 40 nm.

Since these structures assumed by an insoluble copolymer in saline depended upon surface interactions, a series of experiments was designed to characterize the surfaces formed by selected copolymers and to investigate further their interaction with plasma proteins. We developed methods of spreading desired concentrations of copolymer evenly on three supports: 1) five micron beads useful for injection and studies of phagocytosis in vitro, 2) microtiter wells for studies of protein adhesion and macrophage spreading, and 3) flat plastic sheets for contact angle measurements, diffraction and other physiochemical studies. Use of these three supports facilitated quantitative measurements of multiple parameters which provided data for the construction of models of the surfaces formed by each block copolymer at various concentrations, Figure 3. The essential features are that the copolymers spontaneously form highly organized structures at an aqueous surface. We believe that the heterogeniety of

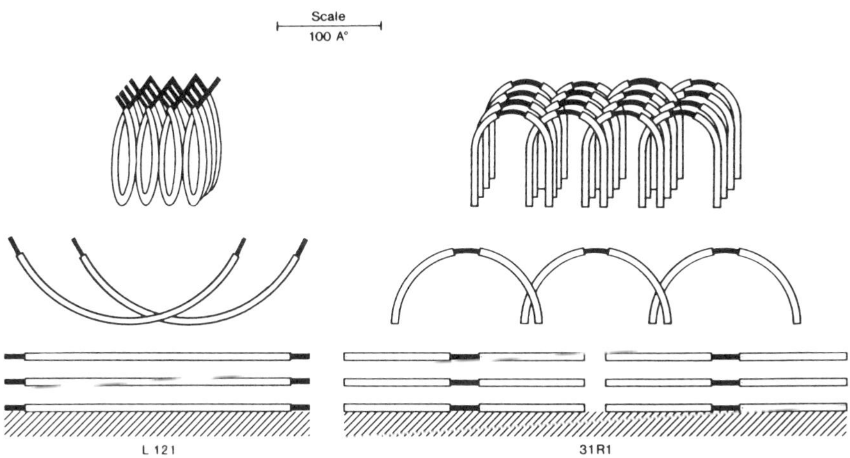

Figure 3, Model of surfaces of copolymers spread at varying concentrations. Triblock copolymer L121 and reverse triblock copolymer 31R1 are drawn to scale with the POE portions black and POP white. At low surface coverages, both copolymers lie flat producing largely hydrophobic surfaces (POP exposed). As the amount of copolymer on the surface increases, the hydrophobicity decreases demonstrating that the molecules become arranged with the POE oriented towards the surface. The surface of thick layers of L121 consists entirely of POE. It is hydrophilic and permits the underlying organizational tendencies of the copolymer to be expressed as fibers. The reverse copolymers are unable to form hydrophilic surfaces because their POE portions are sterically inhibited. This accounts for their formation of spherical oil-like drops in saline. Several lines of evidence suggest that both types of copolymers become arranged in a regular oriented fashion. We propose that this orientation contributes to their biologic activity.

these surface structures contributes to heterogeneity on biologic activity. In particular, the copolymers which are adjuvants in our system form a particular type of hydrophilic adhesive surface. If the blocks of POE are too long, the surface is not sufficiently adsorptive. If the blocks of POP are too short, they are unable to fold to produce a hydrophilic surface.

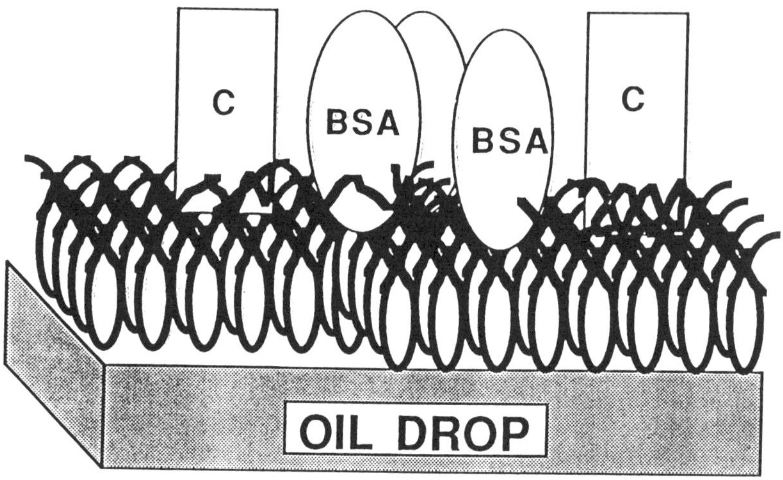

Figure 4, Model of an immunogenic particle. The copolymer L121 folds to form a hydrophilic adhesive surface. Antigen (BSA), complement (C) and mediators bound to the surface are presented to cells of the immune system in a particularly concentrated and effective form.

A model of an active adjuvant preparation of copolymer L121 is shown in Figure 4. The surface of an insoluble polymer which concentrates antigen and activates complement and other mediators would be expected to provide a powerful immunogenic stimulus. The hydrophobic surface of the oil drop is necessary to support the copolymer. The low free energy (hydrophilicity) of the surface allows the generation of a large surface area. The geometry of the molecules and their balance of hydrophilic and hydrophobic properties determine the adhesive properties. Our studies suggest that variation in adhesive properties of the copolymers affects the concentration and conformation of adherent proteins and that this in turn influences the type and intensity of biologic response (Hunter and Bennett, 1986).

The copolymers are effective adjuvants in some situations without oil (Snippe et al, 1981). With sheep red blood cells or other particulates, the copolymer could adsorb to the antigen and produce a similar surface configuration. However, we have recently found preliminary evidence that another mechanism might be involved. The copolymers are adhesive molecules which can promote adhesion of proteins to one another or to cells. The near quantitative retention of BSA in the feet of mice following injection in an emulsion containing L121 is probably due to a polymer mediated adhesion of antigen to cells and structures in the foot (Hunter and Bennett, 1984). Protein injected in a second dose without copolymer is removed from the foot rapidly while that from the first injection remains. These and other data suggested the hypothesis shown in Figure 5. Available evidence suggests that copolymer L121 is able to promote the adhesion of BSA to macrophages.

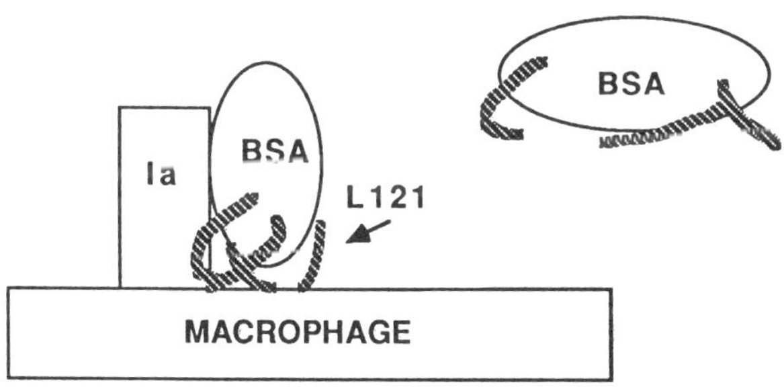

Figure 5, Hypothetical mechanism of antigen presentation mediated by copolymer L121. Being an adhesive molecule, the copolymer is able to mediate adhesion of protein antigens to cells. According to recent experimental evidence, this adhesion would be sufficient to allow effective presentation of antigen to T cells if the antigen were properly juxtaposed to Ia molecules on the surface of potential antigen presenting cell.

Several investigators have demonstrated that antigen adherent to mononuclear cells in the presence of Ia can be presented to T cells. Antigen processing may involve proteolytic cleveage of antigen to produce amphiphilic fragments which adhere to the cell surface. By promoting adhesion of antigen to cell surfaces, the copolymer adjuvants might obviate the need for processing of some antigens.

In Summary, the copolymers are adhesive molecules. Unlike ordinary detergents which disperse lipids and macromolecules, the copolymers which are adjuvants bind them together. Available evidence suggests that this is an essential component of their activity as immunologic adjuvants. As a group, the copolymers display a remarkable diversity of biologic activities. We believe that differences in the strength, solubility and geometry of adhesive domains formed by the copolymers is responsible for most of the heterogeneity of their biologic activities.

REFERENCES

Hunter RL, Strickland F, Kezdy F (1981). Studies on the adjuvant activity of nonionic block polymer surfactants. I. The role of hydrophile-lipophile balance. J Immunol 65:390.

Snippe H, DeReuver MJ, Strickland F, Willers JMN, Hunter RL (1981). Adjuvant effect of nonionic block polymer surfactants in humoral and cellular immunity. Int Arch Allergy Appl Immunol 127:1244.

Hunter RL, Bennett B (1984). The adjuvant activity of nonionic block polymer surfactants II. Antibody formation and inflammation related to the structure of triblock and octablock copolymers. J Immunol 133:1367.

Hunter RL, Bennett B (1986). Structural basis of the activity of surface active adjuvants. In Nervig RM (ed): "Advances in Carriers and Adjuvants for Veterinary Biologics:" Iowa State University Press, p 61.

Hunter RL, Bennett B (1986). The adjuvant activity of nonionic block polymer surfactants III. Characterization of selected biologically active surfaces. Scand J. Immunol 23:287.

Immunopharmacology of Infectious Diseases: Vaccine Adjuvants and Modulators of Non-Specific Resistance, pages 191–201

THE DEVELOPMENT OF AN ADJUVANT FORMULATION THAT ELICITS CELL-MEDIATED AND HUMORAL IMMUNE RESPONSES TO VIRUS SUBUNIT AND OTHER ANTIGENS

Anthony C. Allison and Noelene E. Byars

Institute of Biological Sciences, Syntex Research, 3401 Hillview Avenue, Palo Alto, CA 94304

INTRODUCTION

An immunological adjuvant can be defined as any agent that acts nonspecifically to increase a specific immune response or responses to an antigen. Adjuvants such as aluminium hydroxide and aluminium phosphate have long been used to increase antibody formation against bacterial toxoids in humans, and adjuvants such as saponin are often administered to increase antibody formation against killed virus antigens in domestic animals. Immunization with living viruses presents hazards such as the potential initiation of severe, persistent or transmissible virus infections or malignancy, so that vaccines containing inactivated viruses or virus antigens are now preferred. The production of virus surface subunit antigens by recombinant DNA technology and of synthetic peptide antigens opens a new chapter in the history of immunization. As a rule such antigens elicit protective immune responses only when administered with an adjuvant. Hence the promise of antigens produced by the new technologies will only be realized with the development of an effective adjuvant, able to elicit cell-mediated and humoral immune responses in humans and domestic and farm animals without unacceptable side effects.

For some practical purposes, inducing antibody formation is sufficient. Circulating antibodies, mainly of IgG isotypes interacting with complement and antibody-dependent effector cells, provide effective immunity against bacteria and certain groups of viruses, such as enteroviruses, adenoviruses and arthropod-borne viruses. In contrast, protective immunity against some other viruses, such as herpesviruses, bacteria (Mycobacterium, Listeria, Brucella), protozoa (Plasmodium, Babesia, Theileria, Anaplasma) and several fungi requires cell-mediated immunity.

Freund's adjuvant cannot be used in humans and domestic animals because it produces granulomas at the site of injection, fever and other toxic effects, as well as tuberculin hypersensitivity; moreover, mineral oil is potentially oncogenic. A major practical goal of the research program on adjuvants in our laboratory is to develop an adjuvant formulation that has the desirable effects of Freund's complete adjuvant, namely eliciting potent cell-mediated and humoral immune responses to a wide range of antigens in humans and domestic and farm animals, but lacking the undesirable side effects of Freund's complete adjuvant. The development has been carried out systematically, first defining a potent and non-toxic substitute for mycobacteria and then seeking an efficacious and bland substitute for mineral oil. We have succeeded in laboratory and domestic animals; experimental findings in subhuman primates are encouraging, and toxicology studies suggest that the formulation should also be acceptable for use in humans.

MODE OF ACTION OF ADJUVANTS AND VEHICLES

For a long time studies of adjuvant effects were entirely empirical, and nothing was known of their mode of action. The senior author and his colleagues showed by cell transfer experiments that the primary target cell involved in adjuvant effects is the macrophage (Unanue et al., 1969; Spitznagel and Allison, 1970), and that T-lymphocytes are required for adjuvant effects on antibody formation (Allison and Davies, 1971). These observations suggested that adjuvants induce the production by macrophages or other accessory cells of mediators stimulating the proliferation of helper T-lymphocytes. One obvious candidate for this role is interleukin-1. LPS is a well-known adjuvant and inducer of IL-1 production (Gery et al., 1984), and MDP and silica particles have both activities (Spitznagel and Allison, 1970; Oppenheim et al., 1980; Gery et al., 1984). The term "macrophage" should now be extended to include other antigen-presenting cells, including those of the Langerhans cell lineage that, as interdigitating cells in the T-dependent areas of lymphoid tissues, present antigens to T-lymphocytes, and follicular dendritic cells that present antigens to B-lymphocytes. Adjuvants probably stimulate also the production not only of IL-1 but also of IL-2 and B-cell growth factors by accessory cells. A principal mode of action of adjuvants can thus be defined as inducing the production of lymphocyte growth factors.

In contrast, the role of vehicles seems to be the formation of two-phase systems in which antigens are arranged as a two-dimensional matrix at the interphase. From this large surface area the antigen can be efficiently transferred to the surface of macrophages, Langerhans cells and splenic dendritic cells. If vehicles activate complement, localization of associated antigens on the surface of follicular dendritic cells and the generation of B-lymphocyte memory are increased, as shown for complement activating immune complexes (Klaus et al., 1983). Liposomes and polymer systems that activate complement (e.g. the pluronic polymer formulation discussed below) are found to be better vehicles than those that do not.

TESTS OF EFFICACY

Straightforward assays can be used to ascertain whether an adjuvant increases humoral responses to an antigen. However, as a rule it is necessary not only to maintain a detectable level of antibodies in recipients but also to generate a population of memory B-lymphocytes that will respond to antigenic challenge with a rapid and substantial production of protective antibodies. Furthermore, the isotype of antibodies is often important, both in terms of protection and sensitization. The possible use of adjuvants to elicit selectively the production of antibodies of particular isotypes is discussed below.

Tests for cell-mediated immunity are also established for most species, so that whether adjuvants can elicit this type of immunity can be ascertained. The simplest test is for delayed hypersensitivity, but measuring responses of lymphocytes to antigenic stimulation (proliferation and production of mediators such as interleukin-2 and interferon-γ) is desirable. When syngeneic target cells infected with viruses or protozoa can be used, tests for cytotoxicity provide information that is likely to be correlated with protection. Nevertheless the ultimate test of an adjuvant's efficacy is capacity to elicit immune responses that protect hosts from infections or toxins for a sufficiently long interval to be useful in practice.

UNDESIRABLE EFFECTS OF ADJUVANTS

Potential undesirable effects of adjuvants and adjuvant formulations must be understood, so that only adjuvants which are both efficacious and lacking in side effects are developed (Allison et al., 1986). A list of undesirable side effects of adjuvants includes:

1. Inflammatory, granulomatous, necrotizing or other unacceptable reactions at injection sites.
2. Pyrogenicity.
3. Induction of arthritis.
4. Increased vascular permeability and inflammatory reactions in the eye.
5. Production of vasculitis.
6. Induction of autoimmune responses.

Laboratory animals vary in their sensitivity to side effects. For example, increased vascular permeability and inflammatory reactions in the eye are most easily observed in rabbits and monkeys. Adjuvant arthritis can be elicited in rats but not other species, whereas another type of arthritis can be elicited in the guinea pig by sensitization with bacteria or MDP and challenge with LPS. Some MDPs produce in guinea pigs a distress syndrome with ruffled fur, abnormal behavior and growth impairment. This can be reproduced by injections of culture media from macrophages exposed to toxic, but not non-toxic MDPs, whereas both contain lymphocyte-activating factor activity (Byars, 1984).

Studies in the laboratory of E. Lederer established that N-acetylmuramyl-L-alanyl-D-isoglutamine (MDP) is the minimal structural component of the mycobacterial cell wall able to function as an adjuvant which, when administered with antigens in Freund's incomplete adjuvant, can elicit cell-mediated and humoral immunity (Ellouz et al., 1974). We have recently reviewed the toxic effects of MDP and several analogs (Allison et al., 1986), and Wachsmuth (1986) has discussed the pathogenesis of vasculitis induced by these compounds. Bacterial products such as MDP and lipopolysaccharide (LPS) can induce in susceptible laboratory animals anterior uveitis and arthritis. These are components of Reiter's syndrome, which occurs in genetically predisposed persons (especially of the HLA-B27 haptotype) following infection with gram-negative bacteria (Geczy et al., 1983). Small amounts of bacterial products, or certain drugs such as levamisole, are sufficient to trigger the Reiter's syndrome in genetically predisposed persons.

Hence we have focused attention on achieving separation in MDP analogs of adjuvant activity from side effects - pyrogenicity, capacity to induce uveitis and arthritis, and capacity to increase resistance to infections. Of more than 130 analogs tested, N-acetylmuramyl-L-threonyl-D-isoglutamine [Thr^1]MDP proved to be an excellent adjuvant with the maximum separation so far reported of adjuvant activity from capacity to induce undesirable effects. [Thr^1]MDP was therefore selected as the counterpart of mycobacterial cell walls in an adjuvant formulation.

PLURONIC BLOCK POLYMERS

The next goal of our research program on adjuvants was to obtain an acceptable substitute for the mineral oil component of Freund's complete adjuvant. The most satisfactory of many vehicles tested proved to be pluronic block copolymers, which had been used with mineral oil emulsions by Hunter and colleagues (1981) to increase antibody formation against sheep erythrocytes and dinitrophenylated bovine serum albumin. These non-ionic detergents are single, unbranched chains consisting of a central polymer of polyoxypropylene (POP), which is hydrophobic, flanked by polymers of polyoxyethylene (POE) which is hydrophilic. By varying the overall size of the molecules and the ratios of POE to POP, materials with very different properties can be obtained (Schmolka, 1977). We have found that some of these induce muscle damage at sites of injection whereas others do not. Indeed, some pluronic polyols are among the least toxic surface-active agents, and they are widely used in foods, as well as formulations for drugs and cosmetics (Schmolka, 1977).

Wishing to avoid mineral oil and to obtain a relatively stable pluronic combination for an adjuvant formulation, we have used pluronic L121 (molecular weight 4,400, 10% POE) with squalane and Tween 80. This produces a two-phase system with antigens concentrated at the interphase. The L121 activates complement by the alternative pathway, and C3b on the surface may facilitate the localization of antigen-bearing particles on the surface of antigen-presenting cells such as Langerhans cells as described above. Adding [Thr^1]MDP to the pluronic formulation increases cell-mediated immune responses to antigens, and we designate this combination "Syntex adjuvant formulation-1" or SAF-1.

ACTIVITIES OF SAF-1

Various antigens have been administered to several species of animals in our laboratory and other laboratories. Our standard laboratory animal is the guinea pig. An example of the efficacy of SAF-1 is shown in fig. 1. SAF-1 markedly increases antibody formation against influenza B virus, allowing the use of low antigen doses. We hope that SAF-1 will elicit protective immunity against influenza virus in young children and the elderly in which standard vaccination has not been satisfactory.

The adjuvant formulation is also active in the mouse, although on a mg/kg body weight basis a higher dose of [Thr^1]MDP is required than in the guinea pig. Following administration of antigens with SAF-1 in the mouse most of the antibody formed is of the IgG2a

Figure 1. Primary antibody responses to influenza B virus in guinea pigs using different doses of antigen in saline and in SAF-1.

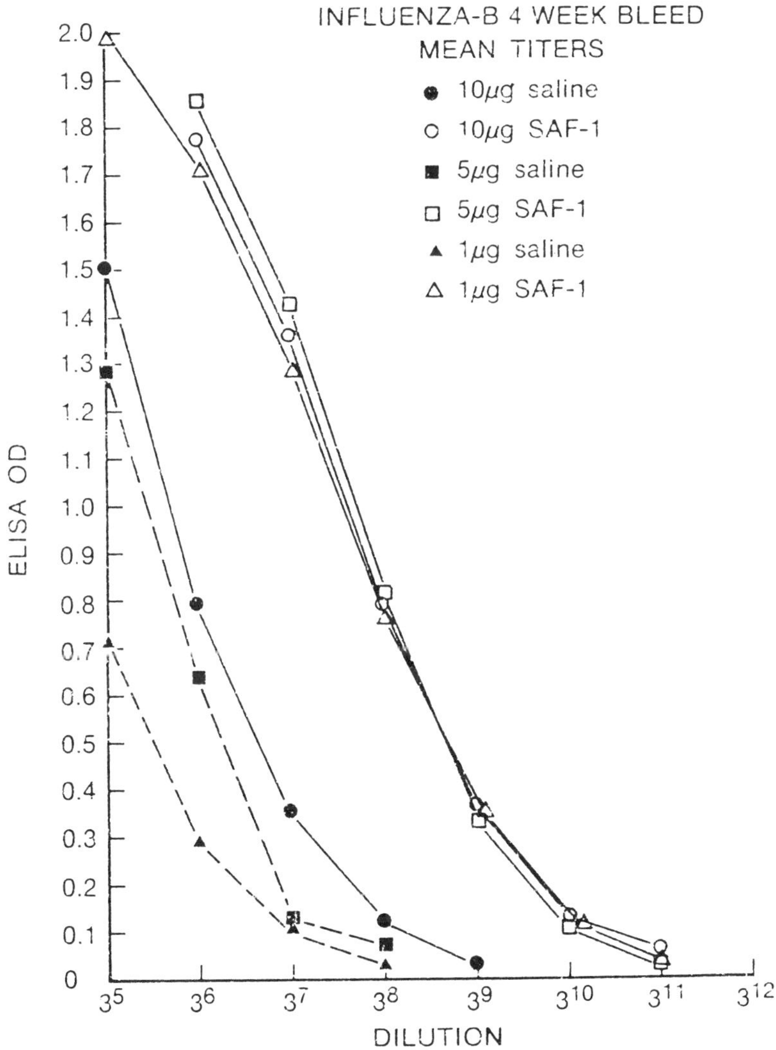

isotype, which activates complement and interacts with antibody-dependent effector cells. Freund's complete adjuvant gives a lower proportion of IgG2a and monophosphoryl lipid A / trehalose dimycolate (used as prescribed by Ribi Immunochemicals Inc.) elicits predominantly IgG1 antibodies. An example of the use of SAF-1 in the mouse is to elicit anti-idiotypic antibodies and specific cytotoxic cells against B-lymphomas (in the laboratory of Ronald Levy, Stanford University). These protect the mice against lymphoma cells bearing the same idiotype. Antigens injected into mice with SAF-1 do not elicit reaginic antibodies, whereas administration with alum, saponin or Bordetella pertussis does. Except in the case of some helminths, elicitation of IgE antibodies would be undesirable in a vaccine.

Our first practical application was immunizing cats against feline leukemia virus using inactivated virus antigen in SAF-1 (Braemer et al., 1984). Excellent protection against viremia following challenge was obtained, and non-viremic cats do not develop lymphosarcomas and other late manifestations of the disease. The adjuvant was the key to success, since the same antigens administered with alum and immune-stimulating complexes based on Quil A provided much less protection. This was the first really effective vaccination against a retrovirus, and raises the exciting possibility of immunization against other retroviruses, including the human immunodeficiency virus (HIV) which can lead to AIDS.

In collaboration with outside investigators, two rhesus monkey models have been studied. One is termed simian AIDS or SAIDS, a type D retrovirus producing a fatal degenerative disease. Monkeys immunized with inactivated SAIDS virus in SAF-1 were protected against viremia following virus challenge and against manifestations of the disease (Marx et al., 1986). The second is termed STLVIII, a lentivirus which depletes the T4 subset of lymphocytes, like HIV. The disease in monkeys has a rapidly fatal outcome. Inactivated virus injected with SAF-1 was found to elicit high titers of antibodies against surface and core antigens of the virus (Letvin et al., 1986). The animals have been challenged with virus and so far remain healthy. Monkeys immunized with the same antigen in Quil A developed lower titers of antibodies against viral antigens and allergic reactions when challenged, suggesting the elicitation of reaginic antibodies.

Many studies with SAF-1 are ongoing in our laboratory and others. A few results can be mentioned to illustrate the possibilities of the system. The cloned surface and core antigens of hepatitis B virus in SAF-1 have elicited high titers of antibodies in experimental animals (K. Murray, University of Edinburgh). The circumsporozoite antigen of the malaria parasite elicits in mice higher titers of antibodies in SAF-1 than any other adjuvant formulation so far used (V. Nussenzweig, New York University). These examples should suffice to indicate the scope of possible applications of SAF-1.

In summary, we have developed an adjuvant formulation with the desired properties, and believe that it will be useful in the coming decades for a new generation of vaccines based on recombinant DNA technology.

ACKNOWLEDGMENTS

We are glad to acknowledge the following collaborators: J. Moffatt, G. Jones, J. Nestor and M. Venuti in the synthesis of MDP analogs; E. Eugui and J. Kenny for information on mediator production and isotypes of antibodies formed; R. Waters and T. Terrell in studies of the toxic effects of adjuvants; and A. Braemer, P. Marx, N. Letvin, K. Murray, V. Nussenzweig, A. Kendal and R. Levy in studies of SAF-1 with several antigens.

REFERENCES

Allison AC, Byars NE, Waters RV (1986) Immunologic adjuvants: efficacy and safety considerations. In Nervig RM et al., ed. "Advances in Carriers and Adjuvants for Veterinary Biologics". Ames, Iowa: The Iowa State University Press, p. 91.

Allison AC, Davies AJS (1971) Requirement of thymus-dependent lymphocytes for potentiation by adjuvants of antibody formation. Nature, Lond. 233:330.

Braemer AC, Peterson M, Renneke G, Bass E, Allison A, Byars N, Fraser D (1984) Effect of inactivated FELV vaccines in the development of persistent viremia. Presentation at 65th Conference of Research Workers in Animal Disease, Chicago.

Byars NE (1984) Two adjuvant active muramyl dipeptide analogs induce differential production of lymphocyte-activating factor and a factor causing distress in guinea pig. Infect. Immunity 44:344.

Ellouz F, Adam A, Ciorbaru R, Lederer E (1974) Minimal structural requirements for adjuvant activity of bacterial peptidoglycan derivatives. Biochem. Biophys. Res. Comm. 59:1317.

Geczy AF, Alexander K, Bashir HV, Edmonds JP, Upfold L, Sullivan J (1983) HLA-B27, Klebsiella and ankylosing spondylitis: biological and chemical studies. Immunol. Revs. 70:23.

Gery I, Lopez-Zuniga JL (1984) Interleukin 1: uniqueness of its production and spectrum of activities. Lymphokines 9:109.

Hunter R, Strickland F, Kedzy F (1981) The adjuvant activity of nonionic black polymer surfactants. I. The role of hydrophile-lipophile balance. J. Immunol. 127:1244.

Klaus GG, Humphrey JH, Kunkl A, Dongworth DW (1983) The follicular dendritic cell: its role in antigen presentation and in the generation of immunological memory. Immunol. Revs. 53:3.

Letvin NL, Daniel NW, Kitoyaki M, Kannagi M, Seghal PK, Arthur LO, Allison AC, Hunt RD, Desrodiers RC (1986) AIDS-like model in macaque monkeys induced by STLV-III: model for AIDS vaccine development. In Chanock R, ed. "Vaccines/AIDS". Cold Spring Harbor Press.

Marx PA, Pedersen NC, Lerche NW, Osborn KG, Lowenstine LJ, Lackner AA, Maul DB, Kwang H-S, Kluge JD, Zaiss CP, Sharpe V, Spinner AP, Allison AC, Gardner MB (1986) Prevention of simian acquired immunodeficiency syndrome with formalin-inactivated type D retrovirus vaccine. J. Virol. (in press).

Oppenheim JJ, Togawa A, Chedid L, Mizel S (1980) Components of mycobacteria and muramyl dipeptide with adjuvant activity induce lymphocyte-activating factor. Cell Immunol. 50:71.

Schmolka IR (1977) A review of block polymer surfactants. J. Am. Oil. Chemists Soc. 54:110.

Spitznagal J, Allison AC (1970) Mode of action of adjuvants retinol and other lysosome-labilising agents as adjuvants. J. Immunol. 104:119.

Unanue ER, Askonas BA, Allison AC (1969) A role of macrophages in the stimulation of immune responses by adjuvants. J. Immunol. 103:71.

Wachsmuth ED (1986) MDP and derivatives II. In Chedid L et al., ed. "Advances in Immunopharmacology" Oxford: Pergamon Press 3:483.

Immunopharmacology of Infectious Diseases: Vaccine Adjuvants and Modulators of Non-Specific Resistance, pages 203–212

VACCINATION BY SYNTHETIC PEPTIDE - MDP CONSTRUCTS

F. Audibert

Department of Pharmacology and Therapeutics,
University of South Florida, College of Medicine,
Tampa, Florida 33612

Muramyldipeptide or MDP(Nac Mur-L-Ala-D-isogln) has been shown to substitute for mycobacteria in Freund's complete adjuvant (Ellouz et al., 1974; Kotani et al., 1975). MDP is adjuvant active when administered in saline and enhances the non-specific immunity against infections. Hundreds of analogs have been now synthesized, they have allowed to demonstrate various immunopharmacological properties of this family of compounds. They have also afforded means to study the relationships between their structure and their biological activities and to segregate some of these activities in view of designing immunomodulatory molecules devoid of side-effects (Chedid et al., 1978; Lefrancier and Lederer, 1981). Most aspects of MDP properties are described by other authors in this same volume. In this paper we will study how the coupling of MDP or of derivatives can influence their immunoadjuvant activity. It will be seen that this coupling enhance their overall biological activity but allows also to modulate it. For example, conjugation of appropriate MDP analogs can influence the isotypic pattern of the antibodies synthetized or modify the immunodominance relationships between the different epitopes present on a conjugate. These various aspects will be discussed mostly in the field of synthetic vaccines and it will be shown that the coupling of MDP could provide efficient synthetic vaccines even in absence of carriers.

Enhancement of MDP activity by covalent linkage to antigens. Several studies using natural macromolecular antigens had indicated that the covalent linkage of MDP could enhance its adjuvanticity. This was observed with laboratory antigens such as bovine serum albumin (Reichert et al., 1980) but also with conventional vaccines such as toxoids (Chedid and Audibert, 1981). The covalent linkage of MDPs to a synthetic copolymer multi-poly (DL-Ala)--poly (L-Lys), hereafter referred as A--L, lead also to an increase in their immunostimulant properties. Two molecules were studied, MDP and its inactive stereoisomer, MDP(DD) (Nac Mur-D-Ala-D-isogln). It was observed that the coupling of MDP to A--L enhanced one hundred fold its capacity to increase nonspecific immunity but more interestingly the coupling of MDP (DD) made it immunostimulant active (Chedid et al., 1979). MDP was also covalently linked to the same A--L bearing synthetic peptidic determinants. In a first study the synthetic poly (L-Tyr, L-Glu)-poly (DL-Ala)--poly (L-Lys) called (T,G) A--L was used. It could be observed that when a MDP (T,G) A--L conjugate was administered to mice in saline, antibodies were elicited; in contrast (T,G) A--L required to be administered in FCA to be immunogenic even in high-responder mice (Mozes et al., 1980). The same result was obtained with a synthetic peptide called P_2 which copies a sequence of the coat protein of the coliphage M_s2. It was observed that a MDP-P_2 - A--L construct was also active in saline and elicited neutralizing anti MS_2 phage antibodies (Arnon et al., 1980). The first example of a totally synthetic molecule capable of eliciting antibodies which protect against a toxin lethal for human was offered by the diphtheria toxin model (Audibert et al., 1981, 1982). In this case it could be even demonstrated that the direct coupling of MPD-Lys to the synthetic peptide without any carrier lead to a copolymer active in saline (Audibert, et al., 1982).

In most cases synthetic peptides representing copies of natural protective antigenic determinants are administered coupled to carriers to obtain high level of immune responses. The covalent linkage of MDP to these peptide carriers conjugates has been shown to provide highly immunogenic constructs. For example, a synthetic peptide copying a protective epitope of the circumsporozoite protein of _Plasmodium knowlesi_ (Gyzin et al., 1984) has been conjugated to tetanus toxoid. This conjugate administered with 100 ug of MDP-Lys evoked the same level of antibodies as a triplicate containing only 1 ug of MDP (Clough et al., 1985a, b). The sera obtained after immunization of mice or guinea-pigs with these conjugates were shown to give highly positive results when tested in the circumsporozoite precipitation assay which is considered as giving a good estimate of the degree of protection (Cochrane et al., 1980). Similar observations have been made using another analog of MDP, amino-caproic-murabutide. This molecule is a derivative of murabutide (Nac-Mur-L-Ala-D-Gln alpha-n-butyl ester) which is currently evaluated in clinical trials (Chedid et al., 1982; Telzak et al., 1986). The coupling of amino caproic murabutide to the conjugate not only enhanced its immunogenicity but induced also modifications of the immunogenic structure of the carrier (Clough et al., 1985b), this observation will be discussed below.

The influence of the linkage of MDP to an antigen was also studied with smaller molecules which are not immunogenic by themselves. The beta chain of HCG (human choriogonadotropin) is considered as a potential contraceptive vaccine (Stevens, 1980; Nash et al., 1982). This natural oligomer of 149 amino acids is not immunogenic and represents an autoantigen. It is generally administered to experimental animals coupled to carriers. MDP-Lys has been directly conjugated to beta-HCG, the copolymer obtained was administered to mice and induced high levels of antibodies. These antibodies were shown to be endowed with biological activity (Schutze et al., unpublished data) when tested in the rat uterine weight assay (Tsong et al., 1985). Similar results have been obtained using amino-caproic murabutide.

It has been mentioned above that a diphtheric peptide of 16 amino acids copolymerized through glutaraldehyde with MDP-Lys had become immunogenic. The same methodology has been successfully applied to other synthetic peptides such as a foot and mouth disease virus peptide (Chedid et al., 1986) or to the decapeptide hormone LH-RH (luteinizing hormone - releasing hormone) (Carelli et al., 1982). LH-RH conjugated to carriers and administered with FCA induced anti-LH-RH antibodies and signs of castration were observed (Fraser, 1980). A similar immunological castration was obtained in male mice when synthetic LH-RH was conjugated directly to MDP-Lys (Carelli et al., 1982).

Influence of the coupling of MDP on its capacity of inducing IL-1. The coupling of MDP to A--L or to other high molecular weight molecules enhanced not only its stimulating activity but also its capacity for inducing interleukin-1 (IL-1) synthesis since it was shown to become highly pyrogenic (Chedid et al., 1979; Carelli et al., 1985). When MDP-Lys was conjugated to LH-RH the resulting molecule was not pyrogenic, showing that under these conditions the pyrogenicity of MDP-Lys had even been decreased (Carelli et al., 1985). Nevertheless, when rabbit macrophages or human monocytes were incubated with LH-RH-Lys-MDP the secretion of endogenous pyrogen could be evidenced as well as the synthesis of LAF (lymphocyte activating factor) (Riveau, 1985). This production of LAF under the influence of a nonpyrogenic MDP-conjugate is interesting since it has been postulated that IL-1 plays a role in the mechanisms of adjuvant activity (Staruch and Wood, 1983).

Influence of the coupling of MDP on the immunogenic structure of a peptide-carrier conjugate. It has been shown above that the coupling of MDP can permit obtaining an immune response after administration in saline of triplicate conjugates containing the haptenic groups and the adjuvant moiety covalently linked to the same back bone (Arnon et al., 1980; Clough et al., 1985, 1985b; Mozes et al., 1980). Further studies have been performed to compare the specificity of the antibodies raised after immunization by such conjugates with built-in adjuvanticity and the specificity of antibodies raised by the corresponding hapten-carrier conjugate mixed with the synthetic adjuvant. Mice received in Freund's Incomplete Adjuvant (FIA) either (T,G) A--L mixed with MDP or MDP(T,G) A--L. The specificity of antibodies was studied by Elisa titration and appropriate inhibition experiments. It was observed that most antibodies were directed against (T,G) after immunization by (T,G) A--L mixed with MDP; on the contrary antibodies bound specifically A--L following immunization by the triplicate. Complementary experiments showed that the T,G motive was as available at the surface of MDP(T,G) A--L as in the (T,G) A--L conjugate (Abehsira-Amar et al., unpublished). Such data demonstrate that the coupling of MDP can deeply modify the immunodominance relationships between the different antigenic determinants present in an immunizing preparation. They indicate that when a chemical modification, even minor, has been introduced in a molecule it is not sufficient to measure the overall antibody response but that an analysis of the specificities is necessary. This is particularly important in the field of synthetic vaccines since the coupling of the adjuvant could impair the expression of protective epitopes.

Nevertheless, the possibility of modulating the structure of the epitopes can be favorable. Carriers are most generally used to enhance the immunogenicity of small peptides but their use can present certain limitations (Audibert and Chedid, 1984). One of them being the risk of hypersensitization following repeated injections of a highly immunogenic molecule. From this viewpoint the use of tetanus toxoid as the only carrier for synthetic vaccines is not devoid of hazards, although it has been used for decades in clinics. It has been reported above that two different triplicates containing _Pl. knowlesi_ peptide linked to tetanus toxoid and MDP-Lys or murabutide can induce high levels of antisporozoites antibodies. In both cases when the antibody response to the carrier has been measured and when MDP-Lys was the adjuvant, very high titers of anti-tetanus toxoid were obtained as compared with controls receiving the peptide tetanus toxoid conjugate alone. In contrast, the murabutide-containing conjugate induced very low levels of anti-tetanus toxoid antibodies (Clough et al., 1985b), indicating that this chemical modification could be useful not only to enhance the response to the synthetic peptide but also to overcome the risk of hypersentization to the carrier.

Influence of the coupling of MDP on the isotypic pattern of specific antibodies. When free MDP has been administered to mice mixed with an antigen the production of IgG_1 antibodies has been most generally reported (Leclerc et al., 1978; Heymer et al., 1978; Lowy et al., 1980). The coupling of certain MDP analogs to an antigen has allowed modulation of the synthesis of IgE antibodies. Mice pretreated by DNP, mycoloyl-muramyl peptides and immunized by DNP-ovalbumin did not develop an anti-DNP IgE response in contrast with their non-pretreated controls (Kishimoto et al., 1979), the anti-DNP IgG response being equivalent in both groups. Similarly, the coupling of MDP-Lys to ovalbumin abolished the IgE response and enhanced the synthesis of IgG_2a and IgG_2b antibodies with no change in IgG levels (Prouvost-Danon et al., 1984).

Enhancement of the adjuvant activity of conjugated MDP by using monoclonal anti-MDP antibodies. Preliminary experiments were performed with a conjugate containing MDP coupled to human albumin (HA). This conjugate was administered to mice in saline either alone or mixed with monoclonal anti-MDP (Bahr et al., 1983) and it could be observed that the use of anti-MDP antibodies could enhance significantly the immunogenicity of HA coupled to MDP (Bahr et al., 1985). Appropriate controls showed that MDP had to be conjugated to the antigen and that the use of an adjuvant-active hapten is necessary. Similar experiments were performed using synthetic antigens such as a streptococcal peptide (Bahr et al., 1985) or a *Plasmodium falciparum* peptide. In the latter case the sixteen amino-acid peptide is (Asn-Ala-Pro-Asn) 4 and copies the major repetitive epitope of the circumsporozoite protein of *P. falciparum*. It was immunogenic and induced high levels of biologically active antibodies when administered coupled to carriers with adjuvants including murabutide (Mazier et al., 1986). MDP-Lys has been conjugated to this peptide and the analytically pure molecule obtained of less than 2500 dalton administered to mice either alone or with monoclonal anti-MDP antibodies. In the first group no anti-peptide antibodies could be detected, in contrast in the second group antibodies were synthetized (unpublished results).

Comparison between the antigenicity and the immunogenicity of MDP after coupling. It was questionable if the coupling of MDPs could affect their antigenic characters. Monoclonal anti-MDP antibodies showed that the MDP as well as the murabutide specific motives were available on their respective conjugates. Surprisingly, even when they were coupled to highly immunogenic carriers they did not induce any antibody response (unpublished results). Thus, even after coupling and although it was fully antigenic MDP was not immunogenic. It should be noted here that in order to obtain polyclonal (Reichert et al., 1980) or monoclonal anti-MDP antibodies (Bahr et al., 1983) the immunizing preparation had to be administered under very intensive conditions.

CONCLUSION

Many results presented here indicate that the covalent linkage of MDP or of its analogs to an immunogenic preparation can enhance its adjuvant activity. Moreover, in several cases not only the quantitative aspect of the immune response but also its characteristics could be modified. For example, it is possible to favor the antibody response to certain epitopes while diminishing the response to others and the synthesis of antibodies of certain isotypes can be favored or diminished. A note of caution has to be added here since the coupling of MDP can enhance some side effects such as pyrogenicity or affect unpredictably the immunogenic structure of a vaccine. Nevertheless, it can be guessed that a better understanding of the relationship between the structure of the conjugates and their biological properties as well as improvement in the control of the coupling reactions will allow using the benefits of the coupling under conditions providing a good therapeutic index.

REFERENCES

Arnon R, Sela M, Parant M, Chedid L (1980). Antiviral response elicited by a completely synthetic antigen with built-in adjuvanticity. 77:6769.

Audibert F, Chedid L (1984). Of antigens adjuvants and carriers in synthetic vaccines. In Chanock RM, Lerner RA (eds): "Modern Approaches to Vaccines, Molecular and Chemical Basis of Virus Virulence and Immunogenicity," Cold Spring Harbor Laboratory, p 397.

Audibert F, Jolivet M, Chedid L, Alouf JE, Boquet P, Rivaille P, Siffert O (1981). Active antitoxic immunization by a diphtheria toxin synthetic oligopeptide. Nature 289:593.

Audibert F, Jolivet M, Chedid L, Arnon R, Sela M (1982). Successful immunization with a totally synthetic diphtheria vaccine. Proc Natl Acad Sci USA 79:5042.

Bahr GM, Eshhar Z, Ben-Yitzhak R, Modabber FZ, Arnon R, Sela M, Chedid L (1983). Monoclonal antibodies to the synthetic adjuvant muramyl dipeptide: Characterization of the specificity. Molec Immunol 20:745.

Bahr GM, Tello D, Chedid L (1985). Marked enhancement in vivo of adjuvant activity of muramyl dipeptide to protein antigens and to synthetic weak immunogens with monoclonal anti-muramyl dipeptide antibodies. Infect Immun 49:312.

Carelli C, Audibert F, Chedid L, Gaillard J (1982). Immunological castration of male mice by a totally synthetic vaccine (LH-RH conjugated to MDP) administered in saline. Proc Natl Acad Sci USA 79:5392.

Carelli C, Ralamboranto L, Audibert F, Gaillard J, Briquelet N, Dray F, Fafeur V, Haour F, Chedid L (1985). Immunological castration by a totally synthetic vaccine: Modification of biological properties of LH-RH after conjugation to adjuvant-active muramyl peptide. Int J Immunopharmac 7:215.

Chedid L, Audibert F (1981). Utilization of muramyl dipeptide derivative as adjuvants of synthetic vaccines. In Yamamura Y, Kotani S, Azuma I, Koda A, Shiba T (eds): "Immunodulation by Microbial Products and Related Synthetic Compounds," Amsterdam-Oxford-Princeton: Excerpta Media, p 241.

Chedid L, Audibert F, Johnson AG (1978). Biological activities of muramyl dipeptide, a synthetic glycopeptide analogous to bacterial immunoregulating agents. Progress in Allergy 25:63.

Chedid L, Carelli C, Audibert F (1986). Use of adjuvants, antigens and carriers in synthetic veterinary vaccines. In Navig M, Cough PM, Kacherle MM, Whestone CA (eds): "Advances in Carriers and Adjuvants for Veterinary Biologies," Ames: Iowa State University Press, p. 48.

Chedid LA, Parant MA, Audibert FM, Riveau GJ, Parant FJ, Lederer E, Choay JP, Lefrancier PL (1982). Biological activity of a new synthetic muramyl peptide adjuvant devoid of pyrogenicity. Infect Immun 35:417.

Chedid L, Parant M, Parant F, Audibert F, Lefrancier P, Choay J, Sela M (1979). Enhancement of certain biological activities of muramyl dipeptide derivatives after conjugation to a multi-poly(DL-alanine)--poly (L-lysine) carrier. Proc Natl Acad Sci USA 76:6557.

Clough ER, Audibert FM, Barnwell JW, Schlesinger DH, Arnon R, Chedid LA (1985). Biologically active antibodies elicited by a synthetic circumsporozoite peptide of Plasmodium knowlesi administered in saline with a muramyl dipeptide derivative. Infect Immun 48:839.

Clough ER, Jolivet ME, Audibert FM, Barnwell JW, Schlesinger DH, Chedid LA (1985). Production of anti-sporozoite antibodies in absence of response to carrier by coupling an MDP derivative to the malaria peptide, tetanus toxoid conjugate. Biochem Biophys Res Comm 131:70.

Cochrane AH, Nussenzweig RS, Nardin EH (1980). Immunization against sporozoites. In Kreier JP (ed): "Malaria in Man and Experimental Animals," New York: Academic Press p 163.

Ellouz F, Adam A, Ciorbaru R, Lederer E (1974). Minimal structural requirements for adjuvant activity of bacterial peptidoglycan derivatives. Biochem Biophy Res Comm 59:1317.

Fraser HM (1980). Inhibition of reproductive function by antibodies to luteinizing hormone releasing hormone. In Hearn JP (ed): "Immunological Aspects of Reproduction and Fertility Control," Lancaster: MTP Press Limited, Falcon House, p 143.

Gyzin J, Barnwell JW Schlesinger DH, Nussenzweig V, Nussenzweig RS (1984). Neutralization of the infectivity of sporozoites of Plasmodium knowlesi by antibodies to a synthetic peptide. J Exp Med 160:935.
Heymer B, Finger H, Wirsing CH (1978). Immunoadjuvant effects of the synthetic muramyl dipeptide (MDP) N-acetylmuramyl-L-alanyl-D-isoglutamine. Zeit Immunitatforsch 155:87.
Kishimoto T, Hirai Y, Nakanishi K, Azuma I, Nagamatsu A, Yamamura Y (1979). Regulation of antibody response in different immunoglobulin classes. VI. Selective suppression of IgE response by administration of antigen-conjugated muramyl peptides. J Immun 123:2709.
Kotani S, Watanabe Y, Shimono T, Narita T, Kato K, Stewart-Tull DES, Kinoshita F, Yokogawa K, Kawata S, Shiba T, Kosumoto S, Tirumi Y (1975). Immunoadjuvant activities of cell walls, their water-soluble fractions and peptidoglycan subunits prepared from various gram-positive bacteria and of synthetic N-acetyl-muramyl peptides. Zeitschrift fur Immunitatsforschung 149:302.
Leclerc C, Audibert F, Chedid L (1978). influence of a synthetic adjuvant (MDP) on qualitative and quantitative changes of serum globulins. Immun 35:963.
Lefrancier P, Lederer E (1981). Chemistry of synthetic immunomodulant muramyl peptides. Progress in the chemistry of organic natural products 40:1.
Lowy I, Theze, J, Chedid L (1980). Stimulation of the in vivo dinitrophenyl antibody response to the DNP conjugate of L-glutamic acid^{60}-L-alanine^{30}-L-tyrosine^{10} (GAT) polymer by a synthetic adjuvant, muramyl dipeptide (MDP): target cells for adjuvant activity and isotypic patterm of MDP-stimulated response. J Immun 124:100.
Mazier D, Mellouk S, Beaudoin RL, Texier B, Druilhe P, Phckmeyer W, Trosper T, Paul C, Charoenvit Y, Young J, Miltgen F, Chedid L, Chirigot JP, Galley B, Brandicourt O, Gentilini M (1986). Effect of antibodies to recombinant and synthetic peptides on Pl. Falciparum sporozoites in vitro. Science 231:156.
Mozes E, Sela M, Chedid L (1980). Efficient genitically controlled formation of antibody to a synthetic antigen [poly(LTy2,LGlu)-poly(DL-Ala)-poly L-Lys)] covalently bound to a synthetic adjuvant (N-acetyl muramyl L-alanyl-D-isoglutamine). Proc Natl Acad Sci USA 77:4933.

Nash H, Talwar GP, Segal S, Luukkainer T, Johansson EDB, Vasquez J, Coutinho E, Sundaram K (1980). Observations on the antigenicity and clinical effects of a candidate antipregnancy vaccine: beta-subunit of human chorionic gonadotropin linked to tetanus toxoid. Fertil Steril 34:328.

Prouvost-Danon A, Bahr GM, Chedid L, Ekwalanga M, Bassot S (1984). In vivo effects of ovalbumin-conjugated muramyl peptides on the anti-ovalbumin IgE and IgG responses in mice. Int J Immunopharmac 6:425.

Reichert CM, Carelli C, Jolivet M, Audibert F, Lefrancier P, Chedid L (1980). Synthesis of conjugates containing N-acetyl-muramylL-Alanyl-D-isoglumine (MDP): Their use as hapten-carrier system. Molec Immunol 17:357.

Riveau G, Carelli C, Chedid L (1985). Relationships between structure and antipyretic activity of LH-RH-Lys MDP. Third International Conference on Immunopharmacology, Florence, May 6-9.

Staruch MJ, Wood DD (1983). The adjuvanticity of interleukin 1 in vivo. J Immunol 130:2191.

Stevens VC (1980). The current status of anti-pregnancy vaccines based on synthetic fractions of HCG. In Hearn JP (ed): "Immunological Aspects of Reproduction and Fertility Control," Lancaster, England: MTP Press Limited, Falcon House, p 143.

Telzak E, Wolff SM, Dinarello CA, Conlon T, El Kholy A, Bahr GM, Choay JP, Morin A, Chedid L (1986). Clinical evaluation of the immuno adjuvant murabutide, a derivative of MDP, administered with a tetanus toxoid vaccine. J Inf Dis 153:628.

Tsong YY, Chang CC, Nash HA (1985). Formulation of a potential antipregnancy vaccine based on the beta-subunit of human chorionic gonadotropin (beta-hCG). I. Alternative macromolecular carriers. J Repr Immun 7:139.

Immunopharmacology of Infectious Diseases: Vaccine Adjuvants and Modulators of Non-Specific Resistance, pages 213–222

COMPARISON OF THE IMMUNO- AND NEUROPHARMACOLOGICAL ACTIVITIES OF MDP AND MURABUTIDE.

Gilles Riveau[§] and Louis Chedid*

[§]Department of Pharmacology & Therapeutics
University of South Florida, College of Medicine
Tampa, Florida; *Immunotherapie Experimentale,
Institut Pasteur, Paris, France

Muramyl dipeptide (MDP) was originally described for its immunoadjuvant properties (Ellouz et al, 1974; Kotani et al, 1975) but it soon appeared that its activity was multifocal (Rev. in Audibert et al, 1986). Besides the adjuvant and immunostimulant activities of MDP, some side effects were described such as pyrogenicity (Kotani et al, 1976). Many derivatives have been prepared in several laboratories with the purpose of selecting effective compounds and establishing correlations between their chemical structure and immunostimulant activity (Chedid et al, 1978;). Among the MDP analogs tested, murabutide was selected (see Figure 1) due to its properties as an immunostimulant and lack of such as pyrogenicity (Chedid et al, 1982).

MDP activity could be explained by its capacity to activate the synthesis of numerous cytokines. Many studies have pointed to the macrophage as playing a major role in MDP-induced immuno- and neuromodulation (Chedid, 1985). Macrophages activated by MDP have been shown to produce biological active mediators such as Interleukin-1 (IL-1) (Oppenheim et al, 1980). The production of this monokine may prove to play a role in the adjuvant activity (Staruch and Wood, 1983) and explain in part the pyrogenicity of the glycopeptide (Dinarello et al, 1978; Riveau et al, 1980). Interestingly, the adjuvant active murabutide, which is not pyrogenic *in vivo*, was found to induce *in vitro* IL-1 production by macrophages. This IL-1, detected by its lymphocyte-activating factor (LAF) activity was devoid of endogenous pyrogen (EP) activity (Damais et al, 1982).

This article will describe:

1) Differences between the actions of MDP and murabutide at the central nervous system (CNS) level.

2) A comparison of the activities of IL-1 induced by MDP and those activities induced by murabutide.

COMPARED EFFECTS OF MDP AND MURABUTIDE ON THE CNS

Influence of MDP and murabutide on body temperature.

MDP represents the minimal active structure responsible for the adjuvant effect ascribed to Freund Complete Adjuvant. It was also demonstrated to be the smallest molecule capable of eliciting the pyrogenic action of bacterial peptidoglycan. Administered intravenously in the rabbit, 30 µg/kg of MDP, induced a rise in body temperature by eliciting EP activity in the plasma (Parant et al, 1980). In contrast, 10 mg/kg of murabutide was shown to be non-pyrogenic via the same route.

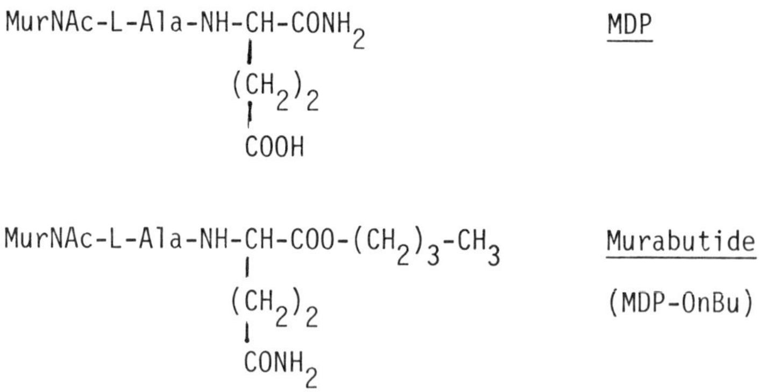

Figure 1. Formula of MDP and of Murabutide.

When intracerebroventricular (icv) injections were performed, a good dose-febrile response curve was obtained. A tremendous increase of sensitivity was shown by the minimal pyrogenic dose (dose inducing an increase in body temperature of 0.6°C) corresponding to 0.13 ng/kg (Figure 2). This dose was 200,000-fold less than that obtained by the intravenous route. Even delivered by the icv route murabutide at a dose of 10 µg/kg was totally ineffective in eliciting a rise in body temperature (Figure 2).

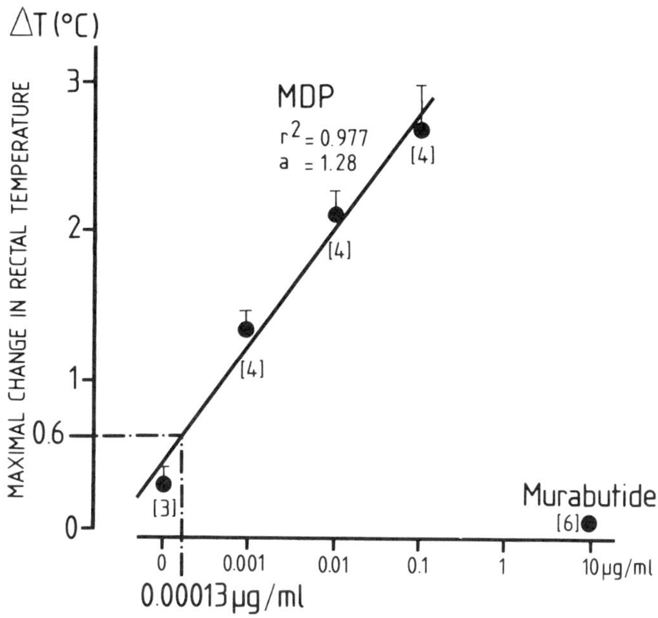

Figure 2. Febrile responses to icv administration of glycopeptide.

Injection of a large dose of MDP by icv route caused a strong and lasting febrile response, although no circulating EP activity could be detected in the plasma or in the cerebrospinal fluid of the rabbit (Riveau et al, 1980). This tremendous potentiation in the pyrogenic effect of MDP observed after icv injection, without detectable EP activity production, suggests that the glycopeptide can be effective by a direct action on the brain structures controlling body temperature. Because murabutide was shown to be apyrogenic after iv and icv injections, it can be postulated that its action differs from that of MDP at the central level. Another neurological effect of MDP, which has been described by Krueger et al (1984), substantiates this hypothesis since MDP infused icv was shown to induce an increase in Slow-Wave Sleep (SWS) while murabutide was inactive.

Influence of MDP and murabutide on the synthesis of prostaglandins within CNS.

The fever elicited by icv administration of MDP can

be inhibited by indomethacin. It was thus very likely that MDP stimulates synthesis and release of prostaglandins (PGs) within the CNS. Masek et al (1985) have shown that the cyclooxygenase pathway in the total brain of the rat could be activated by MDP. These authors observed an increase in the production of prostaglandin E_2 (PGE_2) by the brains of MDP-treated animals. We have observed the amount of PGE_2 in different parts of the rat brain, one hour after treatment with MDP or murabutide. Levels of PGE_2 measured by radio-immunoassay are presented in Table I.

Table I. PGE_2 levels in different parts of the brain, one hour after ip injection of 1 mg of MDP or of murabutide in rats.

	Control	MDP	Murabutide
Cortex	24.1 ± 9.3	25.8 ± 3.0	23.7 ± 12.4
POAH	7.2 ± 1.5	13.8 ± 2.3*	6.8 ± 5.4
Cerebellum	1.9 ± 0.9	0.9 ± 0.2	2.3 ± 0.6
Total Others Regions	13.8 ± 3.8	9.5 ± 2.2	14.1 ± 5.7

Results are expressed by the mean ± SD in ng/100 mg of tissue. * $p < 0.01$. Student's t test (two tailed).

It can be seen that an increase in the PGE_2 level was obtained in the preoptic-antehypothalamic region (POAH) of MDP-treated rats whereas the treatment with murabutide did not induce any change in the level of any studied area. These results seem to confirm that MDP and its nonpyrogenic derivative, differ from one another in their capacity to affect certain brain regulatory mechanisms.

COMPARISON OF THE ACTIVITIES OF IL-1 INDUCED BY MDP OR BY MURABUTIDE.

In vitro experiments have shown that monocytes or macrophages cultured in the presence of MDP could produce pyrogenic IL-1, possessing LAF activity, when tested for its mitogenic effect on mouse thymocytes treated by phytohemagglutinin. Results presented in Table II show that IL-1 produced by macrophages have the same mitogenic effect on mouse thymocytes cultured in the presence of MDP or murabutide.

Table II. Activities of IL-1 produced by macrophages incubated with MDP or murabutide.

	Control	IL-1/MDP	IL-1/MDP-OnBu
EP activity (mean fever rise,°C)	0.06±0.03	0.71±0.05	0.05±0.02
LAF activity (Unit/ml)	12	480	510

(LAF activity in unit (Riveau et al, 1986)

Nevertheless, as it has been described by Damais et al (1982), IL-1/murabutide did not induce a rise in body temperature after iv injection in the rabbit. Moreover, this IL-1 did not provoke fever even by icv administration.

In the following experiments, the influences of MDP and murabutide on macrophages were studied for their ability to induce arachidonic acid (AA) derivatives.

Influence of MDP and murabutide on the synthesis of AA metabolites by macrophages.

The production of AA metabolites by macrophages incubated with MDP or murabutide is presented in Table III.

Table III. Production of prostaglandins and thromboxane B_2 by macrophages incubated with MDP or murabutide.

	PGE_2°	6-keto$PGF_{1\alpha}$°	$PGF_{2\alpha}$°	TxB_2°
Control	2.6±1.6	4.8±1.4	1.5±1.1	4.5±2.4
MDP*	22.9±4.3	53.4±15.6	21.4±1.4	17.5±2.4
Murabutide*	34.1±6.2	48.7±11.1	22.7±1.3	16.4±1.8

° ng/ml of supernatant fluid of macrophage culture (incubation during 18 hr at 39°C). Mean ± SD.

* Macrophages were incubated with 10 ug of glycopeptide per milliliter.

Already described by Wahl et al (1979), the synthesis of PGE_2 by macrophages was increased by the presence of MDP. Similarly, the production of 6-keto-$PGF_{1\alpha}$ (the stable derivative of PGI_2), $PGF_{2\alpha}$ and thromboxane B_2 (TxB_2) were significantly enhanced when rabbit macrophages were incubated with 1 μg/ml of MDP. 6-keto-$PGF_{1\alpha}$ was the major metabolite in these experiments. Murabutide presented the same activity as MDP, showing that this derivative has the capacity to activate the cyclooxygenase pathway in macrophages.

It has been recently observed that MDP did not activate the AA cascade directly (unpublished results). Indeed, it was possible to stimulate the production of 6-keto-$PGF_{1\alpha}$ with a supernatant containing IL-1 from which MDP had been eliminated by dialysis. Interleukin-1 induced by murabutide presented the same activity on prostaglandin synthesis as IL-1/MDP. This synthesis was without delay and macrophages incubated with IL-1/murabutide produced 6-keto-$PGF_{1\alpha}$ level in the range of 20 ng/ml. These results indicated that the production of PGs were dependent on the IL-1 containing supernatant from activated macrophage cultures. It is also evident that the presence of EP activity was not necessary for induction of prostaglandin synthesis.

Influence of MDP and murabutide on plasma metal levels.

Interleukin-1 has been also described as a mediator of a chain of nonspecific host responses such as hypoferremia, hypercupremia and changes in concentration of serum acute-phase proteins (Kampschmidt et al, 1981). Hypoferremia has been regarded as an important defense mechanism whereby the host attempts to limit the availability of essential iron to the invading pathogens. Recently, Chedid et al (1986) described that the combined action of temperature and lowered metal concentration in the serum of MDP-treated rabbit were capable of modifying the virulent phenotype of bacteria. These modifications might be one explanation of the enhancement by MDP of nonspecific resistance to infection.

Intravenous injection of 100 μg/kg MDP in the rabbit induced a rapid decrease in plasma iron concentration to 72% of the original value at 8h. Elevation in plasma copper concentration peaked at 24h with an increase of 71% of the original value. In contrast in these experiments, murabutide did not modify plasma iron and copper concentrations (Table IV).

Table IV. Effect of MDP, murabutide and their IL-1 on plasma metal levels.

	Mean Fall in Iron (%)*	Mean Inc. in Copper (%)°	Mean Fever Rise (°C)	Circul. EP+
PBS	9	9	0.11	-
MDP#	72	71	1.32	+
Murabutide#	9	5	0.12	-
IL-1/MDP¢	70	77	0.72	
IL-1/Murabutide¢	13	10	0.10	

* Mean fall in plasma iron 8 hr after iv injection.
° Mean increase in plasma copper level 24 hrs after injection
\+ Circulating EP detected in plasma of treated rabbit (Riveau et al., 1980)
\# Glycopeptides were injected by iv route. 100 μg/kg.
¢ IL-1 induced by MDP or by murabutide were injected by iv route. 1 ml/kg supernatant fluid.

These modifications could be related to the capacity of the compound to induce production of circulating EP activity. Changes in metal levels were also induced by supernatant from rabbit macrophages cultured with MDP. Injection of this supernatant containing pyrogenic IL-1 (IL-1/MDP, 1 ml/kg) was as effective as an injection of MDP. It has been shown that the effect of IL-1/MDP on plasma iron and copper concentrations were proportional to pyrogenicity (Riveau et al, 1986). Fluid preparations from cell cultures stimulated with murabutide which contained nonpyrogenic IL-1 (IL-1/murabutide) did not affect plasma metal levels. In accordance with the observations of Turchik and Bornstein (1980), recent experiments have shown that hypoferremia and hypercupremia induced by pyrogenic IL-1 can be mediated through the CNS (Riveau et al, 1986).

CONCLUSION

All adjuvant-active muramyl peptides do not have the same degree of pyrogenicity. We have demonstrated that murabutide, although endowed with a comparable immunostimulating activity as MDP, did not induce fever even when administered by the icv route. Other observations indicate that MDP and not murabutide may exert an activity on the thermoregulating centers, such as the POAH region, via increased prostaglandin synthesis. These centers are known to present an important sensitivity to prostaglandins synthesized *in situ*. The somnogenic effect of MDP glycopeptide likewise shows that certain brain functions are sensitive to its structure even when murabutide was not recognized.

In contrast, the capacity of MDP to activate macrophages has been retained with murabutide. Prostaglandins and IL-1 (LAF activity) were produced by macrophages incubated with murabutide. Nevertheless, this IL-1 was non-pyrogenic and unable to induce certain acute-phase reactions.

These results provide further evidence that murabutide is devoid of unwanted neuropharmacological properties of MDP and that a good correlation is observed between the activities of this derivative and those of its IL-1.

REFERENCES

Audibert F, Leclerc C, Chedid L (1985). Muramyl peptides as immunopharmacological response modifiers. In Torrence PF (ed): "Biological Response Modifiers," New York: Academic Press p 307.

Chedid L (1985). Immuno- and neuropharmacological properties of muramyl peptides and Interleukin-1. In Miescher PA, Bolis L, Ghione M (eds): "Immunopharmacology," New York: Raven Press, p 51.

Chedid L, Audibert F, Johnson AG (1978). Biological activities of muramyl dipeptide, a synthetic glycopeptide analogous to bacterial immunoregulating agents. Prog Allergy 25:63.

Chedid LA, Parant MA, Audibert FM, Riveau GJ, Parant FJ, Lederer E, Choay JP, Lefrancier PL (1982). Biological activity of a new synthetic muramyl peptide adjuvant devoid of pyrogenicity. Infect Immun 35:417.

Chedid L, Parant M, Parant F, Riveau G (1986). Nonspecific effects of LPS on bacterial infections. In Szentivanyi A, Nowotny A, Friedman H (eds): "The Immunobiology and Immunopharmacology of Bacterial Endotoxins, Basic and Clinical Aspects," New York: Plenum Press, in press.
Damais C, Riveau G, Parant M, Gerota J, Chedid L (1982). Production of lymphocyte activating factor in the absence of endogenous pyrogen by rabbit or human leukocytes stimulated by a muramyl dipeptide derivative. Int J Immunopharmac 4:451.
Dinarello CA, Elin RJ, Chedid L, Walff SM (1978). The pyrogenicity of the synthetic adjuvant muramyl dipeptide and two structural analogues. J Infect Dis 138:760.
Ellouz F, Adam A, Ciorbaru R, Lederer E (1974). Minimal structural requirements for adjuvant activity of bacterial septidoglycan derivatives. Biochem Biophys Res Com 59:1317.
Kampschmidt RF (1981). Leukocytic endogenous mediator/endogenous pyrogen. In Powanda MC, Canonico PG (eds): "The Physiologic and Metabolic Responses of the Host," Amsterdam: Elsevier/North Holland, p 55.
Kotani S, Watanabe Y, Shimono T, Narita T, Kato K, Stewart-Tull DES, Kinoshita F, Yokogawa K, Kawata S, Shiba T, Kusumoto S, Tarumi Y (1975). Immunoadjuvant activities of cell walls, their water-soluble fractions and peptidoglycan subunits, prepared from various gram-positive bacteria, and of synthetic N-acetylmuramyl peptides. Z Immun-Forsch 149:302.
Kotani S, Watanabe Y, Shimono T, Harada K, Shiba T, Kusumoto S, Yokogawa K, Taniguchi M (1976). Correlation between the immunoadjuvant activities and pyrogenicities of synthetic N-acetylmuramyl peptides or -amino acids. Biken J 19:9.
Krueger JM, Walter J, Karnovsky ML, Chedid L, Choay JP, Lefrancier P, Lederer E (1984). Muramyl peptides. Variation of somnogenic activity with structure. J Exp Med 159:68.
Masek K, Riveau G, Parant M, Chedid L (1985). The involvement of prostaglandin synthetase system in muramyl dipeptide induced fever. IRCS Med Sci 13:151.
Oppenheim JJ, Togawa A, Chedid L, Mizel S (1980). Components of mycobacteria and muramyl dipeptide with adjuvant activity induce lymphocyte activating factor. Cell Immunol 50:71.
Parant M, Riveau G, Chedid L (1980). Influence of indomethacin on various immunopharmacological effects of muramyl dipeptide (MDP). Agents & Actions, AAS 7, p 33.

Riveau G, Masek K, Parant M, Chedid L (1980). Central pyrogenic activity of muramyl dipeptide. J Exp Med 152:869.
Riveau G, Parant M, Damais C, Parant F, Chedid L (1986). Dissociation between muramyl peptide-induced fever and changes in plasma metal levels. Am J Physiol 250:C572.
Staruch MJ, Wood DD (1983). The adjuvanticity of Interleukin-1 in vivo. J Immunol 130:2191.
Turchik JB, Borstein Dl (1980). Role of the central nervous system in acute-phase responses to leukocytic pyrogen. Infect Immun 30:439.
Wahl SM, Wahl LM, McCarthy JB, Chedid L, Mergenhagen SE (1979). Macrophage activation by mycobacterial water-soluble components and synthetic muramyl dipeptide. J Immunol 122:2226.

Immunopharmacology of Infectious Diseases: Vaccine Adjuvants and Modulators of Non-Specific Resistance, pages 223–234

SYNTHETIC LIPID A ANALOGS AS A CANDIDATE FOR USEFUL IMMUNO-MODULATORS

Shozo Kotani,[1] Haruhiko Takada,[1] Tomohiko Ogawa,[1] Masachika Tsujimoto,[1] Ichiro Takahashi,[1] Takako Ikeda,[1] Hidetoshi Shimauchi,[1] Kazuhiro Harada,[2] Haruki Okamura,[3] Toshihide Tamura,[3] Shigenori Tanaka,[4] Yoji Goto[5], Takashi Takahashi,[5] Tetsuo Shiba,[6] and Shoichi Kusumoto[6]

Department of Microbiology and Oral Microbiology, Osaka University Dental School, Suita, Osaka 565[1]; Department of Bacteriology, Osaka Prefectural Institute for Public Health, Higashinari-ku, Osaka 537[2]; Department of Bacteriology, Hyogo College of Medicine, Nishinomiya, Hyogo 663[3]; Tokyo Research Institute, Seikagaku Kogyo Co. Ltd., Higashiyamato, Tokyo 189[4]; Kitasato Institute, Minato-ku, Tokyo 108[5]; and Faculty of Science, Osaka University, Toyonaka, Osaka 560[6], Japan

INTRODUCTION

Several years after the successful synthesis (Kotani et al, 1975; Kusumoto et al, 1976) of *N*-acetylmuramyl-L-alanyl-D-isoglutamine (MDP), the minimal structural unit carrying most of the multifold bioactivities of bacterial cell wall peptidoglycans (Takada and Kotani, 1985), subsequently to but independently of Lederer's group (Ellouz et al, 1974), Shiba started a synthetic study on lipid A portions of endotoxic lipopolysaccharides (LPS) of *Enterobacteriaceae*. One of the purposes of this study is the development of novel compounds with maximal beneficial bioactivities and minimal endotoxic effects, to be used as useful immunomodulators, such as anti-tumor and anti-infectious agents and adjuvants for vaccines. Herein, we report the activities of these synthetic lipid As and their less toxic analogs.

ENDOTOXIC AND RELATED BIOACTIVITIES OF SYNTHETIC COUNTERPARTS OF *E. COLI*-TYPE, *S. MINNESOTA*-TYPE LIPID AS, BIOSYNTHETIC PRECURSOR Ia AND THEIR MONOPHOSPHORYL ANALOGS

Figure 1 shows the acylation patterns of test lipid As

and their analogs. Compound 506 (LA-15-PP) corresponds in structure to *E. coli* Re-mutant F515 lipid A, and is β(1-6)-D-glucosamine 1,4'-bisphosphate that has two β-acyloxyacyl groups at the 2'-amino and 3'-hydroxyl groups (Imoto et al, 1985). Compound 516 (LA-16-PP) corresponds to a major component of the lipid A prepared from *S. minnesota* Re-mutant, R595, and has three β-acyloxyacyl groups at 2- and 2'-amino groups and at 3'-hydroxyl groups of the disaccharide backbone. Compound 406 (LA-14-PP; Imoto et al, 1984) has the structure of the biosynthetic lipid A disaccharide precursor Ia (Hansen-Hagge et al, 1985), which corresponds to IV_A described by Strain et al (1985) and all the four acyl groups of which are (*R*)-3-hydroxytetradecanoic acid. 4'-Monophosphate, 1-monophosphate and dephospho analogs of compounds 506, 516 and 406 have also been synthesized.

Table 1 summarizes the assay results on compound 506, its 4'-monophosphate, 1-monophosphate, and dephospho analogs (compounds 504, 505 and 503, respectively) and compound 406 on endotoxic and related bioactivities when they were administered to animals, and that of the *Limulus* test. Compound 506 exhibited full endotoxic activities identical to, or sometimes stronger than those of a reference F515 lipid A, and almost comparable to *E. coli* LPS, in pyrogenicity, leukopenia-induction in rabbits, body-weight decreasing toxicity in normal mice, lethality in galactosamine (GalN)-loaded mice and chick embryos, and the preparation and provocation of the local

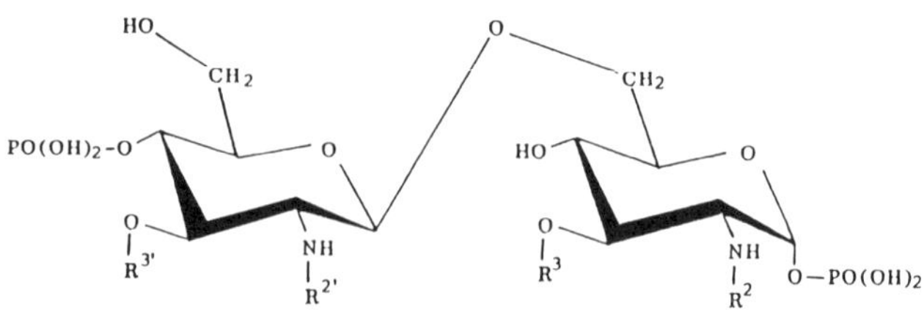

Revised comp. name	Previous comp. no.	$R^{3'}$	$R^{2'}$	R^3	R^2	Type
LA-17-PP	None	C_{14}	C_{14}	C_{14}	C_{14}	
LA-18-PP	None	C_{14}	C_{14}-OH	C_{14}	C_{14}-OH	
LA-14-PP	406	C_{14}-OH	C_{14}-OH	C_{14}-OH	C_{14}-OH	Precursor Ia
LA-15-PP	506	C_{14}-O-(C_{14})	C_{14}-O-(C_{12})	C_{14}-OH	C_{14}-OH	*E. coli*
LA-16-PP	516	C_{14}-O-(C_{14})	C_{14}-O-(C_{12})	C_{14}-OH	C_{14}-O-(C_{16})	*S. minnesota*

Fig. 1. Chemical structure of synthetic lipid As and their analogs with different acylation patterns. C_{14}, tetradecanoyl; C_{14}-OH, (*R*)-3-hydroxytetradecanoyl; C_{14}-O-(C_{12}), (*R*)-3-dodecanoyloxytetradecanoyl; C_{14}-O-(C_{14}), (*R*)-3-tetradecanoyloxytetradecanoyl; C_{14}-O-(C_{16}), (*R*)-3-hexadecanoyloxytetradecanoyl.

TABLE 1. Summary of endotoxic and *Limulus* test of synthetic lipid A, its analogs, and reference bacterial products [a]

Activity (test animal)	Synthetic compound					Bacterial product	
	406 (1,4'-P)	506 (1,4'-P)	504 (4'-P)	505 (1-P)	503 (des-P)	Lipid A[b]	LPS[c]
Pyrogenicity (rabbits)	+	+++	++	++	-	++	+++
Leukopenia (rabbits)	+	+++	+	-	-	++	+++
Toxicity							
Lethality (GalN, C57BL/6)	++±	++±	++	++	-	++	+++
Lethality (chick embryo)	-	+++	++	++	-	+++	++
Body weight loss (ICR)	+	++	++	+	-	++	+++
Shwartzman (rabbits)							
Preparation	-	++±	+	+	-	+++	ND[d]
Provocation	-	+++	ND	ND	ND	+++	ND
Limulus test							
Pre Gel	+++	+++	+++	++	-	+++	+++
Toxicolor	++±	+++	+±	+	±	++±	++

[a] The maximum bioactivity exhibited by test synthetic or bacterial products was scored as +++ (based on the paper of Kotani et al, 1985).
[b] Prepared from *E. coli* O8:K27, Re-mutant (strain F515).
[c] Prepared from *E. coli* O55:B5 (List).
[d] Not determined.

Shwartzman reaction in rabbits. No differences were noted in the *Limulus* test, either the conventional gelation method or the recently developed colorimetric Toxicolor Test, between compound 506 and reference bacterial products. The monophosphoryl analogs, compounds 504 and 505, had considerably weaker bioactivities than the parent bisphosphate molecule, 506. Compound 504 (LA-15-PH in the new nomenclature) corresponds in structure to the major component of detoxified endotoxin, namely monophosphoryl lipid A (MPL) prepared from *S. typhimurium* Re-mutant by Ribi and his collaborators (Qureshi et al, 1982; Ribi et al, 1982 & 1984; Takayama et al, 1984). Compound 504 retained a weak, but definite endotoxicity of the parent bisphosphate compound, 506. Dephospho compound 503 did not show any detectable bioactivities, probably because of its low solubility. Compound 406 was only weakly endotoxic except in GalN-loaded mice.

Table 2 summarizes the possible useful bioactivities of the LA-15 series compounds and compound 406. Compound 506 exhibited adjuvanticity to increase anti-sheep red blood cells (SRBC) hemolytic plaque forming cell (PFC) number in the spleen of mice by intraperitoneal injection with SRBC, and to stimulate both cellular and humoral immune responses of guinea pigs to ovalbumin when administered as a water-in-oil (w/o) emulsion with the antigen. Compound 506 also induced the possible tumor necrosis factor (TNF) and interferons (IFN) α/β

TABLE 2. Summary of possible useful activities of synthetic lipid A, its analogs and reference bacterial products [a]

Activity (test animal)	Synthetic compound					Bacterial product	
	406 (1,4'-P)	506 (1,4'-P)	504 (4'-P)	505 (1-P)	503 (des-P)	Lipid A[b]	LPS[c]
Adjuvant activity							
Increase of anti-SRBC PFC (BALB/c)	++	+++	++	++	-	+++	+++
DTH induction (guinea pigs; w/o)	++	+++±	++	-	-	+	+++
Ab production (guinea pigs; w/o)	++±	+++	++	±	±	±	+
"TNF" induction (BCG-primed ICR)	+++	+++	+	±	-	+++	+++
Interferon induction (*P. acnes*-primed ICR)							
α/β	++	++	ND[d]	ND	ND	++	+++
γ	ND	++	ND	ND	ND	+++	ND

[a] The scoring is the same as in TABLE 1 (based on the paper of Kotani et al, 1985 & 1986 and Takada et al, 1985).
[b-d] The footnotes are the same as in TABLE 1.

and γ in BCG-primed and *P. acnes*-primed mice, respectively. Useful activities of the less toxic compound 406 were not very different from those of fully toxic compound 506. These include the induction of TNF and IFN α/β. The 4'-monophosphate analog, compound 504 also showed definite adjuvanticity and TNF-inducing ability, but these activities were less than those of compounds 506 and 406.

In in vitro assay systems, compound 506 stimulated the lymphocytes, macrophages, polymorphonuclear leukocytes and serum complement cascade in a manner similar to that of bacterial lipid A. Compound 506, its monophosphoryl analogs

TABLE 3. Summary of bioactivities detected by in vitro assays of synthetic lipid A, its analogs, and reference bacterial products [a]

Activity (test animal)	Synthetic compound					Bacterial product	
	406 (1,4'-P)	506 (1,4'-P)	504 (4'-P)	505 (1-P)	503 (des-P)	Lipid A[b]	LPS[c]
Lymphocyte stimulation							
Mitogenicity (BALB/c nu/nu)	++	++	+	++	-	++	+++
(C3H/HeN)	+++	++	±	++	-	++±	+++
(C3H/HeJ)	-	-	-	-	-	-	-
PBA activity (BALB/c)	++	++±	+++	++±	±	++±	+++
Macrophage stimulation (guinea pigs)							
[^{3}H]TdR uptake inhibition	++	++±	++±	++	-	++±	+++
[^{14}C]GlcN uptake increase	++	+++	++	+++	-	+++	+++
Spreading	+	+	±	±	-	+	+
Enhancement of O_2^- generation	+++	+++	+++	++	ND[d]	+++	+++
PMNL stimulation							
Enhanced migration (human)	++	+++	+++	++	+	+++	++
Complement activation via classical pathway (human)	+	+++	+++	+++	-	+++	+

[a] The scoring is the same as in TABLE 1 on general principles (based on the papers of Kotani et al, 1985 & 1986).
[b-d] The footnotes are the same as in TABLE 1.

and compound 406 had similar in vitro bioactivities, but the dephospho analogs, 503 had negligible activity (Table 3).

Table 4 is a summary of the endotoxic and associated bioactivities of compound 516 and its 4'-monophosphate analog (compound 514) whose amide group at the carbon 2 position of the disaccharide backbone is substituted with the (*R*)-3-hexadecanoyloxytetradecanoyl group, namely the third β-acyloxyacyl group, as compared with those of compounds 506 and 406, which have two and no β-acyloxyacyl groups, respectively. Unexpectedly, compound 516, a synthetic counterpart of a major *S. minnesota* R595 lipid A, showed considerably less pyrogenic and leukopenic activities in rabbits and less lethal toxicity in GalN-loaded mice than compound 506. It had negligible preparatory effect on rabbit skin for the Shwartzman reaction and lacked the lethal toxicity in chick embryos. Compound 516 tended to be less active than compound 506 or bacterial *E. coli*-type lipid A in other bioassay systems too, with few exceptions. The 4'-monophosphate analog (compound 514), which corresponds to one of the monophosphoryl lipid As obtained from LPS of *S. minnesota* R595 by Qureshi et al (1985), showed

TABLE 4. Comparison of endotoxic and related bioactivities of synthetic counterparts of biosynthetic precursor Ia (406), *E. coli*-type lipid A (506), *S. minnesota*-type lipid A (516), and 4'-monophosphoryl analog of the latter (514), and bacterial products, F515 and R595 lipid As

Biological activity[a] (Test animal)	Synthetic compound				Bacterial lipid A	
	406	506	516	514	F515	R595
- In vivo assay -						
Lethal toxicity (GalN-loaded C57BL/6 mice)	+++	+++	++	++	++±	++±
(Chick embryos)	-	+++	-	-	+++	+++
Preparatory ability for local Shwartzman reaction (rabbits)	±	+++	+	-	+++	+++
Pyrogenicity (rabbits)	++	+++	++	±	++	++
Leukopenia-inducing activity (rabbits)	+	+++	+	-	++	++
"TNF"-inducing activity (BCG-primed ICR mice)	+++	+++	++	+	+++	+++
IFN-α/β inducing activity (*P. acnes*-primed ICR mice)	+++	+++	++	-	+++	ND[b]
Adjuvant activity: Direct PFC against SRBC (BALB/c mice)	++	+++	++	±	+++	+++
PHA and ELISA against BSA (BALB/c mice)	ND	+++	++	++	+++	+++
- In vitro assays -						
Limulus test: Gelation method (*T. tridentatus*)	+++	+++	+++	++	+++	+++
Colorimetric method (*T. tridentatus*)	++	+++	++	+	+++	+++
Complement activation via classical pathway (Human)	+	+++	+++	+++	+++	+++
Lymphocyte activation: Mitogenicity (BALB/c nu/nu mice)	+++	+++	++	+	+++	+++
(C3H/HeJ mice)	-	-	-	-	-	-
PBA activity (BALB/c mice)	+++	+++	+++	++	+++	+++
Macrophage activation: Increase of GlcN uptake (Guinea pigs)	++	+++	+++	+	+++	+++
Production of O_2^- (Guinea pigs)	+++	+++	+++	++	+++	+++
Production of PGE_2 (ICR mice)	+++	+++	++	±	+++	+++
Generation of IL-1 (DBA/2 mice)	++	+++	+++	+	+++	+++

a The activities of compound 506 (LA-15-PP) were scored as +++ (based on the papers of Kotani et al, 1984, 1985 & 1986 and Takada et al, 1985).
b Not determined.

significantly weaker activity than compound 506 in most of the assays, probably because of of its greater hydrophobicity and consequently lower solubility in assay systems. Judging from Table 4, there is an optimal number of β-acyloxyacyl groups at the glucosamine disaccharide backbone, to exert strong endotoxic activities such as pyrogenicity, lethality in chick embryos and the preparative activity for the Shwartzman reaction. The endotoxic activity was strongest in compound 506, which has two β-acyloxyacyl groups per molecule, and was considerably less in compounds 406 and 516, which have no and three β-acyloxyacyl groups, respectively. The differences between compound 506 and compound 406 or 516 were less apparent in possible beneficial activities such as adjuvanticity, the ability to induce TNF and IFN α/β as well as in the *Limulus* test and stimulatory effects on lymphocytes, macrophages and complement cascade. It is not clear at present whether the observed differences in the endotoxic activities of these three 1,4'-bisphosphorylated diglucosamine compounds are derived directly from the differences in chemical structures or result indirectly from the differences in physical properties. The position as well as the number of β-acyloxyacyl groups at the disaccharide backbone might also be important for expression of the endotoxic activities of the molecule, though experimental evidence is lacking.

POTENTIALLY USEFUL ANALOGS (LA-17-PP and LA-18-PP) OF COMPOUND 406

Based on the above findings, we proceeded to synthesize the LA-17 and LA-18 series compounds whose acylation patterns are shown in Fig. 1. All four acyl groups of LA-17-PP are tetradecanoic acids, and in LA-18-PP the amide-bound acyl groups at the C-2' and C-2 positions are (*R*)-3-hydroxytetradecanoic acids and the ester-bound acyl groups at the C-3' and C-3 positions are tetradecanoic acids.

TABLE 5. Lethal toxicity of LA-17-PP and LA-18-PP and reference synthetic and bacterial products in galactosamine-loaded C57BL/6 mice

Compound	No. of mice / no. of mice tested with the following dose (ng)				LD_{50} (ng)
	1000	100	10	1	
LA-17-PP	9/10	3/5	0/5		≥ 100
LA-18-PP	6/10	4/5	0/5		≥ 126
LA-14-PP		5/5	10/20	0/5	10
LA-15-PP		5/5	4/10	0/5	13
F515 lipid A		5/5	3/10	0/5	16
R595 lipid A		5/5	2/5	0/5	13

LA-17-PP and LA-18-PP exhibited some lethal toxicity in GalN-loaded mice, but their LD_{50} values were about ten times higher than those of compounds 506 and 406 (Table 5). In chick embryos, neither LA-17-PP nor LA-18-PP exerted lethal toxicity at 10 µg per embryo under the experimental conditions in which compound 506 and bacterial lipid A were lethal at a dose of 0.1 µg per embryo (data not shown). LA-17-PP caused a significant febrile response in rabbits only when the highest test dose of 10 µg per kg of body weight was injected; thus the pyrogenicity of this compound was about ten and one thousand fold weaker than those of compounds 406 and 506, respectively. LA-18-PP was non-pyrogenic at doses up to 10 µg/kg (Table 6). Neither LA-17-PP nor LA-18-PP prepared the rabbit skin for provocation of the local Shwartzman reaction by intravenous injection of *E. coli* LPS. In the same three rabbits, compound 506 and bacterial lipid As definitely prepared the injected skin site at a dose less than 2.5 µg per site (data not shown).

TABLE 6. Comparison of the pyrogenicity of LA-17-PP and LA-18-PP with that of reference synthetic compounds in rabbits

Compound	Dose (µg/kg)	Average of maximum increase of temperature (°C)	Positive /tested
LA-17-PP	10	1.40	3/3
	1	0.13	0/3
LA-18-PP	10	0.22	0/3
	1	0.13	0/3
LA-14-PP	10	0.95	1/1
	1	0.80	3/4
	0.1	0.24	0/3
LA-15-PP	1	1.24	4/4
	0.1	1.07	3/3
	0.01	1.23	2/2
	0.001	0.48	0/2

As a possible useful activity, the mice twice immunized by subcutaneous injection of liposomes containing LA-17-PP or LA-18-PP and bovine serum albumin (BSA) at a 4 week interval, showed much higher immune responses than the control mice receiving BSA alone in the liposomes, in terms of highly enhanced production of the serum anti-BSA precipitating antibody of all the IgG, IgM and IgA classes (Table 7). Their adjuvant activity, however, was weaker than that of the reference *E. coli* F515 lipid A. The adjuvanticity of these two less toxic lipid A analogs was confirmed by the enhancement of the antibody production

TABLE 7. Adjuvant activity of LA-17-PP and LA-18-PP as compared with reference bacterial *E. coli*-type F515 lipid A on anti-BSA antibody production of BALB/c mice by subcutaneous injection with BSA in liposomes [a]

Compound	Passive hemagglutination titer ($\log_2$) (mean ± SE)	Enzyme-linked immunosorbent assay (mean ± SE) for: IgG (ratio)[b]	IgM (OD_{405}x100)[c]	IgA (OA_{405}x100)[c]
LA-17-PP	10.86 ± 0.26[d]	78.75 ± 16.79[d]	279 ± 29[f]	142 ± 12[d]
LA-18-PP	10.14 ± 0.46[d]	65.37 ± 20.22[d]	305 ± 37[f]	199 ± 12[d]
F515 lipid A	11.57 ± 0.30[d]	268.58 ± 88.50[d]	468 ± 59[d]	197 ± 17[d]

[a] Groups of eight BALB/c mice were immunized by subcutaneous injection of 100 µg of test adjuvant with 100 µg of BSA in liposomes, and 28 days later they received the second injection of the same mixture. Five days after the booster, the serum anti-BSA antibody level was determined by passive hemagglutination method and enzyme-linked immunosorbent assay. Liposomes consist of L-α-phosphatidylcholine dimyristoyl, cholesterol and dicetyl phosphate in a molar ratio of 2:1.5:0.22.
[b] Ratio of ELISA units in each test group to that in the respective control.
[c] OD_{405}, optical density at 405 nm.
[d] P<0.01.
[f] P<0.05.

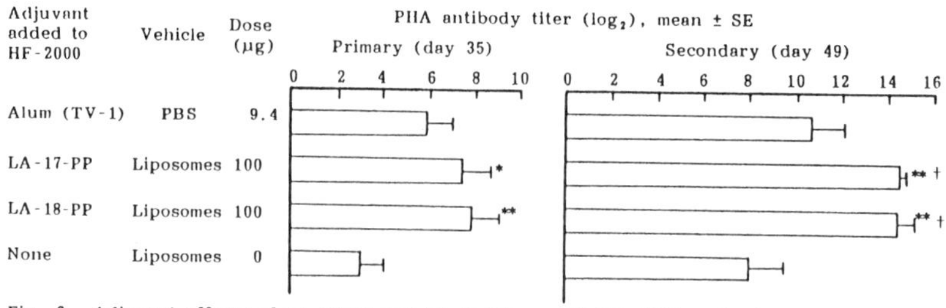

Fig. 2. Adjuvant effects of LA-17-PP and LA-18-PP on anti-HBs PHA antibody production by immunization of BALB/c mice with inactivated HBs antigen (HF-2000). The dose size (per animal) was 1.25 μg of HF-2000 with or without test adjuvant for the primary immunization on day 0 and 1.25 μg of HF-2000 alone for the booster on day 42. Liposomes consist of L-α-phosphatidylcholine dimyristoyl, cholesterol and dicetyl phosphate in a molar ratio of 2:1.5:0.22. Significant difference from none control (*P<0.05; **P<0.01) and from TV-1 control (†P<0.05).

against the inactivated hepatitis B virus surface (HBs) antigen, HF-2000, prepared from the human blood plasma pool. The primary immunization of mice with the HF-2000 antigen with the test synthetic adjuvants and the booster with the antigen alone markedly enhanced the antibody productions in terms of passive hemagglutination (PHA), both in the primary and secondary responses. Their adjuvant effect was significantly higher than that of alum, a reference adjuvant (Fig. 2). Figure 3 shows the activity of LA-17-PP and LA-18-PP to induce the serum factor cytocidal to L929 cells in BCG-primed ICR mice. Both compounds exhibited powerful activity to induce possible TNF, though their activity was weaker than that of bacterial lipid A. Both less toxic analogs are also capable of inducing serum IFN α/β in the mice primed with heat-killed *P. acnes*, but to a lesser extent than the reference synthetic and bacterial lipid As (Table 8).

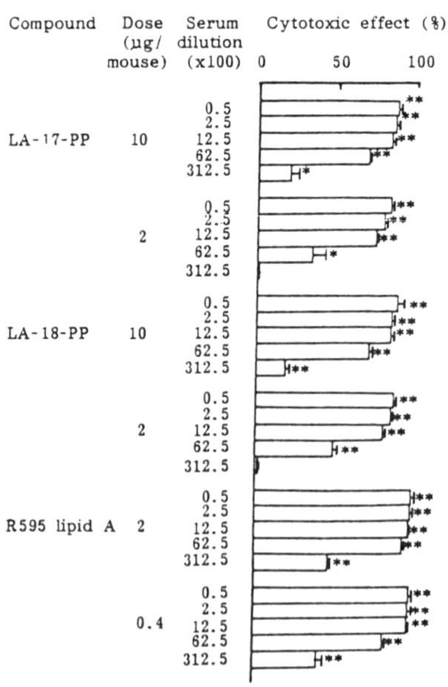

Fig. 3. Cytocidal effects on L929 cells of serum specimens from BCG-primed mice, elicited by intravenous injection of LA-17-PP, LA-18-PP and a reference bacterial lipid A. *P<0.05, **P<0.01.

The biological activities of LA-17-PP and LA-18-PP detected in the in vitro assay systems are summarized in Table 9. The stimulatory effects on murine macrophages and polyclonal B cell activating activity on murine lymphocytes of the test lipid A analogs were not very different from those of the reference synthetic and bacterial lipid As.

TABLE 8. Induction of IFN-α/β in ICR mice primed with *P. acnes* by LA-17-PP and LA-18-PP: Comparison with reference synthetic and bacterial products[a]

Compound	Serum IFN-α/β titer (IU/ml of serum) induced with following dose, μg/mouse (no. of mice tested)				
	10	3.16	1	0.316	0.1
LA-17-PP	800 (2)	ND[b]	480 (2)	ND	100 (2)
LA-18-PP	640 (2)	ND	480 (2)	ND	< 20 (2)
LA-14-PP	3,413 (3)	ND	4,267 (3)	2,133 (3)	226 (3)
LA-15-PP	ND	2,560 (3)	800 (4)	1,920 (2)	360 (4)
F515 lipid A	2,560 (2)	3,840 (2)	960 (4)	1,920 (2)	480 (4)

[a] ICR mice pretreated with *P. acnes* one week before were intravenously challenged with test specimens. The assay results obtained in the same experimental conditions but by separate experiments were combined.
[b] Not determined.

TABLE 9. Summary of bioactivities of LA-17-PP and LA-18-PP as compared with those of reference synthetic and bacterial products [in vitro assays][a]

Compound	*Limulus* test		Human complement activation	Guinea pig macrophages		Murine macrophages Production of		Murine splenocytes	
	Pre Gel Test	Toxicolor Test		GlcN uptake	O_2^- generation	PGE_2	IL-1	Mitogenicity	PBA
LA-17-PP	++	±	+	±	+	+++	++	++	+++
LA-18-PP	+++	+	++	++	++	+++	++	+	+++
LA-14-PP	+++	++	++	++	+++	+++	++	++	+++
LA-15-PP	+++	+++	+++	+++	+++	+++	+++	+++	+++
F515 lipid A	+++	+++	+++	+++	+++	+++	+++	+++	+++
R595 lipid A	+++	+++	+++	+++	+++	+++	+++	+++	+++

[a] The activities of LA-15-PP (compound 506) were scored as +++ (based on the paper of Kotani et al, Infect. Immun., in press).

ANALGESIC ACTION OF LPS AND LIPID A, BACTERIAL AND SYNTHETIC

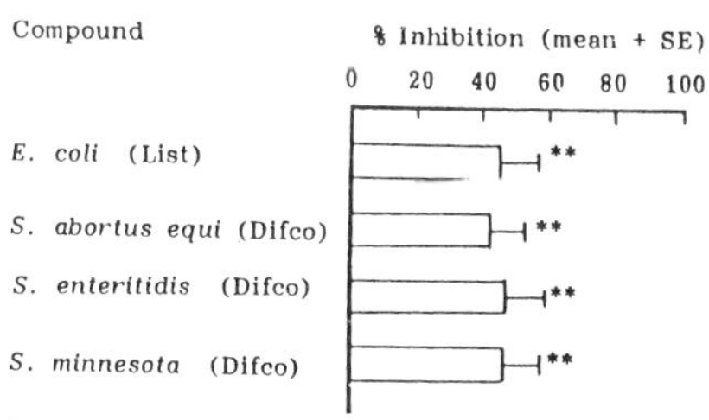

Fig. 4. Analgesic action of bacterial lipopolysaccharides. Test specimens (100 μg/mouse) were given 30 min before acctic acid injection. **P<0.01.

Figure 4 demonstrates that the pretreatment of male ddY mice by subcutaneous injection of several LPS specimens significantly decreased the frequency of writhing movements induced by intraperitoneal injection of aqueous acetic acid. This finding indicates that LPS has analgesic effects just as MDP and its acyl derivatives do (Mašek 1985; Ogawa and Kotani, submitted for publication). The analgesic action, a new neuropharmacological action of LPS, could be reproduced by compound 506 as well as *E. coli* F515 lipid A (data not shown). The analgesic effect was similarly induced by less toxic lipid A analogs, namely compounds 406, LA-17-PP and LA-18-PP as by toxic, synthetic or bacteial lipid As (Fig. 5).

CONCLUSION

Although the results so far obtained seem to be encouraging, none of the lipid A analogs had a strong enough useful bioactivity with minimal undesirable effects to the satisfactory extent. But further cooperative synthetic and biological studies may ultimately provide new types of synthetic immunomodulators that can be useful in clinical and preventive medicine.

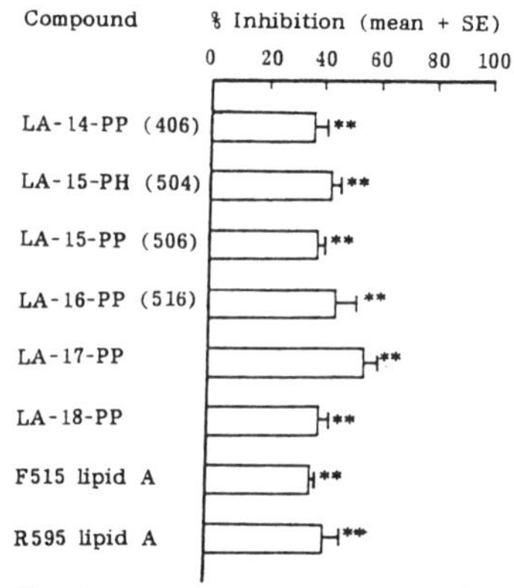

Fig. 5. Analgesic action of synthetic lipid As, *E. coli*- and *S. minnesota*-types, their analogs, and reference bacterial lipid As. Test specimens (100 µg/mouse) were given 30 min before acetic acid injection. **P<0.01.

ADDENDUM

The same preparations of synthetic lipid As and their analogs were examined for their endotoxic and related bioactivities by Freiburg/Borstel groups in West Germany (Galanos et al, 1984 & 1985) and J.Y. Homma's and S. Kanegasaki's groups in Tokyo (Homma et al, 1985; Kanegasaki et al, 1985 & 1986). There are no essential discrepancies among the results obtained by these research groups and ours though the items and systems of bioassays differ somewhat with the group.

REFERENCES

Ellouz F et al (1974). Minimal structural requirements for adjuvant activity of bacterial peptidoglycan derivatives. Biochem Biophys Res Commun 59:1317.

Galanos C et al (1984). Endotoxic properties of chemically synthesized lipid A part structures. Comparison of synthetic lipid A precursor and synbthetic analogues with biosynthetic lipid A precursor and free lipid A. Eur J Biochem 140:221.

Galanos C et al (1985). Synthetic and natural *Escherichia coli* free lipid A express identical endotoxic activities. Eur J Biochem 148:1.

Hansen-Hagge T et al (1985). Isolation and structural analysis of two lipid A precursors from a KDO deficient mutant of *Salmonella typhimurium* differing in their hexadecanoic acid

content. Arch Microbiol 141:353.
Homma JY et al (1985). Structural requirements of lipid A responsible for the functions: a study with chemically synthesized lipid A and its analogues. J Biochem Tokyo 98:395.
Imoto M et al (1984). Chemical synthesis of phosphorylated tetraacyl disaccharide corresponding to a biosynthetic precursor of lipid A. Tetrahedron Lett 25:2667.
Imoto M et al (1985). Total synthesis of *Escherichia coli* lipid A. Tetrahedron Lett 26:1545.
Kanegasaki S et al (1984). Biological activities of analogues of lipid A based chemically on the revised structural model. Comparison of mediator-inducing, immunomodulating and endotoxic activities. Eur J Biochem 143:237.
Kanegasaki S et al (1986). Structure-activity relationship and synthetic lipid A's with different fatty acid compositions. J Biochem Tokyo 99:1203.
Kotani S et al (1975). Immunoadjuvant activities of synthetic *N*-acetylmuramyl-peptides or -amino acids. Biken J 18:105.
Kotani S et al (1984). Immunobiologically active lipid A anlogs synthesized according to a revised structural model of natural lipid A. Infect Immun 45:293.
Kotani S et al (1985). Synthetic lipid A with endotoxic and related biological activities comparable to those of a natural lipid A from an *Escherichia coli* Re-mutant. Infect Immun 49:225.
Kotani S et al (1986). Low endotoxic activities of synthetic *Salmonella*-type lipid A with an additional acyloxyacyl group on the 2-amino group of β(1-6)glucosamine disaccharide 1,4'-bisphosphate. Infect Immun 52:872.
Kusumoto S et al (1976). Chemical synthesis of *N*-acetylmuramy peptides with partial structures of bacterial cell wall and their analogues in relation to immunoadjuvant activities. Bull Chem Soc Jpn 49:533.
Mašek K (1985). The novel pharmacological properties of a synthetic immunomodulators, muramyl dipeptide. Int J Immunother 1:177.
Qureshi N et al (1982). Purification and structural determination of nontoxic lipid A obtained from lipopolysaccharide of *Salmonella typhimurium*. J Biol Chem 257:11808.
Qureshi N et al (1985). Monophosphoryl lipid A obtained from lipopolysaccharides of *Salmonella minnesota* R595. Purification of the dimethyl derivative by high performance liquid chromatography and complete structural determination. J Biol Chem 260:5271.
Ribi E et al (1982). Preparation and antitumor activity of

nontoxic lipid A. Cancer Immunol Immunother 12:91.
Ribi E et al (1984). Lipid A and immunotherapy. Rev Infect Dis 6:567.
Stain SM et al (1985). Location of polar substituents and fatty acyl chains on lipid A precursors from a 3-deoxy-D-*manno*-ocutulosonic acid-deficient mutant of *Salmonella typhimurium*. Studies by ^{1}H, ^{13}C, and ^{31}P nuclear magnetic resonance. J Biol Chem 260:16089.
Takada H et al (1985). Immunopharmacological activities of a synthetic counterpart of a biosynthetic lipid A precursor molecule and of its analogs. Infect Immun 48:219.
Takada H, Kotani S (1985). Immunopharmacological activities of synthetic muramyl-peptides. In Stewart-Tull DES, Davies M (eds): "Immunology of the bacterial cell envelope", Chichester John Wiley & Sons, p 119.
Takayama K et al (1984). Separation and characterization of toxic and nontoxic forms of lipid A. Rev Infect Dis 6:439.

Immunopharmacology of Infectious Diseases: Vaccine Adjuvants and Modulators of Non-Specific Resistance, pages 235–244

MURAMYL PEPTIDES AS ENHANCERS OF HOST RESISTANCE TO BACTERIAL INFECTIONS

Monique A. Parant

Centre National de la Recherche Scientifique, Institut Pasteur, 75724 Paris Cedex 15, France.

INTRODUCTION

Particular host factors are of great importance in determining the outcome of an anti-infectious treatment. Chemotherapy of infections can be unsatisfactory in immunocompromised hosts, since without adequate cellular defences even the most potent antibiotic may be useless, no matter how sensitive the responsible organisms are. So the concept of host defence stimulation comes under renewed and increasing consideration. Actually, immunopotentiating products may turn out to be of major importance in case of problem infections in patients with qualitative and quantitative defects in their immune system. Systemic immunostimulants may therefore be used for the correction of generalized immunodeficiencies resulting for example from the use of drugs or from various chronic diseases, and to enhance the efficacy of chemotherapeutics. A combined therapeutic approach with immunostimulating agents may also be considered against various types of infections to lower the dose of the chemotherapeutic drug that may possess significant inherent toxicity or immunosuppressive effects.

Biological response modifiers (BRMs) can be used either to enhance immunologically specific responses and/or to activate mechanisms of nonspecific host resistance. The diversity and the flexibility of synthetic BRMs may lead to the production of agents displaying only the desired activity. Over the past decade, identification and synthesis of the smallest cell wall structure having the full adjuvant activity of peptidoglycan was decisively achieved (reviewed in Lederer, 1980). The synthesis of MDP (AcMur-L-Ala-D-iGln) or muramyl dipeptide, was followed by the preparation of a large number of analogs (see Lefrancier and Lederer, 1981; Adam, 1985), in an effort to separate desirable activities from adverse effects inherent to the administration of peptidoglycan. Minor chemical modifications have already provided water soluble compounds that do not exhibit untoward side effects (Chedid *et al.*,1982; Allison *et al.*, 1986). For example, Murabutide (AcMur-L-Ala-D-Gln-O*n*Bu) has been selected for development as an adjuvant of vaccines because it has given satisfactory results in several toxicity tests (Chedid *et al.*, 1982a). Several MDP analogs have thus been shown to stimulate specific humoral immunity to a wide variety of natural antigens from bacteria, viruses, and protozoa. They have also been shown to elicit antibodies to numerous synthetic antigens, usually after conjugation to a carrier. In studies related to synthetic vaccines, the use of constructs containing a muramyl dipeptide and antigenic peptides has already revealed some modifications of immune and other biological responses (reviewed in Audibert *et al.*, 1985). One approach has been to couple several different peptides together to create a larger polyvalent molecule capable of eliciting greater responses to each peptide than the response elicited by the individual peptides alone. With this strategy each peptide functions as a carrier for the others (Audibert *et al.*, 1985).

Several muramyl peptides, as well as other adjuvants, have additional effects such as increasing nonspecific immunity to infections or tumors. Many reports on the induction of resistance to bacterial, fungal or parasitic infections have been published (for review, see Parant, 1979; Dietrich *et al.*, 1983a), reflecting the ever-increasing efforts made by several laboratories. Chemically different muramyl peptides were comparatively evaluated, and their effect assessed in a variety of experimental test systems, such as acute infections in adult normal mice or rats, in T-cell depleted mice, in neonates, in mice immunodepressed by irradiation, corticosteroids, or cyclophosphamide treatments, and in mice subjected to chronic protein depletion (Parant, 1979; Kotani *et al.*, 1982; Galland *et al.*, 1982; Dietrich *et al.*, 1983a). Protection by muramyl dipeptides depends on size of the microbial inoculum and the microorganism used, and thereby the small-molecular products are less potent than more complex and heterogenous agents such as BCG (bacillus Calmette-Guérin) or LPS (lipopolysaccharides). In contrast to the other immunostimulants, muramyl dipeptides are not immunogenic unless they are coupled to a carrier, and do not produce a negative phase of higher susceptibility when given simultaneously with the bacterial inoculum (Parant and Chedid 1984). Several modifications physico-chemical of muramyl peptides have been used as means for enhancing anti-infectious effects, such as alteration of hydrophilicity, polymerization, or conjugation to a carrier.

HYDROPHILIC MURAMYL PEPTIDES

Some hydrophilic MDP analogs have shown the greatest separation of immunostimulant effects from side effects so far obtained. Thus, against a bacterial infection, the efficacy of Murabutide is quite comparable to that of MDP, and has also been demonstrated under conditions that make the animal very susceptible to the challenge, as is the case of newborn mice or in adults splenectomized at seven days of age (Chedid *et al.*, 1982a). Its protective activity has shown that an increase in body temperature is not a prerequisite for the immunostimulant properties since, in contrast to MDP, it is exempt of any pyrogenicity, and cannot induce the release of endogenous pyrogen either *in vivo* and *in vitro*.

Hydrophilic muramyl peptides are effective against an infectious challenge under timing conditions that usually lead to a depression of the immune response. Previous data have also shown that animals, which are low-responder to the adjuvant effect of MDP such as Lewis rats and C57Bl/6 mice, are protected against infections as effectively as high-responder animals (Parant, 1979). Moreover, like many immunoadjuvants, some hydrophilic analogs have been shown to generate a T cell-mediated immunosuppressive activity when given in repeated injections of large doses (Leclerc *et al.*, 1982). Such a treatment with MDP or with Murabutide does not impair their protective effect in mice subsequently infected with *Klebsiella pneumoniae* (Parant and Chedid, 1984). These results confirm that the adjuvant effect can be dissociated from the stimulating effect on nonspecific resistance.

LIPOPHILIC MURAMYL PEPTIDES

Several lipophilic MDP derivatives have been prepared to reproduce the anti-tumor activity of bacterial cell walls which have a high lipid content (Petit and Lederer, 1984). Actually, among them, some compounds were significantly effective in causing tumor regression (Kotani *et al.*, 1982; Dietrich *et al.*, 1983b; Phillips *et al.*, 1985). Against bacterial challenges, lipophilic derivatives have often been shown to exhibit a protective activity stronger than the original MDP (Parant *et al.*, 1980; Matsumoto *et al.*, 1981; Dietrich *et al.*, 1983b). Thus, the introduction of a stearoyl group resulted in an increased protective effect as evaluated in mice infected with *Escherichia coli* (Matsumoto *et al.*, 1981). Our data indicate that the presence of a lipophilic chain at the C-terminal peptide end (MDP-L-Ala-glycerol mycolate) resulted in increased effectiveness. The lipophilic compound was more active against *K.pneumoniae* and *Pseudomonas aeruginosa* infections, as was shown to elicit a significant degree of protection in mice challenged with a virulent strain of *Streptococcus pneumoniae*, whereas MDP was inactive. This compound is of particular interest since it has been shown to induce delayed-type hypersensitivity to a protein antigen in the absence of Freund's incomplete adjuvant (Parant *et al.*, 1980).

With another lipophilic MDP derivative MDP-GDP or MDP-dipalmitoyl-*sn*-glycerol (Phillips *et al.*, 1985), the protective effect was not markedly increased when the compound was administered as a suspension in saline. However, the incorporation of MDP-GDP in liposomes resulted in an enhanced protective activity in animals infected with *K.pneumoniae*, the effective dose being 1,000-fold lower. Similar potentiation has been reported when another encapsulated MDP derivative was administered in mice subsequently infected with *Candida albicans* or in hamsters with a localized *P.aeruginosa* skin infection (Eppstein *et al.*, 1986). The series of derivatives coupled with the dipalmitoyl-glycerol lipid moiety has revealed some interesting observation. Thus, free MDP(D,D)-GDP was a potent stimulator of host immunity, whereas the hydrophilic MDP(D,D) or AcMur-D-Ala-D-iGln was inactive. In contrast, the lipophilic derivatives of inactive muramyl tripeptides (obtained by linking of D-Ala or NMeAla) were still ineffective against infections.

OLIGOMERS AND CONJUGATES

A change in the physicochemical properties by polymerization may serve as a mean for enhancing anti-infectious activities of muramyl dipeptides by reducing the rapid excretion (Parant *et al.*, 1979) and by probably modifying the affinity for the target cells (Parant *et al.*, 1978).

The conjugation procedure with an appropriate carrier, natural or synthetic, immunogenic or non-immunogenic, was also used for increasing the size and efficiency of MDP and of some analogs. Thus, the anti-infectious activity was potentiated to a considerable extent when MDP or MDP(Lys) was linked to a synthetic carrier, multi-poly(DL-Ala)--poly (L-Lys), hereafter abbreviated as A--L, to BSA (bovine serum albumin), tetanus toxoid, or to viral subunits (Chedid *et al.*, 1986; Parant *et al.*, 1986). With the A--L chain, it has been shown that the inactive MDP stereoisomer, MDP(D,D), could acquire some potency against various bacterial infections (*Klebsiella*, *Pseudomonas*, and *Listeria*) after coupling though it remained inactive as immunoadjuvant (Chedid *et al.*, 1979). Other carriers such as Influenza viral subunits have been used to prepare conjugates endowed with a similar protective activity, i.e. effective at a very low dosage level of MDP. Even more interesting is the fact that such a conjugate prepared with viral subunits may enhance the mouse resistance against an unrelated viral infection when administered intranasally, whereas free MDP was inactive (Parant *et al.*, 1986). This type of investigation has a potential for developing antibacterial and antiviral agents endowed with both specific and nonspecific activities. In some cases, the pyrogenicity of the glycopeptide was increased after conjugation (Chedid *et al.*, 1982b), but the effective dose is far smaller than with free MDP, and the same procedure could be repeated with non-pyrogenic MDP analogs.

INFLUENCE OF INDOMETHACIN

Treatment with indomethacin prevents the febrile responses to free or conjugated MDP derivatives but does not affect immunoadjuvant effects. The enhancement of nonspecific resistance to infectious challenges elicited by MDP or derivatives was not antagonized by the anti-pyretic drug, in most cases it was even increased. Thus, a synergistic effect could be demonstrated against *Listeria* or *Klebsiella* infections when indomethacin was administered with a low dose of MDP-A--L; ineffective by itself (Parant *et al.*, 1980). So, neither pyrogenicity nor increased prostaglandin levels appeared to be necessary for stimulation of the resistance by muramyl peptides. However, indomethacin does not decrease MDP-induced release of endogenous pyrogen *in vivo* or *in vitro* and is even known to potentiate IL1 production in some cases (Damais *et al.*, 1982). Such macrophage-derived factors could be implied in resistance to infections. Moreover, the effect of indomethacin may be related to enhanced phagocytosis of particles and O_2^- generation (Gay *et al.*, 1985) and to suppress the negative feedback of arachidonic acid metabolites on factor production.

COMBINED USE OF MURAMYL PEPTIDES AND ANTI-MICROBIAL AGENTS

Several studies were undertaken to evaluate the therapeutic usefulness of an antibiotic-immunostimulant combination against infection. The potential importance of these treatments has stimulated the evaluation of muramyl peptides with regard to their possible synergistic, and/or additive effect with antibiotics. In normal mice, the first observation has been reported with soluble glycopeptides administered subcutaneously, MDP or nor-MDP, and a cephalosporine derivative given orally. It was shown that in many types of acute infections (*K.pneumoniae, Pasteurella multocida,* and *Salmonella typhimurium*), the median effective dose of antibiotic was lowered by muramyl dipeptide treatment (Dietrich *et al.*, 1981). With a single subcutaneous injection of gentamicin administered two hours after a Klebsiella challenge, we observed a synergistic effect with MDP. To minimize the protection elicited by the glycopeptide alone, the challenge dose of bacteria was increased, and the combined treatment with MDP and the antibiotic resulted in a significant increase in the number of survivors. The efficacy of the non-pyrogenic Murabutide and of the lipophilic derivative MDP-GDP was evaluated in the same experimental model and found quite comparable. With another lipophilic derivative (6-O-stearoyl-MDP), Osada *et al.* (1982) have also reported a marked increase in average survival time as compared with mice receiving either the stearoyl-MDP or the antibiotic alone. This effect was demonstrated with cefazolin and gentamicin against various types of infection (Osada *et al.*, 1982). *Candida albicans* is considered to be an important nosocomial pathogen, its establishment in patients being facilated by corticoids, antitumor agents, tissue damage, and impaired cellular immunity. Against an experimental murine candidiasis lipophilic MDP derivatives were superior (Osada *et al.*, 1982; Eppstein *et al.* 1986), and their efficacy was enhanced by the simultaneous administration of anti-fungal agents. In our assays, the protective effect of MDP-GDP was assessed by the increase in survival time after a severe challenge that killed almost all the controls within 5 days. Administration of amphotericin B in a single injection was successful in increasing the protective activity. Various combinations of antibiotics and MDP derivative should still be examined, and their efficacy evaluated in both normal and immunodepressed animals.

SYNERGISM BETWEEN MDP AND LPS

As for BCG, there exists a toxic synergism between MDP and LPS which was first reported by Ribi *et al.*,(1979). Like with BCG and LPS, it is also possible to produce the production of TNF (tumor necrosis factor) by administering MDP and LPS simultaneously (Chedid *et al.*, 1986). Moreover, such a combination was shown to be very potent in inducing necrosis and regression of grafted tumors in mice (Bloksma *et al.*, 1984). Against a bacterial infection (*K.pneumoniae*) we observed that a low dose of LPS (1 ng) could potentiate the protective effect of MDP or Murabutide in mice challenged with a large bacterial inoculum. Both the effect against tumors and against infection could be related to the production of TNF.

COMBINED USE OF MURAMYL PEPTIDES AND CYTOKINES

The first example of a synergistic combination between MDP and a cytokine has been provided by Sone and Fidler (1980). By incorporating both MAF (macrophage-activating factor) and MDP in liposomes, they could synergistically stimulate the tumoricidal activity of rat alveolar macrophages *in vitro* and they obtained a therapeutic effect against cancer metastases (Sone and Fidler, 1980; Fidler and Schroit, 1984). Recombinant human TNF was used against a diverse range of experimental infections and was shown to reproduce the marked protective effect previously demonstrated by us with TNF serum prepared in mice (Parant *et al.*, 1980), indicating that TNF could represent an important mediator in nonspecific immunity (Chedid *et al.*, 1986; Parant *et al.*, 1986). To evaluate a possible potentiation by muramyl peptides, mice were infected with a severe challenge of *C.albicans*. The survival was considerably increased (about 50 % on day 30) by the combined treatment with rTNF and MDP-GDP, which could only produce a significant delay in mortality when given alone.

The production of endogenous mediators by recombinant DNA technology should permit further investigations regarding their role against bacterial, viral, and parasitic infections. By the combined use of muramyl peptides, the effective dose of recombinant molecules -and thereafter their untoward toxicity- could be reduced. Efforts should be directed toward improving combined treatments.

REFERENCES

Adam A (1985). "Synthetic Adjuvants". New York: John Wiley & Sons, 239 pages.

Allison AC, Byars NE, Waters RV (1986). Immunologic adjuvants : efficacy and safety considerations. In Nervig RM, Gough PM, Kaeberle ML, Whetstone CA (eds): "Advances in Carriers and Adjuvants for Veterinary Biologics", Ames: The Iowa University Press, p 91.

Audibert F, Leclerc C, Chedid L (1985). Muramyl peptides as immunopharmacological response modifiers. In Torrence PF (ed): "Biological Response Modifiers", Orlando: Academic Press, p 307.

Bloksma N, Hofhuis FMA, Willers JMN (1984). Endotoxin-induced antitumor activity in the mouse is highly potentiated by muramyl dipeptide. Cancer Letters 23:159.

Chedid L, Parant M, Parant F, Audibert F, Lefrancier P, Choay J, Sela M (1979). Enhancement of certain biological activities of muramyl dipeptide derivatives after conjugation to a multi-poly(DL-Ala)--poly(L-Lys) carrier. Proc Natl Acad Sci USA 76:6557.

Chedid L, Parant M, Audibert F, Riveau G, Parant F, Lederer E, Choay J, Lefrancier P (1982a). Biological activity of a new synthetic muramyl peptide adjuvant devoid of pyrogenicity. Infect Immun 35:417.

Chedid L, Parant M, Riveau G (1982b). Immunopharmacological activities of MDP. In Webb DR (ed): "Immunopharmacology and the Regulation of Leukocyte Function", New York: Marcel Dekker, p 159.

Chedid L, Parant M, Parant F, Riveau G (1986). Nonspecific effects of LPS on bacterial infections. In Szentivanyi A, Nowotny A, Friedman H (eds): "The Immunobiology and Immunopharmacology of Bacterial Endotoxins, Basic and Clinical Aspects", New York: Plenum Press, in press.

Damais C, Riveau G, Parant M, Gerota J, Chedid L (1982). Production of lymphocyte-activating factor in the absence of endogenous pyrogen by a rabbit or human leukocytes stimulated by a muramyl dipeptide derivative. Int J Immunopharmac 4:451.

Dietrich FM, Sackmann W, Zak O, Dukor P (1981). Synthetic muramyl dipeptide immunostimulants; protective effects and increased efficacy of antibiotics in experimental bacterial and fungal infections in mice. In Nelson JD, Grassi G (eds): "Current Chemotherapy and Infectious Diseases", Am Soc Microbiol p 1730.

Dietrich FM, Sackmann W, Mitchell GH, Voller A (1983a). Modulation of resistance to infections by synthetic low molecular-weight compounds endowed with immunostimulatory properties : experimental results and potential role in human medicine. In Anand N, Sen AB (eds): "Chemotherapy and Immunology in the Control of Malaria, Filariasis and Leishmaniasis", New Delhi: Tata McGraw-Hill Publ, p 277.

Dietrich FM, Lukas B, Schmidt-Ruppin KH (1983). MTP-PE (synthetic muramyl peptide) : prophylactic and therapeutic effects in experimental viral infections. 13th Int Cong Chemotherapy, p 1730.

Eppstein DA, Van der Pas MA, Fraser-Smith EB, Kurahara CG, Felgner PL, Matthews TR, Waters RV, Venuti MC, Jones GH, Metha R, Lopez-Berestein G (1986). Liposome-encapsulated muramyl dipeptide analogue enhances non-specific host immunity. Int J Immunother 11:115.

Galland RB, Trachtenberg LS, Rynerson N, Polk HC (1982). Non-specific enhancement of resistance to local bacterial infection in starved mice. Arch Surgery 117:161.

Gay JC, English D, Lukens JN (1985). Stimulation of neutrophil oxidative metabolism by indomethacin. Agents Actions 16:336.

Kotani S, Takada H, Tsujimoto M, Kubo T, Ogawa T, Azuma I, Ogawa H, Matsumoto K, Siddiqui WA, Tanaka A, Nagao S, Kohashi O, Kanoh S, Shiba T, Kusumoto S (1982). Nonspecific and antigen specific stimulation of host defence mechanisms by lipophilic derivatives of muramyl dipeptides. In Jeljaszewicz J, Pulverer G, Roszkowski W (eds): "Bacteria and Cancer", London: Academic Press, p 67.

Kotani S, Takeda H, Tsujimoto M, Ogawa T, Mori Y, Koga T, Iribe A, Tanaka S, Nagao S, McGhee JR, Michalek SM, Morisaki S, Kawata T, Shiba T, Kusumoto S (1983). Lipophilic muramyl peptides and synthetic lipid A analogs as immunomodulators. In Yamamura Y, Tada T (eds): "Progress in Immunology V", Tokyo: Academic Press, p 1359.

Leclerc C, Bourgeois E, Chedid L (1982). Demonstration of muramyl dipeptide (MDP)-induced T suppressor cells responsible for MDP immunosuppressive activity. Europ J Immunol 12:249.

Lederer E (1980). Synthetic immunostimulants derived from the bacterial cell wall. J Med Chem 23:819.

Lefrancier P, Lederer E (1981). Chemistry of synthetic immunomodulant muramyl peptides. In Herz W, Grisebach H,Kirby GW (eds): "Progress Chem Org Nat Prod, vol 40", New York: Springer Verlag, p 1.

Matsumoto K, Ogawa H, Kusama T, Nagase O, Sawaki N, Inage M, Kusumoto S, Shiba T, Azuma I (1981). Stimulation of nonspe-

cific resistance to infection induced by 6-O-acyl muramyl dipeptide analogs in mice. Infect Immun 32:748.
Osada Y, Mitsuyama M, Matsumoto K, Une T, Otani T, Ogawa H, Nomoto K (1982). Stimulation of resistance of immuno-compromised mice by a muramyl dipeptide analog. Infect Immun 37:1285.
Parant M (1979). Biologic properties of a new synthetic adjuvant, muramyl dipeptide (MDP). Springer Semin Immuno-pathol 2:101.
Parant M, Parant F, Chedid L, Yapo A, Petit JF, Lederer E (1979). Fate of the synthetic immunoadjuvant, muramyl dipeptide (^{14}C-labeled) in the mouse. Int J Immunopharmac 1:35.
Parant M, Riveau G, Parant F, Dinarello CA, Wolff SM, Chedid L (1980). Effect of indomethacin on increased resistance to bacterial infection and on febrile responses induced by muramyl dipeptide. J Infect Dis 142:708.
Parant M, Audibert F, Chedid L, Level M, Lefrancier P, Choay J, Lederer E (1980). Immunostimulant activities of a lipophilic muramyl dipeptide derivative and of desmuramyl peptidolipid analogs. Infect Immun 27:826.
Parant M, Parant F, Chedid L (1980). Enhancement of resistance to infections by endotoxin-induced serum factor from *Mycobacterium bovis* BCG-infected mice. Infect Immun 28:654.
Parant M, Chedid L (1984). Stimulation of nonspecific resistance to infections by synthetic immunoregulatory agents. Infection 12:230.
Parant M, Masihi KN, Lange W, Brehmer W,Parant F, Jolivet M, Chedid L (1985). Enhancement of nonspecific resistance to bacterial and viral infections by MDP conjugated to tetanus toxoid or viral subunits. Infect Immun, in press.
Parant M, Parant F, Vinit MA, Chedid L (1986). Tumor necrosis factor, an endotoxin-induced monokine, as mediator of non-specific antimicrobial immunity. EOS J Immunol Immuno-pharmac 6:5234.
Petit JF, Lederer E (1984). The structure of the mycobacterial cell wall. In Kubica GP, Wayne LG (eds): "The Mycobacteria", New York: Marcel Dekker, p 301.
Phillips NC, Moras ML, Chedid L, Lefrancier P, Bernard JM, (1985). Activation of alveolar macrophage tumoricidal activity and eradication of experimental metastases by freeze dried liposomes containing a new lipophilic muramyl dipeptide derivative. Cancer Res 45:125.
Ribi EE, Cantrell JL, Von Eschen KB, Schwartzman SM (1979). Enhancement of endotoxic shock by N-acetyl-muramyl-L-alanyl-(L-seryl)-D-isoglutamine (muramyl dipeptide). Cancer Res 39:4756.

Immunopharmacology of Infectious Diseases: Vaccine Adjuvants and Modulators of Non-Specific Resistance, pages 245–254

STIMULATION OF HOST DEFENSE MECHANISMS WITH SYNTHETIC MDP AND CHITIN DERIVATIVES AGAINST VIRAL INFECTION IN MICE

Ichiro Azuma, Joji Iida, Keiko Nishimura, Chiaki Ishihara and Yuichi Yamamura*

Institute of Immunological Science, Hokkaido University, Sapporo 060, and *Osaka University, Suita 565, Japan

INTRODUCTION

It has been reported that the immunoadjuvants stimulate not only immune responses but also host-resistance against cancer and bacterial and viral infections. The authors have reported the immunological properties of various kinds of bacterial fractions such as the cell-wall skeletons (CWS) of *Mycobacterium bovis* BCG, *Nocardia rubra*, *Propionibacterium acnes* and *Listeria monocytogenes* (Azuma *et al*., 1985). Especially BCG-CWS and *N. rubra*-CWS were shown to be effective for the prolongation of survival periods of cancer patients and for the protection against viral infections. Recently, synthetic immunoadjuvants such as the analogs and derivatives of N-acetylmuramyl-L-alanyl-D-isoglutamine (MDP), cord factor (trehalose dimycolate, TDM), lipid A and chitin, were chemically synthesized and examined their immunological properties in our laboratory collaborating with several research groups in Japan.

In this symposium, the authors will summarize our recent results on the stimulation of host-resistance with synthetic stearoyl-MDP derivatives and chitin derivatives against viral infection in mice.

MATERIALS AND METHODS

Adjuvant

N-Acetylmuramyl-L-alanyl-D-isoglutamine (MDP), 6-O-stearoyl-N-acetylmuramyl-L-alanyl-D-isoglutamine (L18-MDP) and N^{α}-acetylmuramyl-L-alanyl-D-isoglutaminyl-N^{ε}-stearoyl-L-lysine [(MDP-Lys(L18)] (Fig. 1) were synthesized by the procedure described previously (Kusumoto et al., 1976, 1978, 1979). Chitin was prepared from queen crab shells according to the method of Hackman (1954). Partially (70%) deacetylated chtins (DAC-70) was prepared from chitin by deacetylation in suitable alkaline conditions as reported previously (Nishimura et al., 1984). Carboxymethyl-chitin (CM-chitin) was prepared by the carboxymethylation of 6-O position of chitin (Tokura et al., 1983) and N-methylated DAC-70 [DAC-70(Me)] was synthesized from DAC-70 by N-methylation (Fig. 2). These polysaccharides were dissolved by homogenizing in saline at a concentration of 2.5 mg/ml and sterilized by heating at 60°C for 30 min just before use.

Animals

Specific pathogen-free, male inbred BALB/c slc mice of 4-6 weeks of age were obtained from Shizuoka Cooperative for Experimental Animals, Hamamatsu, Japan. Water and pelleted diets (Nihon Nosan Kogyo Co., Ltd., Yokohama, Japan) were supplied ad libitum.

Protection against Sendai Virus Infection

Mice were intranasally (in) administered 0.02 ml of the adjuvant solution under light Ketamine (Ketalar-50, Sankyo Co., Ltd., Tokyo, Japan) anesthesia. The 0.2 ml of the adjuvant preparation was also administered through infra-orbital venous plexus or through intraperitoneal route. The Sendai strain of parainfluenza type I virus was purchased from Flow Laboratories Inc., Rockville, MD, U.S.A. and passed for 10 generations in suckling C3H/He mice before storing. Mouse lungs of the 10th passage were homogenized in PBS, and the supernatant fluid was dispersed in ampoules in 1 ml lots, frozen and stored as stock virus suspension at -70°C until used. For each experiment, an ampoule was thawed, and 0.03 ml of the stock virus suspension was infected intranasally under light Ketamine anesthesia. The infectious inoculum was $10^{4.4}$ virus when determined by haemadsorption in LLCMK2 cells. The protective effect of adjuvants was represented as percent of survivors recorded 21 days after Sendai virus infection.

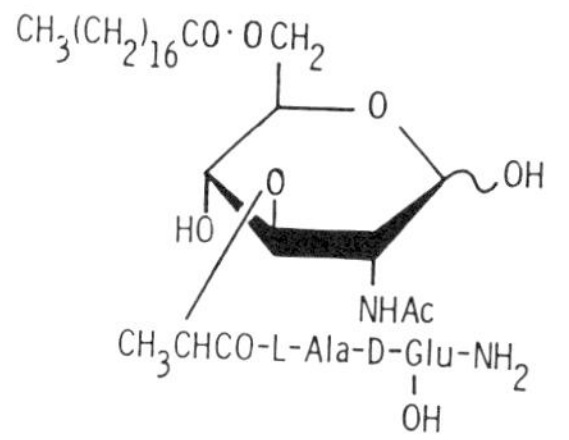

L18-MDP

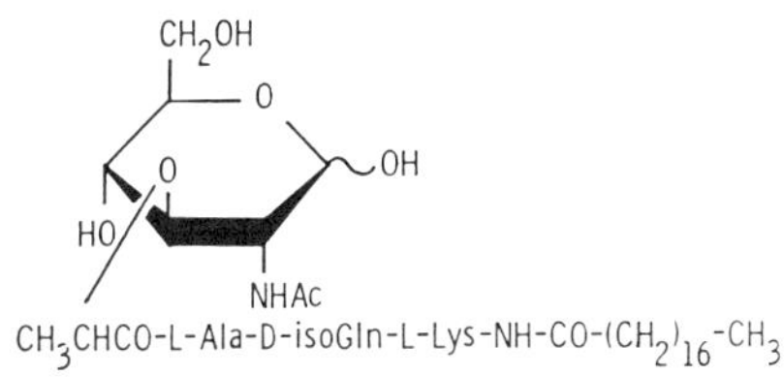

MDP-Lys-L18

Figure 1. Stearoyl derivatives of N-acetylmuramyl-L-alanyl-D-isoglutamine (MDP).

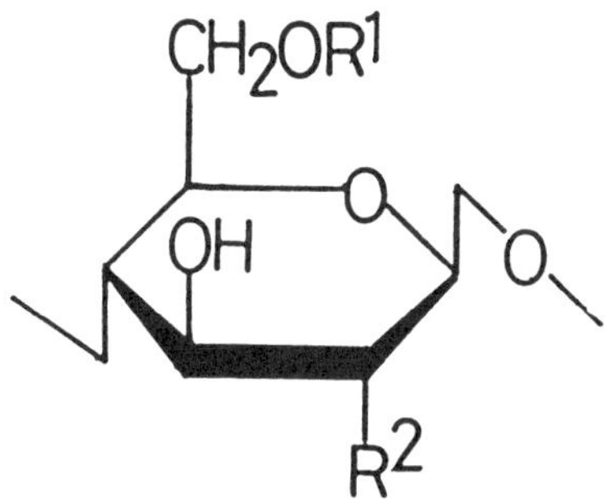

R^1= H	R^2= $NHCOCH_3$	: 0.3	70% deacetylated chitin (DAC-70)
	NH_2	: 0.7	
R^1= H	R^2= $NHCOCH_3$	: 0.3	N-methylated DAC-70 (DAC-70(Me))
	$N^+(CH_3)_3$	: 0.7	
R^1= CH_2COOH	R^2= $NHCOCH_3$		Carboxymethyl chitin (CM-chitin)

Figure 2. Chitin derivatives.

RESULTS

Effect of MDP-Lys(L18) on Host Resistance against Sendai Virus Infection in Mice

Intranasal pretreatment with MDP, L18-MDP and MDP-Lys-(L18) dissolved in PBS augmented the nonspecific resistance to intranasal infection with Sendai virus in mice. Intranasal administration of MDP-Lys(L18) and L18-MDP gave 100% and 88% survival rates, respectively. MDP also showed 71% survival rate. The survival rate of control group was 38%. Intranasal administration of MDP-Lys(L18) (10 μg) 3 days and 1 day before intranasal challenge with Sendai virus resulted in 100% survival rates; however, administration of MDP-Lys-(L18) 1 day after the infection was 20% and control group was 20%, in this experimental condition. It was also shown that intranasal administration of 10μg and 1μg of MDP-L18(L18) showed 86% and 83% survival rate, respectively, but the survival rate of the group treated with 0.1 μg of MDP-Lys(L18) was 29% and control group was 29%. The effect of administration route of MDP-Lys(L18) was examined by using the same experimental model. Intranasal administration of MDP-Lys(L18) was highly effective even at a dose of 10 μg per mouse (100% survival rate). When mice were treated with a 100 μg dose of MDP-Lys(L18) by intravenous or intraperitoneal route, the survival rates were 60% and 67%, respectively. The survival rate of control mice was 20%. Subcutaneous injection of MDP-Lys(L18) was not effective (33%) for the protection against Sendai virus infection in comparison with that of control group (20%). The details of this experiment have been reported and discussed previously (Ishihara _et al_., 1985).

Effect of Chitin Derivatives on Resistance against Sendai Virus Infection in Mice

The protective effect of chitin derivatives, DAC-70, CM-chitin, DAC-70(Me), on the Sendai virus infection was examined by using the same experimental model described above. MDP-Lys(L18) was used as positive control. As shown in Fig.3, intranasal administration of DAC-70 (50 μg), DAC-70(Me) (50 μg) and MDP-Lys(L18) (10 μg) 1 day before infection was effective for the prevention against Sendai virus infection. However, intranasal administration of CM-chitin was ineffective in this experimental condition. By the dose response

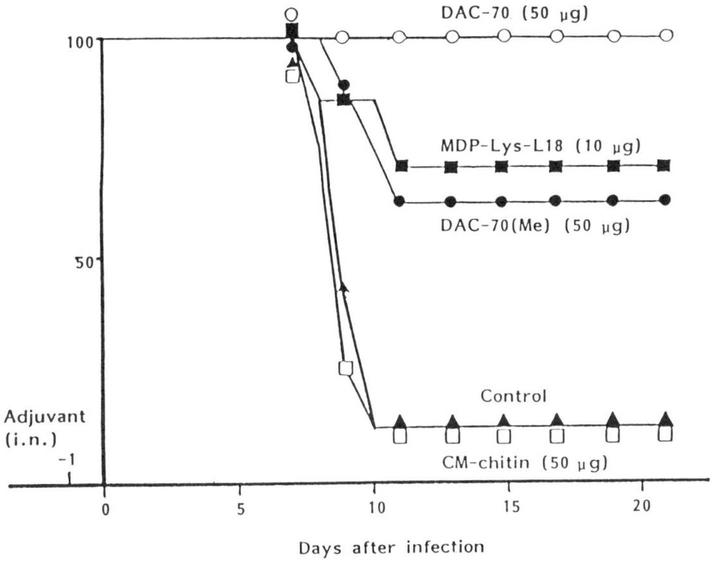

Figure 3. Preventive effect of chitin derivatives given intranasally (in) against Sendai virus infection in mice.

test, it was shown that the survival rates of mice treated with 50, 10, 1, 0.1 μg of the DAC-70 1 day before infection and of control mice were 100%, 83%, 67%, 57% and 14%, respectively. DAC-70 was effective even at dose of 0.1 μg in comparison with control. The survival rate of MDP-Lys(L18) (at 10 μg) was 71%. The experiment on the interval between DAC-70 treatment and Sendai virus infection indicated that the intranasal administration of 50 μg of DAC-70 7, 3 and 1 days before the infection showed 100% of survival rate, however, the administration of DAC-70 1 day after the infection was not effective. Multiple administration intranasally of 50 μg of DAC-70 1, 2 and 3 days after the infection showed no effect on survival rate compared with control mice. The effect of the route of administration of DAC-70 on resistance against Sendai virus infection was examined. Intranasal administration 1 day before infection of DAC-70 was most effective at a dose of 50 μg (100% survival rate). Intravenous administration of DAC-70 (100 μg) showed 67% survival rate, however, intraperitoneal and subcutaneous administrations of DAC-70

(100 μg) revealed no protective activity (25% and 33% respectively) in comparison with control group (0%). As shown in Table 1, lung washings collected 24 h after Sendai virus infection from MDP-Lys(L18)- or DAC-70- treated mice contained high titers of α/β interferon. However, DAC-70 treatment without infection produced no interferon not only in the lung washings but also in the serum. Only low titer of interferon was detected in the lung washings of the control group.

TABLE 1. Induction of Interferon in DAC-70-treated and Sendai Virus-infected Mice

Treatment	Mean interferon titer (U/ml)	
	serum	lung washings
DAC-70 alone	<20	17
DAC-70 + infection	<10	1585
MDP-Lys(L18) + infection	38	1278
Infection alone	<20	208

Mice were treated intranasally with 50 μg of DAC-70 1 day before infection of $10^{4.4}$ HAD Sendai virus.

DISCUSSION

After the first report by Ellouz *et al*. (1974) on MDP, various kinds of biological activities have been reported (Adam and Lederer, 1984). Chedid *et al*. (1977) have reported that MDP stimulated host-resistance against *Klebsiella pneumoniae* infection in mice. Matsumoto *et al*. (1981a, 1981b, 1983) have also examined 64 acyl-MDP derivatives as adjuvants for the stimulation of host-resistance against nonspecific bacterial infection by using sepsis type infection model with *Escherichia coli* in mice, and selected 2 candidates, L18-MDP and MDP-Lys(L18). The stimulatory effects of both stearoyl-MDP derivatives were examined in detail (Matsumoto *et al*.,

1983; Okuda et al., 1986; Osada et al., 1982a, 1982b, 1982c, 1982d). Both stearoyl-MDP derivatives were shown to be effective for stimulation of host-resistance against infection with *E. coli*, *Staphylococcus aureus*, *Pseudomonas aeruginosa* and *Candida albicans*, but not effective for infections with *Salmonella typhimurium* and *Listeria monocytogenes*. It was also shown that both stearoyl-MDP derivatives stimulated the hosts which were immunosuppressed by the treatment with cyclophosphamide, x-irradiation, cortisone or by aging in mice, rats and guinea pigs. Both stearoyl-MDP derivatives were shown to have a synergistic effect on combination with antibiotics such as cephazolin, gentamicin and amphotericin B. On the mechanism of stimulation of the host with stearoyl-MDP derivatives, Osada et al. (1982c) have shown that functions such as migration, phagocytosis and production of superoxide of polymorphonuclear cells were stimulated by the administration of stearoyl-MDP derivatives. The authors have also shown that both L18-MDP and MDP-Lys(L18) are effective for host stimulation against opportunistic infection with *C. kutscheri* infection in mice (Ishihara et al., 1984).

Chitin, β-(1→4)-poly-N-acetyl-D-glucosamine, is widely distributed in nature, e.g. in crustaceans, insects, mushrooms and the cell walls of bacteria, and is characteristic of rigid crystalline structure through intra- and intermolecular hydrogen bonds. The authors have reported the chemical synthesis of chitin which was purified from queen crab shells and examined the immunological properties in detail (Nishimura et al., 1984, 1985, 1986a). Among these chitin derivatives, DAC-70 was shown to have the most potent immunoadjuvant activity on the murine macrophage activation, induction of delayed type hypersensitivity and production of circulating antibody in guinea pig, and induction of allogeneic killer T cells, activation of natural killer (NK) cells, induction of cytokines such as IL-1 and CSF in mice. DAC-70 was also shown to have activities for the suppression of murine tumor, Meth A in BALB/c mice, and stimulation of host-defense mechanism against *E. coli* infection in mice. More recently, the authors reported that the multi-porous beads prepared from 80% deacetylated chitin (DAC-80) was effective for the activation of murine peritoneal macrophage *in vivo* (Nishimura et al., 1986b). The usefulness of the multi-porous beads of DAC-80 as the unique carrier of drugs such as anticancer chemotherapeutics and hormones is now being investigated in our laboratory. The details of anti-infectious activity of chitin derivatives will be reported elsewhere.

Although further investigation will be required to clarify the mechanism of stearoyl-MDP derivatives and chitin derivatives on the immune cells, especially on macrophages and polymorphonuclear cells, these synthetic compounds may play very important roles as the non-specific immunoadjuvants for the protection of bacterial and viral infections.

In conclusion, the authors would like to emphasize that nonspecific immunostimulation of host-defense mechanisms, especially on immunocompromized hosts such as cancer patients will be important subjects in the future, and immunoadjuvants will be one of the most useful tools in this field.

SUMMARY

The authors described the experimental approaches for the stimulation with synthetic immunoadjuvants of host-defense mechanism against Sendai virus infection in mice. Stearoyl-MDP derivatives and chitin derivatives, especially MDP-Lys(L18) and DAC-70, were shown to be effective for the protection against Sendai virus infection in BALB/c mice. It was shown that at 1 day after infection high titer of α/β-interferon was detected in the lung washing of mice treated with MDP-Lys(L18) or DAC-70 1 day before infection. The effectiveness as immunoadjuvant for the host stimulation of MDP-Lys(L18) and DAC-70 was also discussed.

ACKNOWLEDGMENT

This work was supported in part by Grants-in-Aid for Cancer Research from the Ministry of Education, Science and Culture, Japan; from the Ministry of Health and Welfare for Comprehensive 10-Year Strategy for Cancer Control, Japan; and also for Scientific Research from the Ministry of Education, Science and Culture, Japan.

REFERENCES

Adam A, Lederer E (1984). Muramyl peptides immunomodulators, sleep factors, and vitamins. Medicinal Res Rev 4: 111-152.

Azuma I, Yamamura Y (1985). Stimulation of host-defense mechanisms with immunoadjuvants. In Reichard S, Kojima M (eds): "Macrophage Biology: Progress in Leukocyte Biology Vol.4," New York: Alan R. Liss, 597.

Chedid L, Parant M, Lefrancier P, Choay J, Lederer E (1977). Enhancement of nonspecific immunity to Klebsiella pneumoniae infection by a synthetic immunoadjuvant (N-acetylmuramyl-L-alanyl-D-isoglutamine) and several analogs. Proc Natl Acad Sci USA 74: 2089-2093.

Ellouz F, Adam A, Ciorbaru R, Lederer E (1974). Minimal structural requirement for adjuvant activity of bacterial peptidoglycan derivatives. Biochem Biophys Res Commun 59: 1317-1325.

Hackman RH (1954). Chitin. I. Enzymic degradation of chitin and chitin esters. Aust J Biol Sci 7: 168-178.

Ishihara C, Hamada H, Yamamoto K, Iida J, Azuma, I (1985). Effects of muramyl dipeptide and its stearoyl derivatives on resistance to Sendai virus infection in mice. Vaccine 3: 370-374.

Ishihara C, Yamamoto K, Hamada N, Azuma I (1984). Effect of stearoyl-N-acetylmuramyl-L-alanyl-D-isoglutamine on host resistance to Corynebacterium kutscheri infection in cortisone-treated mice. Vaccine 2: 261-264.

Kusumoto S, Ikenaka K, Shiba T (1979). Synthesis of several muramyl peptides in relation to chemical structures of less immunoadjuvant bacterial cell wall. Bull Chem Soc Jpn 52: 1655-1671.

Kusumoto S, Okada S, Yamamoto K, Shiba T (1978). Synthesis of 6-O-acyl derivatives of immunoadjuvant active N-acetyl-muramyl-L-alanyl-D-isoglutamine. Bull Chem Soc Jpn 51: 2122-2126.

Kusumoto S, Tarumi Y, Ikenaka K, Shiba T (1976). Chemical synthesis of N-acetylmuramyl peptides with partial structures of bacterial cell wall and their analogs in relation to immunoadjuvant activities. Bull Chem Soc Jpn 49: 533-539.

Matsumoto K, Ogawa H, Kusama T, Nagase O, Sawaki N, Inage M, Kusumoto S, Shiba T, Azuma I (1981a). Stimulation of non-specific resistence to infection induced by 6-O-acyl muramyl dipeptide analogs in mice. Infect Immun 32: 748-758.

Matsumoto K, Ogawa H, Nagase O, Kusama T, Azuma I (1981b). Stimulation of nonspecific resistance to infection induced by muramyl dipeptides. Microbiol Immunol 25: 1047-1058.

Matsumoto K, Otani T, Une T, Osada Y, Ogawa H, Azuma I (1983). Stimulation of nonspecific resistance to infection induced by muramyl dipeptide analogs substituted in the γ-carboxy group and evaluation of N^{α}-muramyl dipeptide-N^{ϵ}-stearoyl-lysine. Infect Immun 39: 1029-1040.

Nishimura K, Ishihara C, Ukei S, Tokura S, Azuma I (1986a). Stimulating effect of 70% deacetylated chitin on the production of cytokines in mice. Vaccine (submitted).

Nishimura K, Nishimura S, Nishi N, Numata F, Tone Y, Tokura S, Azuma I (1985). Adjuvant activity of chitin derivatives in mice and guinea pigs. Vaccine 3: 379-384.

Nishimura K, Nishimura S, Nishi N, Saiki I, Tokura S, Azuma I (1984). Immunological activity of chitin and its derivatives. Vaccine 2: 93-99.

Nishimura K, Nishimura S, Seo H, Nishi N, Tokura S, Azuma I (1986b). Macrophage activation with multi-porous beads prepared from partially deacetylated chitin. J Bio Mat Res (in press).

Okuda T, Endo N, Zen-Yoji H, Osada Y (1986). Restoration by N^{α}-(N-acetylmuramyl-L-alanyl-D-isoglutamine)-N^{ε}-stearoyl-L-lysine from the decomplement state in mice induced by cobra venom factor, followed by acquisition of resistance to bacterial infections. J Jap Associ Infect Dis 60: 204-209 (in Japanese).

Osada Y, Mistuyama M, Matsumoto K, Une T, Otani T, Ogawa H, Nomoto K (1982a). Stimulation of resistance of immunocompromised mice by a muramyl dipeptide analog. Infect Immun 37: 1285-1288.

Osada Y, Mitsuyama M, Une T, Matsumoto K, Otani T, Satoh M, Ogawa H, Nomoto K (1982b). Effect of L18-MDP(Ala), a synthetic derivative of muramyl dipeptide, on nonspecific resistance of mice to microbial infections. Infect Immun 37: 292-300.

Osada Y, Otani T, Sato M, Une T, Matsumoto K, Ogawa H (1982c). Polymorphonuclear leukocyte activation by a synthetic muramyl dipeptide analog. Infect Immun 38: 848-854.

Osada Y, Otani T, Une T, Ogawa H, Nomoto K (1982d). Enhancement of non-specific resistance to Pseudomonas pneumoniae by a synthetic derivative of muramyl dipeptide in immunosuppressed guinea pigs. J Gen Microbiol 128: 2361-2370.

Tokura S, Nishi N, Tsutsumi A, Somorin O (1983). Studies on chitin. VIII. Some properties of water soluble chitin derivatives. Polymer J 15: 485-489.

Immunopharmacology of Infectious Diseases: Vaccine Adjuvants and Modulators of Non-Specific Resistance, pages 255–265

MODULATION OF NON-SPECIFIC RESISTANCE BY MTP·PE

Peter Dukor and Gebhard Schumann

Research Department, Pharmaceuticals Division,
CIBA-GEIGY Limited, CH-4002 Basel, Switzerland

INTRODUCTION

As for any other group of drugs, the beneficial use of immunomodulators depends on their therapeutic window, i.e. the margin between wanted pharmacological effects and unwanted side effects. Drug prototypes are often unsatisfactory in this respect: their efficacy is either to small or toxicity to high.

There are three classical strategies of improvement: The synthesis of derivatives, the diligent choice of altered schedules and routes of administration and the development of suitable delivery forms. Muramylpeptides provide a case in point. Through the pioneering work of Lederer (Ellouz et al., 1974), Kotani (Kotani et al., 1975), Chedid (Chedid et al., 1978) and their associates, MDP (N-acetyl-muramyl-L-alanyl-D-isoglutamine) has become the essential reference compound in immunostimulation. However, a number of well-known shortcomings have limited or prevented its clinical use: MDP is rapidly eliminated and has only moderate effects on cell-mediated immunity and non-specific resistance to many bacterial pathogens, and to viruses or tumor cells. Moreover, it is pyrogenic and leads to generalized inflammatory reactions at higher dose levels in sensitive species (Wachsmuth and Dukor, 1981).

Three main avenues have been pursued in the search for second generation derivatives of MDP: Analogs with decreased pyrogenic and phlogogenic properties such as GIRPI's murabutide (Chedid et al., 1982) and Syntex' threonyl-MDP (Jones et al., 1978), antigen-conjugated MDPs as vaccines with intrinsic adjuvanticity (Leclerc et al., 1983), and lipophilic MDPs, of which several representatives have been reviewed in this book. Increased lipophilic properties ought to provide a prolongation of plasma-half life, slow release from lipophilic binding sites and compartments, decreased plasma peaks, altered penetration into tissue compartments, facilitated insertion into biomembranes, stable incorporation into liposomes, and hence a qualitatively different biological profile.

In this contribution, we will restrict ourselves to a brief review of MTP·PE (N-acetyl-muramyl-L-alanyl-D-isoglutaminyl-L-alanine-2-(1',2'-dipalmitoyl-sn-glycero-3'-hydroxy-phosphoryl-oxy)-ethylamide-mono-sodium salt) (Tarcsay et al., 1981), which in a liposomal formulation has recently entered clinical trials in the U.S..

BIOLOGICAL PROFILE OF HYDROPHILIC AND LIPOPHILIC MDPs

There are distinct differences between the biological profiles of hydrophilic and lipophilic MDPs that can mostly be attributed to differential pharmacokinetics (Schumann and Dukor, 1986).

MDP and nor MDP (desmethyl-MDP) are cleared from blood and tissues within minutes, while MTP·PE has a much longer plasma half-life. In terms of acute tolerability, MTP·PE is less pyrogenic, particularly if injected s.c. or i.m.. MTP·PE also has a smaller tendency to induce slow-wave-sleep and the so called guinea-pig distress syndrome. Probably due to its physicochemical characteristics, MTP·PE may induce delayed-type hypersensitivity (DTH) to simultaneously administered peptide antigens even if given without lipid vehicles. As an inducer of non-specific resistance, MTP·PE displays longer-lasting prophylactic effects, particularly against fungi and viruses. Moreover, its antiviral and anti-tumor properties are more pronounced than those of the watersoluble parent compounds.

However, early observations by Fidler, Poste and others indicated, that liposome-entrapped immunostimulants could be targeted to macrophages (Poste et al., 1979; Schroit et al.,

1983), thus enhancing the induction of tumor cytotoxicity. In this context, MTP·PE appeared to be particularly well-suited for stable incorporation into multilamellar vesicles (MLV). In this way, it was hoped to simultaneously achieve increased efficacy and a decrease of systemic toxicity, thus widening the therapeutic window of MTP·PE.

EFFECT OF LIPOSOME ENCAPSULATION ON PHARMACOKINETICS, TOLERABILITY AND BIOLOGICAL PROFILE OF MTP·PE

The liposome technology used by our group (Fankhauser and van Hoogevest, 1986) is based on fully synthetic endogenous lipids: palmytoyl oleyl phosphatidyl choline (POPC) and dioleyl phosphatidylserine (OOPS) in a 7:3 weight ratio. They are combined with MTP·PE in an organic solvent usually in a proportion of 1:250 w/w. Proprietary methods are used to achieve a dry lipid preparation, which can be mass produced and stored. The formulation is constituted into liposomes prior to use by adding Ca^{++} and Mg^{++}free PBS, and by vortexing, and yields MLV with an average size of 2.3μ. They remain stable in suspension for several weeks. Using ^{14}C-labelled lipid and ^{3}H-labelled drug it was found that MTP·PE - in contrast to hydrophilic MDP or nor MDP - remains firmly associated with the liposomes. Any vesicles or aggregates greater than 7μ are removed by filtration during injection.

Both, lipophilic substitution and liposome-entrapment, dramatically change the distribution and fate of radiolabelled MDP. In a systematic study, Fogler et al. (1985) compared the pharmacokinetics of free and liposome-encapsulated ^{3}H-nor MDP and ^{3}H-MTP·PE following i.v. administration in mice. The initial plasma half-life of the hydrophilic nor MDP is about 2.5 minutes, and within 1 hour 75% of the injected radioactivity is recovered in the urine as intact molecules. Only low levels of radioactivity are retained in the organs.

In contrast, free MTP·PE is eliminated much more slowly, with some 20% of the injected dose remaining in the circulation one hour later. At 24 hours, appreciable levels of radioactivity are still distributed to all organs, with significant accumulation in the liver and still more than 3% of the initial dose in the blood. Radioactivity is almost exclusively associated with intact MTP·PE and its two main metabolites MDP and lyso-MTP·PE.

Liposome-entrapped MTP·PE one hour after injection is found to have distributed to the lung, where levels stay relatively elevated over 24 hours. Blood levels remain remarkably constant throughout the observation period and do not show the initially very high concentrations that are seen with free MTP·PE.

The findings indicate that liposome-entrapped MTP·PE may remain longer available to relevant compartments than hydrophilic nor MDP, but avoids excessive exposure of the circulatory system that may be characteristic for the free lipophilic compound. Indeed, as shown repeatedly in independent studies in three different institutions by Graepel (1986), Kanter (1986) and Fidler et al. (1985), liposome-encapsulation markedly reduces the systemic toxicity of MTP·PE.

We reported earlier that free MTP·PE given parenterally in high doses to rabbits or dogs is prone to induce generalized inflammatory lesions (Braun et al., 1984). Thus, free MTP·PE given to dogs at a dose of 0.1 mg/kg/day i.v. for only two weeks leads to the development of epi- and pericarditis, to synovitis and to characteristic vascular lesions in small arteries (subintimal and medial cell infiltration). In contrast, liposome-encapsulated material in the same daily dose, but given for a period of 3 months, fails to elicit any of these pathological manifestations. Apart from the elevation of $alpha_2$- and $beta_1$-globulins, and of fibrinogen, from an accelerated sedimentation rate and transient increases in monocytes and neutrophils, no changes in general symptomatology are observed (Graepel, 1986).

Similar results are obtained in rabbits and guinea pigs, and 0.1 mg/kg/day is now considered to represent a no toxic effect level for prolonged administration of liposome-encapsulated MTP·PE.

On the other hand, liposome-encapsulated muramylpeptides clearly display enhanced pharmacological activity in many model systems. Mere lipophilic substitution of the MDP-moiety is already conferring a markedly higher potency to the parent molecule. Fogler and Fidler recently compared the macrophage-activating potency of different forms and formulations of MDP. As measured by the induction of tumoricidal properties, free lipophilic MTP·PE is approximately 40 times more potent than nor MDP in a human monocyte system. As was shown separately, this is directly related to a greater uptake of MTP·PE (Fogler and Fidler, 1986 b).

If nor MDP is entrapped in MLV, about 400 x less MDP is required to reach the same level of monocyte cytotoxicity as with the free nor MDP. Again, this is due to a proportionally greater cellular uptake of the liposome-encapsulated material (Fogler and Fidler, 1986 a).

However, for the already highly cytotropic MTP·PE liposome-entrapment leads merely to a further 4 x increase in potency. Indeed, liposomal MTP·PE is even considerably less potent than liposome-entrapped water-soluble nor MDP. This is not surprising, since nor MDP is released rather rapidly from the liposomes, while the tightly bound MTP·PE stays associated with the lipid vesicles for a prolonged time (Fogler and Fidler, 1986 b). This may also explain the significantly longer persistence of MTP·PE liposome-induced monocyte cytotoxicity.

These findings in vitro translate into increased efficacy of lipid-substituted and of liposomal MTP·PE in suitable models of non-specific resistance in vivo. This is particularly striking in some fungal systems: While prophy lactic induction of resistance to C. albicans infections by hydrophilic MDPs is only very short-lasting, MTP·PE induces resistance for up to two weeks (Sackmann and Dietrich, 1986). However, the efficacy of MTP·PE in this model is apparently not further enhanced by liposomal entrapment.

Several groups have reported that lipophilic MDPs administered in free form via different routes or entrapped in MLV have also pronounced protective or even therapeutic effects in a variety of viral infections.

Thus i.n., s.c. or i.v. administered free MTP·PE was shown to exert prophylactic effects in mice infected with influenza A, B, parainfluenza 1 or herpes simplex type 1 (HSV 1) viruses (Dietrich et al., 1986). Again, MTP·PE affords a more marked and clearly longer duration of protection than watersoluble MDPs.

In several models of viral disease, resistance is further enhanced by the use of liposome-encapsulated MTP·PE. In a series of experiments by Gangemi et al. (1986), survival of C3H/HeN mice with an otherwise lethal HSV-1 pneumonitis could be significantly increased by MTP·PE using different treatment schedules. Liposome-encapsulated MTP·PE in each instance proves to be more effective than free i.v. drug. Protection is highly significant if 100μg of encapsulated material is given 3 x i.v. on days -3, 0, and +2 relative to nasal infection.

These data support earlier findings by Koff in HSV-2 infections, where an increased rate of survival was obtained in mice treated with 40μg of liposomal MTP·PE i.v. 2 days before,simultaneously with and 2 days after an i.p. or i.v. viral challenge (Koff et al., 1985). Analogous results were reported by Kende et al. (1983), who achieved prophylactic and even therapeutic effects in murine Rift Valley fever infections in mice treated i.v. with MTP·PE in liposomes, and by Acevedo (1986), who observed considerable prolongation of survival in Friend leukemia virus-infected SJL mice following s.c. pretreatment with liposome-encapsulated MTP·PE. Parenteral application of free MTP·PE was less effective in all these systems.

However, the antiviral efficacy of MTP·PE has not remained uncontroversial, since some of the results proved to differ with different laboratory conditions (Morahan et al., 1986). Clearly, rigorous standardization of models, materials and procedures is called for in order to further clarify the therapeutic potential of this compound.

Moreover, the mechanism of the antiviral effects of MTP·PE is not yet fully understood. In vivo, MTP·PE given by itself is not an inducer of interferon (IFN), does not change the kinetics of serum or lung IFN during viral infections, but enhances IFN levels in tissues and plasma if given prior to an IFN inducer such as Tilorone (Dietrich et al., 1986). In vitro, on the other hand, MTP·PE fails to prime for IFN synthesis, and, on the contrary even inhibits the induction of IFNs by a variety of inducing agents (Meyer et al., 1986).

Possibly, much of the antiviral activity of MTP·PE must

be attributed to the induction of macrophage cytotoxicity. Indeed, in vitro free and liposome-encapsulated MTP·PE was shown by Koff et al. (1984) to render monocytes selectively cytotoxic to HSV2-infected, but not to uninfected normal target cells.

As is the case in several viral infections, liposome-encapsulation greatly increases the biological efficacy of MTP·PE also in various tumor systems. In the classical model originally introduced by Fidler (1980), C57Bl/6 mice are injected with melanoma cells into a footpad and the tumor bearing leg is amputated some 4 weeks later. Even if i.v. therapy with free MTP·PE is initiated in doses up to 2.5mg/kg within days after amputation, almost all mice succumb to lung and lymph node metastases. On the other hand, as little as 10µg of encapsulated MTP·PE is sufficient to eradicate metastases in a high proportion of animals (Schumann and Dukor, 1986).

Liposome composition is critical in this and several other models. Delivery to macrophages, macrophage activation and anti-metastatic activity in vivo are greatly enhanced by the phosphatidyl serin component (Schroit and Fidler, 1982; Fidler 1985): While MTP·PE in POPC liposomes is virtually ineffective, MTP·PE encapsulated in 7 parts POPC and 3 parts of either OOPS or dimyristoyl phosphatidyl serine leads to apparent cures in a high percentage of melanoma-inoculated and surgically treated mice (Schumann and Dukor, 1986). Indeed, as has been suggested by Tanaka and Schroit (1983), PS exposed in the plasma membrane of aged RBC may provide a signal for their recognition by macrophages.

Of course, the anti-metastatic activity in the melanoma model also critically depends on the treatment schedule. In a recent systematic study by Fidler (1986) it was determined that 2 x weekly treatment for 4 weeks gives nearly optimal results (10µg/dose), while 1 x weekly for 8 weeks is clearly less effective and 1 x weekly for 4 weeks does not provide significant benefits at all.

MTP·PE in appropriately constituted MLV displays tumor therapeutic properties also in other models including growth inhibition of autochthonous UV-induced skin carcinoma and sarcoma by systemic i.v. 2 x weekly administration of MTP·PE in MLV. In this way, host survival is prolonged significantly (Talmadge et al., 1986).

However, biological response modifiers including MTP·PE may eventually become clinically useful only if used in appropriate combination with other agents. A large body of evidence, mainly from Fidler and Sone and their associates, indicates a striking synergism between muramylpeptides and macrophage-activating lymphokines (MAF, gammaIFN) (Sone and Fidler, 1980; Saiki and Fidler, 1985; Saiki et al., 1985). This is exemplified by a recent experiment by Sone et al. (1986), where human monocytes are rendered cytotoxic in vitro by incubation with threshold doses of liposomal MTP·PE and increasing concentrations of rhugammaIFN, which by itself confers only minimal cytotoxicity.

As was originally shown by Ruco and Meltzer (1978), the activation of macrophages to the tumor cytotoxic state requires at least 2 activation steps in a defined sequence: lymphokine priming followed by a bacterial triggering signal. In the case of gammaIFN and MTP·PE, gammaIFN primes the monocytes to respond to MTP·PE, which then triggers the expression of macrophage cytotoxicity.

While in vivo combination of gammaIFN with liposomal MTP·PE may have considerable promise, combination of MDP-mediated macrophage activation with more conventional cytoreductive therapy could be a modality of choice. Recent data of Saiki et al. (1986) provide a good example: C_3Hf/Kam mice are injected i.v. with 10^5 fibrosarcoma cells which localize in the lung. Five days later the mice are treated with low dose local thoracic irradiation (5 or 8 Gy) followed by 10μg MTP·PE in MLV, given i.v. twice weekly for 4 weeks. This regimen leads to significant survival of mice (which at day 140 are sacrificed and can be shown to be tumor-free). Treatment with irradiation alone or MTP·PE-MLV alone is significantly less effective. Clearly, administration of MTP·PE-MLV after reduction of the total tumor burden by classical therapeutic regimens may have clinical potential.

EFFECT OF BACTERIAL COMPONENTS AND MTP·PE ON IMMUNOGLOBULIN ISOTYPE EXPRESSION

In addition to, but possibly still linked to macrophage activation, there is yet another property of muramylpeptides that may have profound effects on host resistance: modulation of immunoglobulin isotype expression of lymphoid cells.

As discovered by Durkin et al. (1981) Peyer's patches (PP) of germfree (GF) rats and conventional rats differ strikingly. GF rat PP contain high numbers of surface IgE-bearing cells (20% of total), 1/2 of which simultaneously display sIgA, while $sIgE^+$ cells are absent from PP of conventional rats. GF rat PP also contain elevated numbers of $sIgA^+$ cells and decreased numbers of $sIgM^+$ cells.

Exposure to components of normal gut flora was found to dramatically affect the cellular composition of gut associated lymphoid tissue (Durkin et al., 1986): Within 18 hours after feeding GF rats with certain bacteria or after oral, but not i.v. treatment with murein, MDP or MTP·PE, $sIgE^+$ B cells are eliminated and the other surface isotypes normalized. On the other hand, LPS, core lipid A, and E. coli lipoprotein are ineffective. The component-induced changes are paralleled by shifts in the number of suppressor T cells (Thy 1^+ phenotype) which are greatly elevated in GF rat PP. Feeding with appropriate bacteria or oral murein, MDP or MTP·PE, but not with the other bacterial components, eliminates the suppressors and elevates the helper cells.

After each treatment, there is no evidence of cell division in PP or of a redistribution of $sIgE^+$ or Thy 1^+ cells to bone marrow, other lymphoid organs or blood. On the other hand, cell transfer studies indicate that purified $sIgE^+IgA^-$ cells acquire the $sIgE^+IgA^+$ and $sIgE^-IgA^+$ phenotypes in conventional, but not GF rats (Durkin et al., 1986).

Taken together, the data suggest that components of gut flora, in particular murein and muramylpeptides influence IgE to IgA isotype switching in PP B-cells possibly through the mediation of macrophages and sThy 1^+ regulatory cells. Since on a dose-effect base MTP·PE is even more potent than murein or MDP in stimulating these effects, isotype regulation by MTP·PE may prove to have clinical significance in a variety of conditions including the modulation of host defense to mucosal infections.

REFERENCES

Acevedo H (1986). In preparation.
Braun DG, Dukor P, Lukas B, Schumann G, Tarcsay L, Court H, Schaffner JC, Skripsky T, Fischer M, Graepel P (1984). In "International Seminar on the Immunological System as a Target for Toxic Damage", Luxembourg, Commission of the European Communities.
Chedid L, Audibert F, Johnson AG (1978). In "Progr Allergy", Basel:Karger, p.63.
Chedid L, Parant MA, Audibert FM, Riveau GJ, Parant FJ, Lederer E, Choay JP, Lefrancier PL (1982). Infect.Immun. 35:417.
Dietrich FM, Hochkeppel HK, Lukas B (1986). Int J Immunopharmac (in press).
Durkin HG, Bazin H, Waksman BH (1981). J exp Med 154:640.
Durkin HG, Chice SM, Bazin H, Tarcsay L, Dukor P (1986). Sixth Int Congr Immunol, Abstract (Toronto, Canada).
Ellouz F, Adam A, Ciorbaru R, Lederer E (1974). Biochem Biophys Res Commun 59:1317.
Fankhauser P, van Hoogevest (1986). In preparation.
Fidler IJ (1980). Science 208:1469.
Fidler IJ (1985). Cancer Res 45:4714
Fidler IJ (1986). Cancer Immunol Immunother 21:169.
Fidler IJ, Brown NO, Hart IR (1985). J Biol Response Modifiers 4:298.
Fogler WE, Fidler IJ (1986a). J Immunol 136:2311.
Fogler WE, Fidler IJ (1986b). Int J Immunopharmac (in press).
Fogler WE, Wade R, Brundish DE, Fidler IJ (1985). J Immunol 135:1372.
Gangemi JD, Nachtigal M, Barnhart D, Krech L, Jani P (1986). J Infect Dis (in press).
Graepel P (1986). In preparation.
Jones GH, Moffatt JG, Nestor Jr JJ (1978). USP-4,082.736.
Kanter P (1986). In preparation.
Kende M, Schroit AJ, Rill W, Canonico P (1983). ICAAC Abstract (Las Vegas, Nevada), p 108.
Koff WC, Fidler IJ, Showalter SD, Chakrabarty MK, Ceccorulli LM, Kleinerman ES (1984). Science 224:1007.

Koff WC, Showalter SD, Hampar B, Fidler IJ (1985). Science 228:495.
Kotani S, Watanabe Y, Kinoshita F, Shimono T, Morisaki I, Shiba T, Kusumoto S, Tarumi Y, Ikenaka K (1975). Biken J 18:105.
Leclerc C, Morin A, Chedid L (1983). In Thompson RA, Rose NR (eds) "Clinical Immunology", Edinburgh:Churchill Livingstone 3:187.
Meyer T, Dietrich FM, Walker MR, Hochkeppel HK (1986). J Interferon Res 6:183.
Morahan PS, Leake ER, Tenney DJ, Bit M (1986). This volume.
Poste G, Kirsh R, Fidler IJ (1979). Cell Immunol 44:71.
Ruco LP, Meltzer MS (1978). J Immunol 121:2035
Sackmann W, Dietrich FM (1986). In preparation.
Saiki I, Fidler IJ (1985). J Immunol 135:684.
Saiki I, Sone S, Fogler WE, Kleinerman ES, Lopez-Berestein G, Fidler IJ (1985). Cancer Res 45:6188.
Saiki I, Milas L, Hunter N, Fidler IJ (1986). Cancer Res 46:4966.
Schroit AJ, Fidler IJ (1982). Cancer Res 42:161.
Schroit AJ, Hart IB, Madsen J, Fidler IJ (1983). J Biol Response Modifiers 2:97.
Schumann G, Dukor P (1986). In preparation.
Sone S, Fidler IJ (1980). J Immunol 125:2454.
Sone S, Tandon P, Utsugi T, Ogawara M, Shimizu E, Nii A, Ogura T (1986). Int J Cancer (in press).
Talmadge JE, Lenz BF, Klabansky R, Simon R, Riggs C, Guo S, Oldham RK, Fidler IJ (1986). Cancer Res 46:1160.
Tanaka Y, Schroit AJ (1983). J Biol Chem 258:11335.
Tarcsay L, Baschang G, Hartmann A, Stanek J (1981). EP-A-0025495.
Wachsmuth ED, Dukor P (1981). In Yamamura Y, Kotani S (eds): "Immunomodulation by microbial products and related synthetic compounds", Amsterdam:Excerpta Medica, p. 60.

Immunopharmacology of Infectious Diseases: Vaccine Adjuvants and Modulators of Non-Specific Resistance, pages 267–278

PROTECTIVE EFFECTS OF A NEW IMMUNOMODIFIER, LF 1695, ON BACTERIAL AND PARASITIC INFECTIONS IN NORMAL RODENTS

Marc Pascal, Phillippe Lagrange and Michel Joseph

Laboratoires Fournier, Research Center, Daix, 21121 Fontaine les Dijon, France (MP), Institut Pasteur, 25 Rue du Dr Roux, 75724 Paris-Cedex 15, France (PL), Institut Pasteur, 15 rue Camille Guerin, 59019 Lille-Cedex, France (MJ).

INTRODUCTION

Evaluation of an immunomodifier in experimental infection models is often a difficult task for the following reasons:

a) Most of the models used deal with animals possessing a normal immune status. Thus compounds with immunorestorative potential may not demonstrate their efficacy in such models.

b) Immune resistance differs from one model to another. Depending on the host and the microorganisms different types of cells and mechanisms are involved. Therefore results may vary greatly from one model to another.

c) Models usually involve acute infection and may not be representative of the potential usefulness of an immunomodifier in chronic infection.

Conflicting and even disappointing results can be obtained with immunomodifiers, especially those acting on acquired cellular immunity. Such compounds can stimulate or suppress immune responses depending on their targets and on the treatment protocol used. A reasonable approach would be to use well documented models for which resistance mechanisms are well understood and which would be compatible with the presumed properties of the compound. This should permit a better understanding of the effect of the compound and its potential usefulness as an antiinfective agent in humans.

LF 1695 [5 amino-2-(4 methyl-1-piperidinyl)-phenyl]-(4 chlorophenyl)-methanone, is a new immunomodifier which has been shown to modulate mouse and human proliferative responses to lectins, and to induce differentiation of bone marrow T precursor cells (Othmane et al., 1985). Besides its action on T lymphocytes, LF 1695 has been shown to activate mouse peritoneal macrophages in a specific way (Pascal and Derrepas, 1986). As with certain products derived from microorganisms, LF 1695 induces interleukin 1 (IL-1) synthesis and secretion and potentiates phagocytosis. However, by contrast with microbially derived products, prostaglandin E2 (PGE2) synthesis was not induced but was inhibited when stimulated by lipopolysaccharide (LPS) or calcium ionophore A23187. Leukotriene B4 (LTB4) synthesis, on the other hand, was induced to high levels indicating that arachidonic acid metabolism was activated and directed toward lipoxygenase product information through prostaglandin inhibition. Such results indicate that LF 1695 activates macrophages to generate positive signals (IL-1, LTB4) for T cells but inhibits negative signals such as PGE2.

Recent data demonstrate that the differentiating activity of LF 1695 was not restricted to T cells: leukemic promyelocytic cells (HL 60) or histiocytic lymphoma cells (U 937) differentiate into functionally mature granulocytes and into macrophage-like cells, respectively (unpublished data).

In view of these properties of LF 1695 investigations were made using four experimental infection models. The models were chosen in relation to the mechanism of resistance described for them, and their relevance to what is known concerning their compound targets.

LISTERIA MONOCYTOGENES INFECTION IN MICE

In mice, host resistance to <u>Listeria monocytogenes</u> appear to be mediated by different cell populations. During the first 2 days of infection, resistance is mediated by radioresistant resident macrophages providing a non-T-cell-mediated protection (Mitsuyama et al., 1978). Thereafter acquired cellular immunity, as demonstrated by adoptive transfer experiments or infection in T-cell-deprived mice, permits clearance of remaining bacteria (Nomoto et al., 1983, Mackaness, 1969, Lane and Unanue, 1972). This T cell dependent mechanism of resistance correlates with delayed-type hypersensitivity (DTH) to Listeria (Kaufman and Hahn, 1982).

Moreover a T cell-independent acquired resistance that is particularly enhanced in nude mice, mediated by radiosensitive monocyte derived macrophages, has been described (Newborg and North, 1980).

When LF 1695 was administered by the intraperitoneal route at a dose of 5 mg/kg, 3 hours before or 3 hours after infection, growth curves of Listeria monocytogenes in the spleen and liver (Figure 1) indicated that bacterial counts were reduced in treated compared to control animals only after 48 and 72 hours of infection.

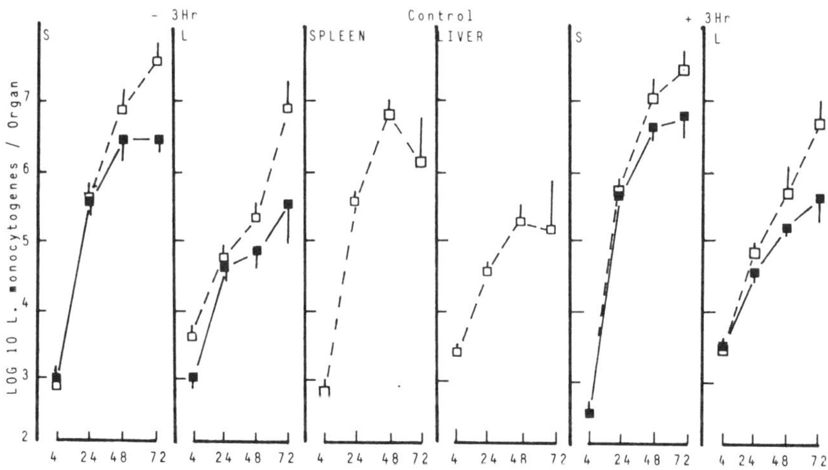

Fig 1 : Growth of L.monocytogenes (2.7×10^4/mouse) in Spleen (S) and in Liver (L) inoculated I.V in normal mice (Control) and in mice which received one single I.P injection of 0.5 ml of LF 1695 (■) (5 mg/kg) or the same volume of diluent (□). 3 hours before (- 3Hr) or 3 hours after (+ 3Hr) the challenge. Mean of 5 mice $\pm$ SEM.

The resistance index measured 72 hours after infection was maximally enhanced in mice treated with LF 1695 48 hours before infection (Figure 2) indicating that the drug had a preventive action. However, a slight increase in the resistance index was observed in mice treated after infection.

The growth curves suggest that LF 1695 is acting on late acquired resistance. If innate resistance were involved, an effect of the compound should have been observed in the first 48 hours of infection. Furthermore, evidence that acquired immunity is implicated in the preventive effect of LF 1695 comes from experiments demonstrating enhanced DTH to Listeria antigens measured at day 7 after infection (Figure 3).

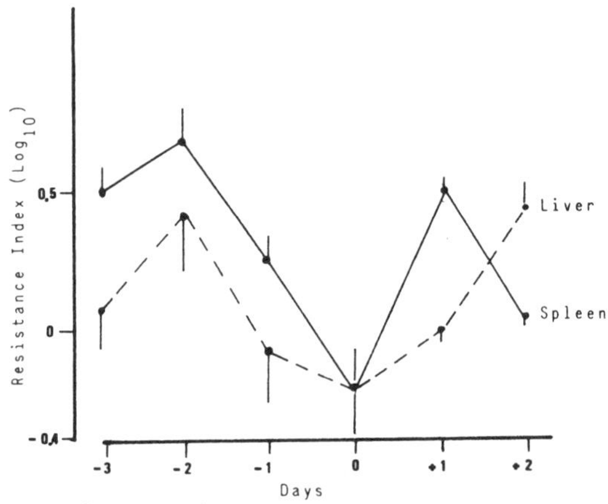

Fig 2 : Resistance Index in Spleen and liver expressed 72 hours after one I.V injection of 3.5×10^4 L.monocytogenes in mice which received one I.P injection of 0.5 ml of LF 1695 (5 mg/kg) or the same volume of diluent at varying time Intervals before or after the challenge given at To. Mean of 5 mice $\pm$ SEM.

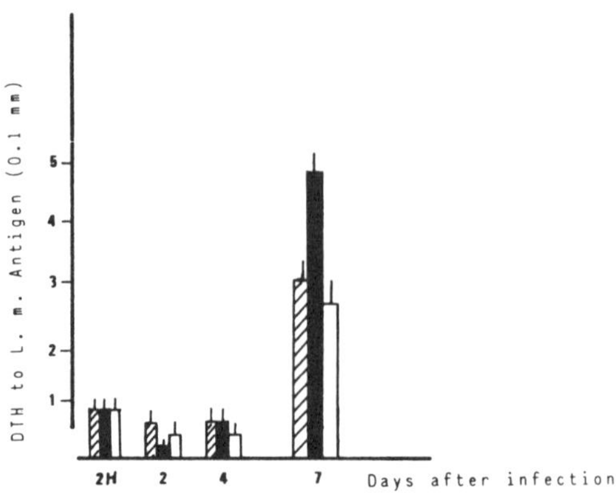

Fig 3 : Levels of 24 H DTH to 33 ug of L.monocytogenes antigens developped in listeria monocytogenes infected mice on day 0 : hatched bar, control group, black bar, mice treated with one IP injection of LF 1695 (5 mg/kg), two days prior infection, open bar, mice treated with diluent only.
Mean of 5 mice $\pm$ SEM

No effect of LF 1695 could be observed in irradiated or dextran sulfate treated animals suggesting that radiosensitive monocytes are implicated, although T cell participation cannot be excluded.

The results obtained with LF 1695 are clearly different from those described for microbially derived products such as *Corynebacterium parvum*; in the latter case, resident macrophage-mediated innate resistance was enhanced, bacterial counts in organs being reduced as early as 24 hours after infection (Miyata et al., 1980). However, DTH was suppressed by *Corynebacterium parvum* treatment indicating a reduced acquired immunity.

Increased resistance to *Listeria* monocytogenes infection by LF 1695 could be due to potentiation of T cell activation by LF 1695 or to increased monocytosis as already observed in rodents (non-published data). Alternatively, inhibition of prostaglandin synthesis by LF 1695 may be implicated as the suppression of acquired resistance to *Listeria monocytogenes* has been shown to be mediated by prostaglandins (Petit et al., 1985).

CANDIDA ALBICANS INFECTION IN MICE

Infection by *Candida albicans* usually develops in individuals with depressed immunity where Candida specific cellular immunity response is often altered, suggesting that T lymphocytes and macrophages are involved (Rogers and Balish, 1980). In mice infected with low doses of *Candida albicans*, resistance appears to be mediated by T cells. However, when high doses are used ($>10^6$ *Candida albicans*/mice) death occurs rapidly, and resistance is only mediated by polymorphonuclear cells (Hurtrel et al., 1980). LF 1695 activity was investigated in this latter model in order to assess its capacity to activate phagocytic polymorphonuclear cells. As shown in Figure 4, LF 1695 treatment did not modify survival time.

MYCOBACTERIUM BOVIS INFECTION IN MICE

In mice infected intravenously with *Mycobacterium bovis* (BCG strain), the bacteria proliferate in various organs during 12 to 21 days. Thereafter proliferation ceases and a progressive elimination of bacteria occurs concomitantly with the establishment of a specific cellular response

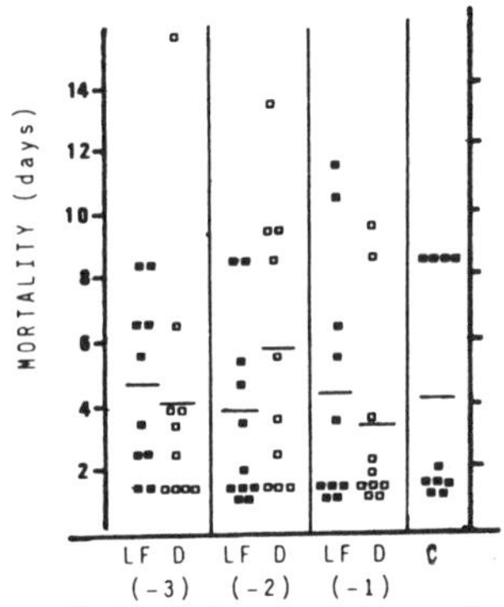

Fig 4 : Individual Survival time of normal mice (C) or mice which received one single I.P injection of 0.5 ml of LF 1695 (5mg/kg) or the same volume of diluent (D), three (-3), two (-2) or one (-1) day before the I.V injection of 10^6 C.albicans. 10 mice/group.

(North et al., 1972). Acquired resistance appears to be mediated by resident macrophages, monocytes and T lymphocytes. This type of infection has a more chronic pattern compared to Listeria monocytogenes infection and should be more appropriate for the study of compounds acting on acquired resistance.

As shown on Figure 5, growth of Mycobacterium bovis in the spleen was inhibited in OF1 mice treated continously with LF 1695 administered in the drinking water. The effect was dependent on the strain of mice used, and was observed only during the first three weeks. There was no difference in bacterial counts at a time where acquired immunity is required for bacterial elimination. This could also be due to depressed DTH to tuberculin observed after 3 weeks of infection in LF 1695 treated animals (Figure 6). The rapid onset of LF 1695 protective activity in this model suggests that the compound acts on the innate ability of non-immune macrophages to kill or inhibit the growth of the organisms during the first two weeks after infection. This resistance mechanism is under genetic control (Lagrange et al., 1982), thereby providing an explanation of strain differences in LF 1695 action. Inhibition of specific cellular immunity observed at 3 weeks may be due to the treatment protocol used. Long continuous treatment by the oral route may lead to immunosuppression in mice. Alternatively, as shown by Lagrange et al., 1982, and Forget et al., 1981, bacterial multiplication is a prerequisite for the production of specific DTH, therefore LF 1695 inhibition of Mycobacterium bovis growth during the first phase of infection may suppress the DTH response.

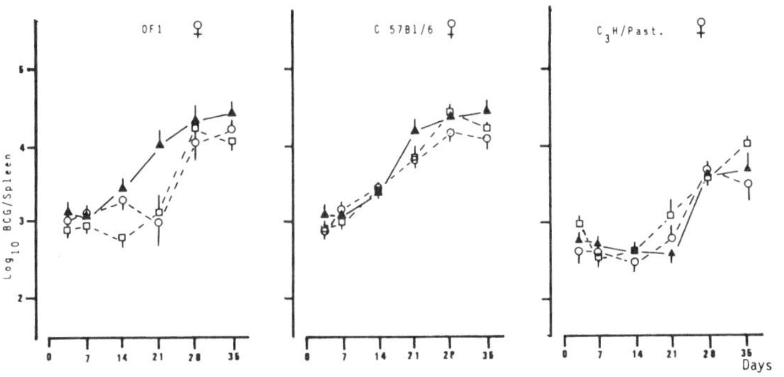

Fig 5 : Growth curves of BCG in spleen after one single intravenous inoculation of 1 x 10^4 viable BCG in normal mice (▲——▲) and in mice receiving the LF 1695 treatment in the drinking water at two concentrations, 20 mg/l (○——○) or 100 mg/l (□- - - -□). Mean of 10 Mice ± SEM.

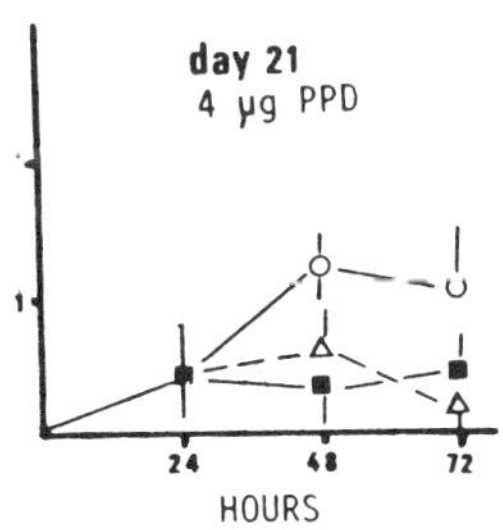

Fig 6 : Delayed type hypersensibility (DTH) to 4 μg of tuberculin developped 21 days after one IV injection of 1 x 10^4 BCG in normal mice (○——○) and in mice receiving the LF 1695 treatment in the drinking water at two concentrations, 20 mg/l (■——■) or 100 mg/l (△- - -△).
Mean of 10 mice ± SEM.

SCHISTOSOMA MANSONI INFECTION IN RATS

Antibody dependent cell cytotoxicity has been described as a major mechanism of immune defence against metazoan parasites and more particularly schistosomes (Captron et al., 1982). In man and rats, eosinophils, macrophages, and platelets have been shown to have cytocidal properties towards the larvae of Schistosoma mansoni, with the essential involvement of parasite-specific IgE antibody (Capron et al., 1983).

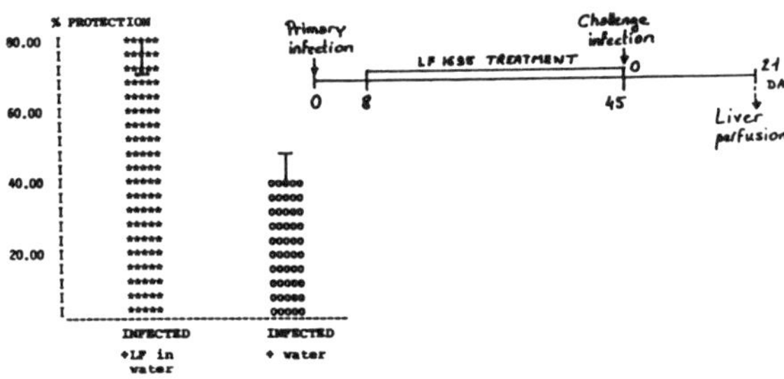

Fig 7 : In vivo efficiency of LF 1695 oral treatment of rats in acquired immunity against S. MANSONI
LF 1695 was administrated by the drinking water (20 mg/l)

As shown in Figure 7, acquired immunity to Schistosoma mansoni was clearly enhanced in rats treated with LF 1695 by the oral route. IgE-dependent antischistosomal cytotoxicity of rat peritoneal macrophages and rat blood platelets was also enhanced 3 and 4 days after an intraperitoneal injection of LF 1695 (Figure 8). Furthermore, LF 1695 treatment could increase the cytocidal activity of immune sera incubated with normal rat macrophages (Figure 9) indicating that LF 1695 acts at two levels: increasing the cytocidal activity of cells, and probably increasing the levels of immune IgE in serum. LF 1695 was also found to enhance Candida phagocytosis by rat peritoneal macrophages.

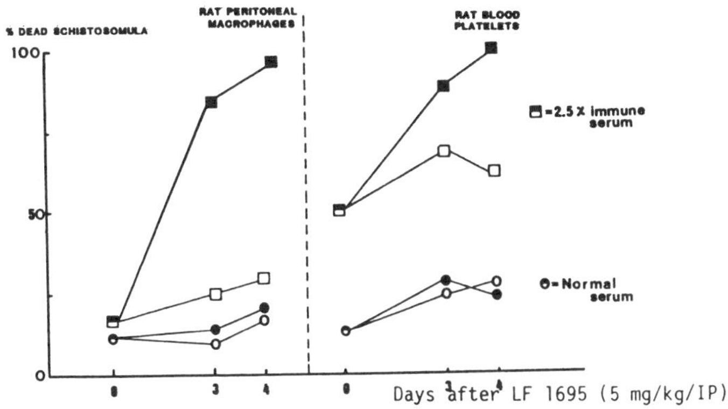

Fig 8 : IgE-DEPENDENT ANTISCHISTOSOME CYTOTOXICITY
AFTER I.P. INJECTION OF LF 1695

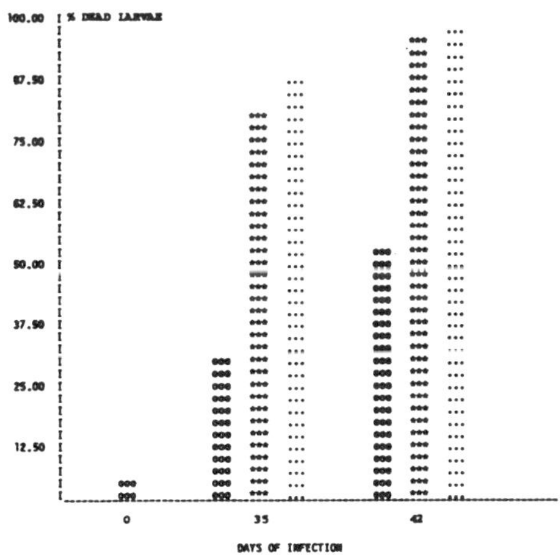

Fig 9 : LF 1695 activity in acquired immunity : serum efficiency on normal rat macrophages. 000, control rats, *** LF 1695 IP treatment, ... LF 1695 oral treatment. LF 1695 was injected IP in weekly doses of 3 mg/rats between the 7th and the 35 th day after infestation with 1 000 cercariae or given orally (20 mg/l driking water) during the same period. Sera were collected on day 42;

CONCLUSIONS

The results presented here demonstrate that LF 1695 can increase resistance to infection by a number of different mechanisms. The antibacterial effect of LF 1695 involves principally the mononuclear phagocyte system. Depending upon the type of infection considered, different subpopulations of T cells may participate in LF 1695 modification of cell mediated immunity. The antibacterial effect may be the consequence of the ability of LF 1695 to activate macrophages and to induce differentiation of cells of the monocyte/macrophage type. LF 1695 was also shown to be effective in enhancing protective immunity to *Schistosoma mansoni* by IgE and non-IgE dependent mechanisms.

It remains to be shown whether such effects are relevant to the human situation. Protective effect in chronic infection may be obtained if resistance in man is primarily mediated by the mechanisms by which LF 1695 has been shown to be active and provided that appropriate treatment schedules can be devised.

REFERENCES

Capron A, Dessaint JP, Capron M and Joseph M, (1983). Effector mechanisms against schistosomes, in: Yamamura Y, Tadat T, ed., 5th International Congress of Immunology, "Progress in Immunology, V," New York: Academic Press: pp. 1305-1316.

Capron A, Dessaint JP, Hague A and Capron M (1982). Antibody dependent cell mediated cytotoxicity against parasites. Prog Allergy 31: 234-267.

Forget A, Skamene E, Gros P, Miailhe AC, Turcotte R (1981). Differences in response among inbred mouse strains to infection with small doses of *Mycobacterium bovis* BCG. Infect Immun 32:42-47.

Hurtrel B, Lagrange PH, Michel JC. (1980) Systemic candidiasis in mice. II. Main role of polymorphonuclear leukocytes in resistance to infection. Ann Immunol (Inst. Pasteur) 131C: 105-118.

Kaufmann SHE, Hahn H (1982). Biological functions of T cell lines with specificity for the intracellular bacterium Listeria monocytogenes, in vitro and in vivo. J Exp Med 155:1754-1765.

Lagrange PH, Hurtrel B and Thickstun PM (1979). Immunological behaviour after mycobacterial infection in selected lines with high or low antibody responses. Infect Immun 25(1):39-47.

Lane FC, Unanue ER (1972). Requirement of thymus (T) lymphocytes for resistance to listerosis. J Exp Med 135:1104-1112.

Mackaness GB (1969). The influence of immunologically committed lymphoid cells on macrophage activity in vivo. J Exp Med 129:973-992.

Mitsuyama, M, Takeya K, Nomoto, K, Shimotori S (1978). Three phases of phagocyte contribution to resistance against Listeria monocytogenes. J Gen Microbiol 106:165.

Miyata H, Nomoto K and Takeya K (1980). Characteristics of resistance to Listeria monocytogenes enhanced by Corynebacterium parvum in mice. Immunology 40:33-39.

Newborg MF, North RJ, (1980). On the mechanism of T cell independent anti-Listeria resistance in nude mice. J Immunol 124(2);571-576.

Nomoto K, Shimamoto Y, Taniguchi K, Kubo C, Kawauchi H, Mitsuyama M, Takeya K (1983). Development of immunity against Listeria monocytogenes in athymic versus neonatally thymectomized mice. Cellular Immunol 75:134-143.

North RJ, Mackaness GB, Elliott RW (1972). The histogenesis of immunologically committed lymphocytes. Cell Immunol 3:680-694.

Othmane O, Touraine JL, Sanhadji K and Pascal M (1985). A new immunomodulator, LF 1695-I: In vitro effects on the T lymphocyte lineage in man. Int J Immunopharmacol 7(4):543-548.

Pascal M and Derrepas P (1986). Increased interleukin 1

and modulation of interleukin 2 production by murine macrophages and lymphocytes treated with LF 1695. Int J Immunopharmacol 8(5):499-508.

Petit JC, Burghoffer RB, Dauget GL (1985). Suppression of cellular immunity to Listeria monocytogenes by activated macrophages: Infec Immun 49(2):383-388.

Rogers TJ and Balish E (1980). Immunity to Candida albicans. Microbiol Rev 44:660-682.

Immunopharmacology of Infectious Diseases: Vaccine Adjuvants and Modulators of Non-Specific Resistance, pages 279–289

MECHANISMS OF IMMUNOSTIMULATION BY PYRIMIDINONES

Daniel E. Tracey and Karen A. Richard

Department of Hypersensitivity Diseases Research, The Upjohn Company, Kalamazoo, Michigan 49001

INTRODUCTION

Pyrimidinones are synthetic compounds with multiple, potent, immunomodulatory activities which may account for their broad range of antiviral, antitumor, and antiinflammatory properties (Wierenga et al., 1980; Stringfellow, 1981; Fast et al., 1982; Skulnick et al., 1986). Although over one hundred chemical analogs have been synthesized, the most active compounds are 5-halo-6-arylpyrimidinones. The structures of the three most intensively studied compounds in this series, ABPP, AIPP, and ABmFPP, are shown in Figure 1.

Some of the immunomodulatory and therapeutic activities of pyrimidinones in animal models are listed in Table 1. Most of these activities were seen in rodents, particularly in mice. The immunological activities were all measured *in vivo* or *ex vivo*. The therapeutic activities were all measured *in vivo*. In fact, neither antiviral nor antitumor activities of pyrimidinones have been observed *in vitro* (Stringfellow, 1981), suggesting that these compounds act primarily by stimulating host defense mechanisms. In some studies, a direct role for natural killer (NK) cells and/or activated macrophages was found for the antitumor activity of ABmFPP, for example (Li et al., 1985).

The current studies are focused on the mechanisms involved in NK cell activation by several pyrimidinones. In particular, the role of the cytokines interferon (IFN), interleukin-1 (IL-1), and interleukin-2 (IL-2) will be evaluated.

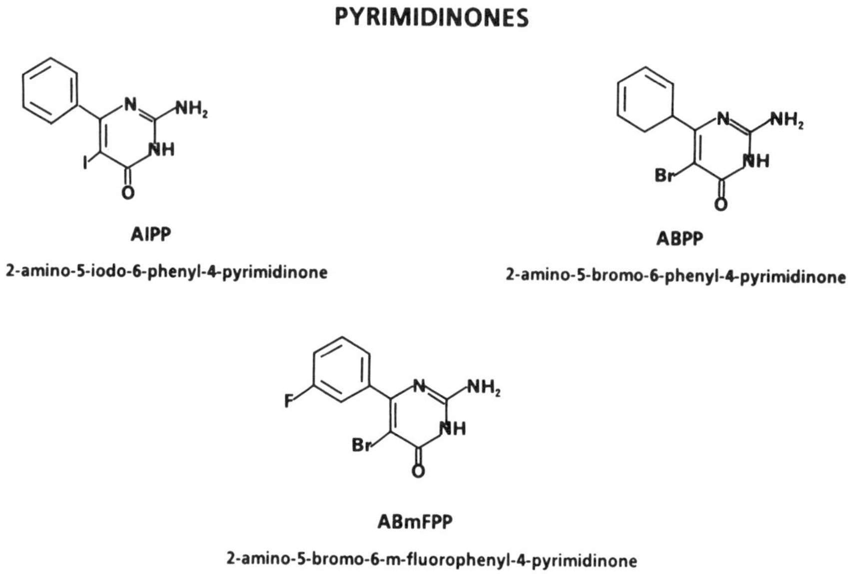

FIGURE 1. Chemical structures of three pyrimidinones.

TABLE 1. Some biological activities of pyrimidinones.

IMMUNOMODULATORY ACTIVITIES	THERAPEUTIC ACTIVITIES
NK Cell Activation	Antiviral
Macrophage Activation	RNA Viruses
Polyclonal B Cell Activation	DNA Viruses
Enhanced Antibody Production	Antitumor
Decreased Delayed Type Hypersensitivity	Antiinflammatory
Enhanced Bone Marrow CFU	Adjuvant Arthritis
	Reversed Passive Arthus Reaction

RESULTS AND DISCUSSION

NK Cell Activation by Pyrimidinones

All of the 5-halo-6-arylpyrimidinones which have been tested were found to enhance murine splenic NK activity in *ex vivo* experiments. Two intensively studied compounds,

ABPP and AIPP, were potent NK augmenting agents when administered as single injections of 50-400 mg/kg i.p. or s.c., but only ABPP was active when administered p.o. (Loughman et al., 1980; Lotzova et al., 1983). The timecourse of induction of splenic and peritoneal NK activities by ABPP and AIPP are shown in Figures 2 and 3. Both splenic and peri-

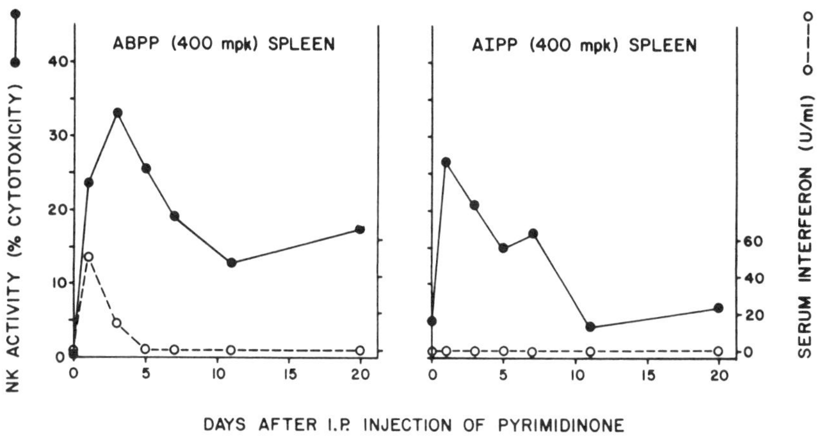

FIGURE 2. Timecourse of augmentation of CBA mouse splenic NK activity by ABPP and AIPP. Spleen cells from i.p. injected mice were assayed for NK activity in a 3-hour ^{51}Cr-release assay using YAC-1 tumor cells as targets. Serum IFN was measured in a VSV plaque reduction assay with L929 target cells.

toneal NK activities were significantly enhanced 24 hours after ABPP or AIPP injection and the enhancement persisted for at least 20 days, especially in the peritoneal cells. A similar timecourse of pyrimidinone enhanced NK activity was also seen using an <u>in vivo</u> NK cell assay which measures the NK-dependent elimination of intravenously injected, radiolabeled YAC-1 tumor cells from the lungs of A/J mice (Richard et al., 1986).

Previous studies with another NK-stimulatory agent, *Mycobacterium bovis*, strain BCG, showed a requirement for macrophages in the NK cell augmentation by BCG (Tracey, 1980). A similar macrophage dependence of NK stimulation by ABPP and AIPP is shown in Table 2. Silica, known to be

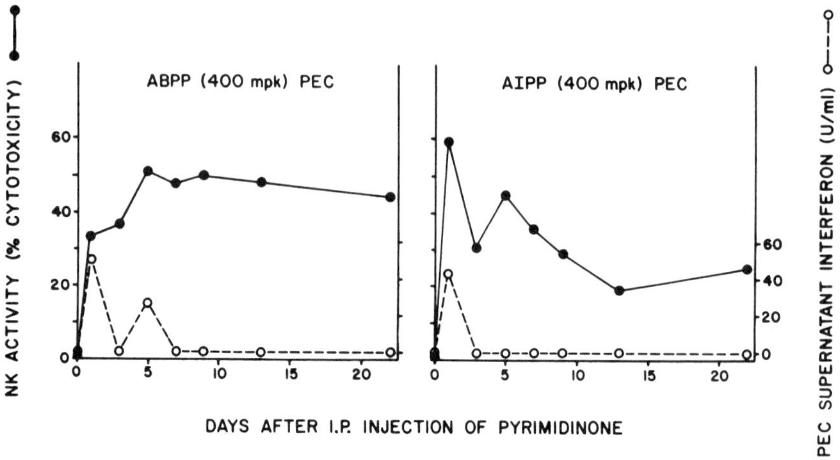

FIGURE 3. Timecourse of augmentation of CBA mouse peritoneal exudate cell (PEC) NK activity by ABPP and AIPP. The NK assay was done as in Figure 2. IFN was measured in 24-hour supernatants of cultured PEC.

selectively toxic to macrophages, abrogated the NK enhancement induced by the pyrimidinones as well as the positive control, BCG.

Since macrophages may be involved in NK cell augmentation via production or induction of cytokines, we investigated the roles of various cytokines in pyrimidinone induced NK cell augmentation. It is known that IFN (alpha, beta and gamma), IL-2, and possibly IL-1 in synergy with IFN and IL-2, can augment NK activity (Herberman and Holden, 1978; Henney et al., 1981; Dempsey et al., 1982).

Involvement of Interferons in NK Augmentation by Pyrimidinones

Originally, the pyrimidinones were recognized as potent IFN inducers (primarily IFN alpha and beta) and it was felt that IFNs played a key role in the biological activities of these compounds (Stringfellow,et al., 1980). Several studies have shown good correlation between IFN induction and protection against Semliki Forest Virus infection or antiinflammatory activities among a series of pyrimidinones (Skulnick

TABLE 2. Silica abrogates the induction of peritoneal NK activity by pyrimidinones.*

INJECTIONS		PERITONEAL NK ACTIVITY ON DAY 4
Day 0	Days -1, +1	($LU_{10}/10^7$ Cells)
PBS	-	0
	RPMI	250
	Silica	0
ABPP	-	19,979
	RPMI	13,556
	Silica	177
AIPP	-	13,414
	RPMI	21,473
	Silica	1,581
BCG	-	4,137
	RPMI	5,442
	Silica	3

* CBA/J mice were injected i.p. with 400 mg/kg ABPP or AIPP, 10^8 BCG organisms, 150 mg/kg silica particles (5 microns) in RPMI medium, or RPMI medium alone on the days indicated. On day 4, NK activities of the PEC were measured as in Figure 2 and are expressed as lytic units (LU) at 10% lysis.

et al., 1985). However, pyrimidinone-induced protection against Herpes Simplex Virus infections or various murine tumors or the induction of NK activity in mice was not directly correlated with serum IFN levels in treated mice (Skulnick et al., 1985; Figure 2). Although AIPP is an excellent NK enhancing agent and is a poor serum IFN inducer (Figure 2), some IFN could be detected in AIPP-induced PEC culture supernatants soon after injection (Figure 3 and Lotzova et al., 1986). A low level of peritoneal IFN may be sufficient to enhance NK activity, since a recent article showed abrogation of AIPP-induced NK activity with anti-IFN treatment of the mice (Lotzova et al.,1986). Thus, it seems likely that IFN plays a role in pyrimidinone mediated NK augmentation, but discrepancies between IFN and NK levels suggest an additional role for other cytokines.

Involvement of IL-1 in NK Augmentation by Pyrimidinones

The fact that pyrimidinones have adjuvant activity, and induce macrophage and polyclonal B cell activation, suggests that IL-1 may be induced by these compounds. Indeed, we have found that several pyrimidinones induced IL-1 *in vitro* and *in vivo*. When ABmFPP, ABPP, or the well known IL-1 inducer, zymosan, were added to murine P388D$_1$ macrophages, human peripheral blood leukocytes (PBL), or murine peritoneal cells *in vitro*, IL-1 was readily detected in cell-free supernatants and cell sonicates (Figure 4). Similar results were also obtained with AIPP with each of these cells (not shown).

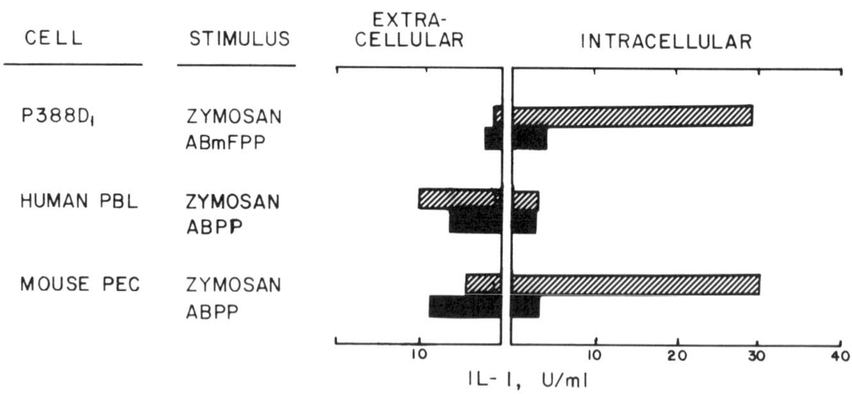

FIGURE 4. Induction of IL-1 by pyrimidinones *in vitro*. Cells were cultured with 100 µg/ml ABmFPP, 500 µg/ml ABPP or zymosan for 48 - 72 hours. Extracellular IL-1 was measured in cell-free supernatants and intracellular IL-1 was measured in cell sonicates using a murine LBRM-33-1A5 cell/HT-2 cell assay (Gillis and Mizel, 1981). None of the cells produced any measurable IL-1 without stimulation.

Ex vivo experiments, in which pyrimidinones were injected i.p. into mice and peritoneal fluids and peritoneal cells were examined for IL-1 content in vitro, also demonstrated that ABPP and ABmFPP induced IL-1 (Figure 5). The intra-

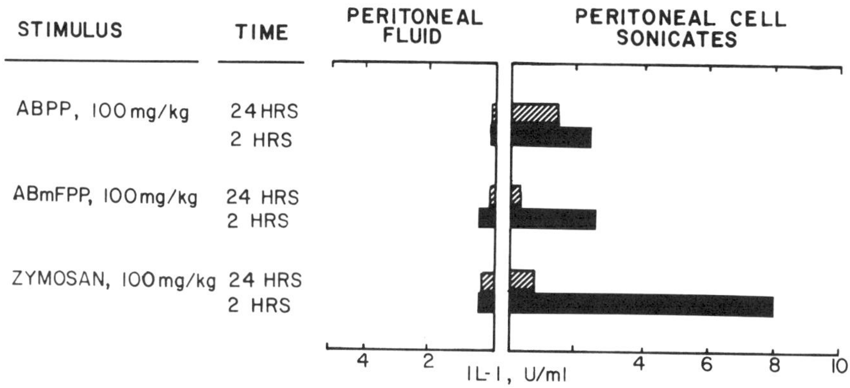

FIGURE 5. Pyrimidinones induce IL-1 in the murine peritoneal cavity. Stimuli were injected i.p. into CBA mice and IL-1 was measured ex vivo (LBRM-33-1A5/HT-2 cell assay) in the peritoneal fluid and in sonicates of PEC removed from the peritoneum at 2 or 24 hours after injection. No IL-1 was detectable in peritoneal fluids or cells from unstimulated mice.

cellular levels of IL-1 were induced very rapidly (<2 hours) with ABPP, ABmFPP and zymosan and had waned by 24 hours. Although IL-1 in the peritoneal fluids was detectable, the levels were quite low at both timepoints. When pyrimidinone induced PEC were further stimulated with LPS in vitro, they continued to produce intracellular IL-1, but at levels far below those achieved with unstimulated or PBS-induced PEC (Figure 6). It appears that pyrimidinone-induced PEC were refractive to further IL-1 induction by LPS, a further indication that they had been induced to produce IL-1 in vivo.

Direct evidence for in vivo induction of IL-1 by pyrimidinones was obtained by measuring serum IL-1 levels in mice given i.p. injections of pyrimidinones (Richard et al., 1986). For example, Table 3 shows the timecourse of IL-1 induction by ABPP in A/J mice as compared with the potent IL-1 inducer,

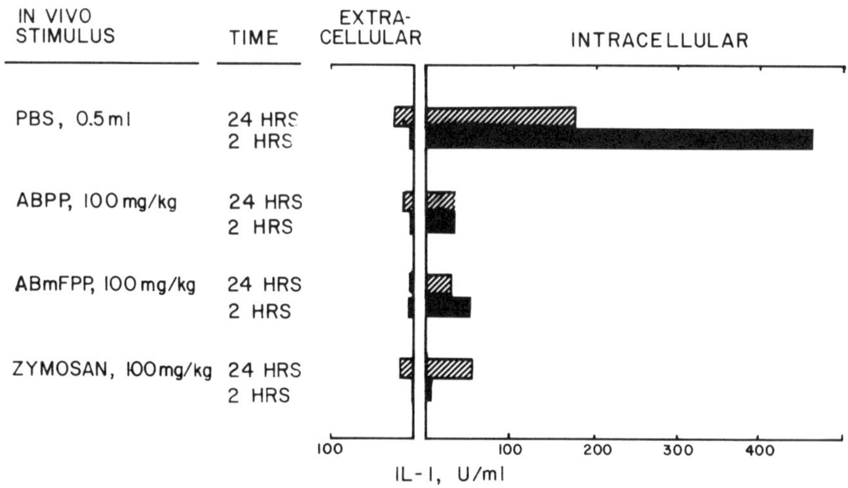

FIGURE 6. Peritoneal cells from CBA mice injected i.p. 2 or 24 hours previously with various stimuli were cultured *in vitro* with 10 μg/ml *E. coli* lipopolysaccharide (LPS). After 24 hours, the levels of IL-1 in the supernatants (extracellular IL-1) or sonicates (intracellular IL-1) were measured in the LBRM-33-1A5/HT-2 cell assay.

TABLE 3. Serum IL-1 and IL-2 levels after ABPP injection.*

Time After Injection (Hours)	Serum IL-1 (U/ml)		Serum IL-2 (U/ml)
	ABPP	LPS	ABPP
0	4.3	4.3	0.0
1	2.3	4.9	0.0
2	1.0	17.1	0.0
4	12.4	65.8	0.0
8	2.9	0.8	0.0
24	2.4	0.7	0.0

* Sera were obtained from A/J mice after i.p. injection of 200 mg/kg ABPP or 2.5 mg/kg LPS. IL-1 was measured in 1:500 diluted sera. IL-2 was measured with HT-2 cells on 1:10 sera.

LPS. In addition, significant elevation in the acute phase protein, serum amyloid P, in these mice was seen (Richard et al., 1986). Since serum acute phase protein levels increase in response to IL-1, this provides further evidence that ABPP induces IL-1 systemically in mice.

Involvement of IL-2 in NK Cell Augmentation by Pyrimidinones

We previously reported that several pyrimidinones, especially AIPP, potentiated IL-2 production by LBRM-33-1A5 cells stimulated with IL-1 and PHA *in vitro* (Tracey et al., 1985). This effect has been seen, however, in only six of ten experiments with 10^{-4} or 10^{-5}M AIPP or ABPP. Given this variability and the *in vitro* nature of these experiments, we sought to determine whether pyrimidinones induced IL-2 *in vivo*. As shown in Table 3 using an extremely sensitive assay which could detect IL-2 in spiked sera, no IL-2 was found in sera at any timepoint after ABPP injection. Furthermore, spleen cells from ABPP or AIPP treated mice did not produce increased levels of IL-2 spontaneously or when stimulated with the mitogen Concanavalin A (Table 4).

TABLE 4. Con A induced IL-2 production by spleen cells from pyrimidinone stimulated mice.*

Treatment of Mice	IL-2 (U/ml) in Spleen Cell Supernatants	
	Unstimulated	Con A (2.5 ug/ml)
None	0.0	2.6
ABPP 400 mg/kg	0.0	2.6
AIPP 400 mg/kg	0.0	1.7

* A/J mice were injected i.p. with pyrimidinones 48 hours prior to removal of spleen cells. Spleen cells were cultured at 5 x 10^6 cells/ml with or without Con A for 48 hours. Supernatants were harvested and the IL-2 content was measured in an HT-2 cell proliferation assay.

The augmentation of NK activity by pyrimidinones *in vivo* appears not to require T-cell derived lymphokines, including

IL-2. Augmentation of NK activity by ABPP in athymic nude mice (Loughman et al., 1980) or athymic rats (Lotzova et al., 1984) suggests an IL-2 independent mechanism. Furthermore, when mice were pretreated with cyclosporin A, a drug known to block the production of several T-cell derived lymphokines, no diminution in ABPP-induced NK augmentation *in vivo* was observed (Richard et al., 1986). These observations collectively suggest that products of activated T cells are not involved in ABPP-induced NK augmentation, but they do not rule out the possibility that IL-2, IFN-gamma or other "T-cell derived lymphokines" are induced directly in non-T-cell populations, such as large granular lymphocytes (LGL).

In summary, several pyrimidinones could be shown to augment NK cell activity and to induce IFN and IL-1, but not IL-2 *in vivo*. Since the magnitude of the NK augmentation by various pyrimidinones did not correlate with serum IFN levels, and IFN and IL-1 have each been shown to augment murine NK activity *in vivo* (Richard et al., 1986), it is possible that IFN and IL-1, and possibly other cytokines, act synergistically to augment NK activity. Such immunomodulatory properties of pyrimidinones may contribute to their wide range of host defense and antiinflammatory activities *in vivo*.

REFERENCES

Dempsey RA, Dinarello CA, Mier JW, Rosenwasser LJ, Allegretta M, Brown TE, Parkinson DR (1982). The differential effects of human leukocyte pyrogen/lymphocyte activating factor, T cell growth factor and interferon on human natural killer cell activity. J. Immunol. 129:2504.

Fast PE, Hatfield CA, Sun EL, Stringfellow DA (1982). Polyclonal B-cell activation and stimulation of specific antibody responses by 5-halo-pyrimidinones with antiviral and antineoplastic activity. J. Biol. Resp. Mod. 1:199-215.

Henney CS, Kuribayashi K, Kern DE, Gillis S (1981). Interleukin-2 augments natural killer cell activity. Nature 291:335.

Herberman RB, Holden HT (1978). Natural cell mediated immunity. Cancer Res. 27:305.

Gillis S, Mizel SB (1981). T-cell lymphoma model for the analysis of interleukin-1 mediated T-cell activation. Proc. Nat. Acad. Sci. (USA) 78:1133-1137.

Li LH, Wallace TL, Richard KA, Tracey DE (1985). Mechanism

of antitumor action of pyrimidinones in the treatment of B16 melanoma and P388 leukemia. Cancer Res. 44:2841-2847.
Lotzova E, Savary CA, Stringfellow, DA (1983). 5-halo-6-phenyl pyrimidinones: new molecules with cancer therapeutic potential and interferon-inducing capacity are strong inducers of murine natural killer cells. J. Immunol. 130: 965-969.
Lotzova E, Savary CA, Khan A, Stringfellow, DA (1984). Stimulation of natural killer cells in two random-bred strains of athymic rats by interferon-inducing pyrimidinones. J. Immunol. 132:2566-2570.
Lotzova E, Savary CA, Lowlachi M, Murasko DM (1986). Cytotoxic and morphologic profile of endogenous and pyrimidinone-activated murine NK cells. J. Immunol. 136:732-740.
Loughman BE, Gibbons AJ, Taggart MT, Renis HE (1980). Modulation of mouse natural killer cell activity by interferon and two antiviral isocytosines. In Nelson JD, Grassi C (eds): "Curr. Chemother. Infect. Dis., vol 2" Washington D.C., Am. Soc. Microbiol. pp 1398-1400.
Richard KA, Mortensen RF, Tracey DE (1986). Cytokines involved in the augmentation of natural killer cell activity by pyrimidinones in vivo. (Submitted).
Skulnick HI, Weed SD, Eidson EE, Renis HE, Stringfellow DA, Wierenga W (1985). 2-Amino-5-halo-6-aryl-4(3H)-pyrimidinones: interferon-inducing antiviral agents. J. Med. Chem. 28:1864-1869.
Skulnick HI, Ludens JH, Wendling MG, Glenn EM, Rohloff NA, Smith RJ, Wierenga W (1986). N-substituted-6-phenylpyrimidinones and pyrimidinediones with diuretic/hypotensive and antiinflammatory activity. J. Med. Chem. (in press).
Stringfellow DA (1981). 6-arylpyrimidinols: interferon inducers, immunomodulators, antiviral and antineoplastic agents. Progr. Cancer Res. Ther. 16:215-228.
Tracey DE (1980). The requirement for macrophages in the augmentation of natural killer cell activity by BCG. J. Immunol. 123:840-845.
Tracey DE, Richard KA, Davis JW, Koehneke EM (1985). Induction of interleukin-1 and interleukin-2 secretion in murine cell lines by pyrimidinones. Agents Actions 16:628.
Wierenga W, Skulnick HI, Stringfellow DA, Weed SD, Renis HE, Eidson EE (1980). 5-substituted 2-amino-6-phenyl-4(3H)-pyrimidinones. Antiviral and interferon-inducing agents. J. Med. Chem. 23:237-239.

Immunopharmacology of Infectious Diseases: Vaccine Adjuvants and Modulators of Non-Specific Resistance, pages 291–301

NON-SPECIFIC RESISTANCE AGAINST MICROBIAL INFECTIONS INDUCED BY POLYRIBONUCLEOTIDE COMPLEXES.

Arthur G. Johnson

Department of Microbiology, University of Minnesota, School of Medicine, Duluth, Minnesota 55812

Agents which increase non-specific resistance against multiple infectious microorganisms have been sought since Rowley (1956, 1964) and others (Landy, 1956) focussed attention on this phenomenon. These studies established that injection of bacteria or their products prior to challenge with unrelated microorganisms protected prophylactically against infection by a variety of different bacterial genera. Bacterial endotoxins were exploited initially since they were one of the most potent inducers of resistance (Landy, 1956), and they had been found to have a profound effect on immune regulation (Morrison and Ryan, 1979). However, their toxicity in extremely small doses led gradually to diminished interest. Recently, endotoxins of markedly reduced toxicity have demonstrated activity in this respect (Takayama et al., 1984), and they are now receiving renewed attention.

A second category of microbial products which could effect resistance against unrelated agents emerged when ribonucleotides were synthesized and polymerized in a search for defined compounds which might mimic the capacity of certain viruses to induce interferon. No polyribonucleotide alone was capable of this effect; however, when polymers of the opposite base pairs, polyinosinic acid and polycytidylic acid (poly I·poly C) were mixed, the resulting double helical complex was found to be a potent inducer of interferon (Field et al., 1967), but it too was toxic. A second complex, resulting from combining polyadenylic acid with polyuridylic acid (poly A·poly U), was a very poor inducer of interferon but was non-toxic. Further experimentation showed both these complexes to be potent immunomodulating agents (Johnson, 1979), and when tested for their capacity to induce non-specific increase in resistance to various unrelated microbial challenges, this activity was also found to be a property of both. Most of the experimentation in this area occurred 10-15 years ago after which activity has waned. Accordingly, with the renewed interest in this area selected examples of the action of these homoribopolymer complexes which highlight their capacity to increase non-specific increase in resistance will be reviewed with discussion as to how some mechanisms might or might not be explanatory.

RESULTS

The homoribopolymer complexes exhibit several major properties relative to events encompassing the total immune response. First the capacity to induce interferon (in species other than man) is well known, albeit quantitative differences exist between selected complexes (Field, et al., 1967). Second, the immunomodulating activities of both poly I·poly C and poly A·poly U on antibody synthesis and cell mediated immunity have been documented extensively and the data have been reviewed in a number of publications to which the reader is referred (Johnson, 1979; Cone, 1980; Braun et al., 1971). The broad range of effectiveness of these compounds is readily apparent from Table 1, and renders them suitable candidates as adjuvants for inclusion in human vaccines.

TABLE 1. Immunomodulatory properties of polynucleotide complexes.

Enhances or suppresses both humoral and cell-mediated immunity.
Double stranded complex is required.
Inactivated by RNase and normal serum.
Effective with a variety of antigens, routes, and species.
Protects against microbial challenge.
Affects multiple cell types.
Induce interferon and interleukin 1.
Repairs deficiencies in neonates, aged, and genetically low responder mice.

The third property, that of inducing non-specific resistance to a variety of infectious agents is described vide infra. Although it is reasonable to postulate at the outset that the first two, interferon induction and/or an increase in humoral and cell mediated immunity, may rationally explain the third, cogent arguments will be advanced which suggest that other unknown mechanisms are operative.

Initial experiments describing the ability of the polyribonucleotides to induce protection against infectious agents followed their synthesis in 1967 (Field et al., 1967). Resistance against vesicular stomatitis virus was induced in vitro by exposure of primary rabbit kidney monolayers to the homoribopolymer complexes. Presumably this was mediated by the stimulus of interferon. Noteworthy findings were (a) the low effective doses of each (<1.3 ng/ml poly I·poly C and 1.5 ng/ml poly A·poly U, (b) the efficacy of poly A·poly U, a very poor interferon inducer, and (c) the requirement for the helical complex for this activity, the individual homopolymers being inactive.

In vivo protection of 80-90% against the murine viruses, Columbia SK and pneumonia virus of mice, also was induced by microgram amounts of poly I·poly C (Field et al., 1967). An absolute need for the complex form was demonstrated as well in this in vivo study, poly I alone or poly C alone being inactive. In addition, mice were protected by small amounts of poly I·poly C against foot and mouth disease virus (FMDV), 100% surviving after 150 μg and 50% surviving when given 1.5 μg poly I·poly C 18 hr before challenge (Richmond and Hamilton, 1969). The time constraints were found to be quite restrictive in that the homoribopolymer complex induced no protection when given at -3 or +1 days. A correlation was noted between interferon titers at 1.5 hr and number of subsequent survivors. However, poly A·poly U, the poor interferon inducer, also was found to protect against FMDV, raising the question as to whether interferon induction was a cause and effect relationship. In a related publication (Hamilton et al., 1969), evidence was tabulated that poly A·poly U also protected against Herpes induced cytopathology and keratoconjunctivities in rabbit eyes. Thus, if interferon were involved as the protective mediator, it need not be present in high titers.

The temporal restrictions of the polynucleotide complex relative to efficacy was again demonstrable using Herpes simplex virus-1 as challenge organism in C58 mice (Martinez et al., 1980). Thus poly I·poly C was an effective prophylactic when given 1 day before challenge, while a single injection on day +1 was ineffective. Therapeutic effects however, did become partially manifest with 5/10 survivors occurring if multiple (5) injections were begun on day +1 or +2. In experiments designed by these same investigators (Martinez et al., 1980) to determine the cellular target of poly I·poly C, mice were injected 1 day before poly I·poly C with either silica to inactivate macrophages, cyclophosphamide to destroy lymphocytes, or adult thymectomy plus antithymocyte serum to selectively deplete T lymphocytes. Only the silica treatment abolished the typical prophylactic efficacy of poly I·poly C given a day before challenge. Thus, the macrophage was implicated as necessary for this action of poly I·poly C.

Of interest are the recent findings by Kende (1985) reporting both prophylactic and therapeutic efficacy of poly I·poly C stabilized with poly-L-lysine and carbomethylcellulose (poly I·C-LC) against infection with Rift Valley fever virus (RVFV). Optimum efficacy was determined to be injection of poly I·poly C-LC 3 times on days -4, +1, and +6 relative to challenge with LD_{100} RVFV. Protection was also evident when poly I·poly C-LC was injected 24 hrs after challenge. In addition a high degree of therapeutic synergism was achieved when the polynucleotide complex was combined with the anti-viral drug ribavirin as late as 48 hr post-infection. Thus, efficacious dosages of poly I·C-LC below toxic levels could be utilized.

Poly I·poly C also was effective in a different species, protecting rabbits against infection with rabies street virus (Fenje and Postic, 1970). In this system, poly I·poly C was protective when given iv either 24 hr before, together with, or up to 24 hr after challenge with 25 LD_{50} rabies virus. On rechallenge of the survivors 35 days after the original infection, none succumbed. Such long range protection must be assigned another mechanism than interferon. Retention of the virus may have been sufficient to induce active immunity via memory cells, resulting in an effective secondary response.

Using a different approach, Woodhour et al., (1969) incorporated the polynucleotide complexes into a second base adjuvant, termed adjuvant 65, containing a metabolizable peanut oil, aluminum monostearate and mannide monooleate together with influenza vaccines. Under these conditions, both poly I·poly C and poly A·poly U were effective at increasing antibody associated with protection of guinea pigs and monkeys over that elicited by adjuvant 65 alone.

The above demonstrations of polynucleotides preventing viral infections clearly establish these compounds as efficacious in this respect. This efficacy could be attributable to interferon, with the caveat that the small amount of interferon released locally by poly A·poly U was sufficient in this respect. However, this logical hypothesis is open to question since poly I·poly C and poly A·poly U both have been shown to protect in like manner against Gram negative and Gram positive bacterial infections (Weinstein et al., 1970). The same temporal condition prevailed in these experiments also in that the complexes needed to be given 1 day before challenge. Thus, poly I·poly C at the 1 μg level protected 5/6 mice against E. coli, and a like number against Streptococcus pyogenes, as well as 4/6 mice following challenge with either Klebsiella pneumoniae, Pseudomonas aeruginosa, or Staphylococcus aureus. The data from our laboratory employing poly A·poly U as a deterrent of bacterial infections are shown in Table 2, and illustrate the efficacy of this compound in both neonatal and young adult mice against Pseudomonas aeruginosa and Streptococcus pneumoniae respectively. Whether or not interferon gamma by activating macrophages might be the effective mediator is at present unknown.

Earlier results establishing the ability of poly A·poly U to subvert bacterial infections were published by Cheers and Cone (1974). In these experiments 250 μg of poly A·poly U were injected ip at -1 hr, -48 hr and -96 hr and the $\log_{10}$ of the number of organisms counted in the spleen on day 8. A highly significant reduction was achieved when the polynucleotide was injected 1 hr before infection. A lesser, but still significant reduction was seen when given at -48 hr and at +1 hr. There were no data given for -1 day, the most effective time period found by other investigators. A requirement for complexing of the poly A·poly U was also evident in these experiments. The bacterial count decreased by 1½ logs when the complex was given versus no change when

TABLE 2

Non-Specific Resistance Induced by Poly A Poly **U** Against Infections.

Ages of Mice	Challenge Organism	Adjuvant Injected*	No. Survivors** / No. Injected	% Survival
7 days	Pseudomonas aeruginosa (2×10^5, SC)	None	2/31	7
		Poly A·Poly U (10γ, SC)	3/12	25
		Poly A·Poly U (100γ, SC)	12/30	40
4 months	Streptococcus pneumoniae (2×10^2, iv)	None	1/8	13
		LPS, 10γ iv	8/8	100
		Poly A·**U**, 100γ iv	7/8	88

*Injected one day before challenge.

**Counted on day 15.

either poly A alone or poly U alone was injected (Madraso and Cheers, 1978).

DISCUSSION

From the data presented in the above examples, it is concluded that the polyribonucleotide complexes can effectively prevent the establishment of a variety of infectious microorganisms in the host. Although prophylaxis was induced routinely, therapeutic regiments were rarely effective. The time interval of approximately 1 day after introduction of the polynucleotides found repeatedly to be necessary to develop optimal resistance against both viral and bacterial pathogens suggests activation of host cells is necessary, probably for the synthesis and secretion of mediating endogenous factors. If the pathogen is introduced prior to the completion of this interval, the organism becomes established and infectivity is favored. An early stimulation of opsonic antibody appears not to be a mechanistic event, inasmuch as the 1 day interval is too short and more importantly, injection of the polynucleotide complexes 1 day before antigen results in a profound suppression of antibody synthesis (Johnson, 1979).

The nature of the cells and mediators postulated to be operative in vivo is as yet only speculative. Of prime consideration is the demonstrable activation of macrophages which reaches its optimum 18-24 hr after exposure to the polynucleotide complexes. Similarly T cells undergo activation by these complexes (Johnson, 1979). Natural killer cells, a heterogeneous population, are also activated by the polynucleotide complexes probably through the interferon pathway. Evidence exists that these cells can be effector cells in resistance against certain disease entities (Baccarini et al., 1985). However, they have been described recently by Abruzzo and Rowley (1983) as down regulators of the immune system. It is now well known that a considerable number of mediators are secreted by both macrophages and T lymphocytes. Which mediators, if any, are effective in heightening resistance is unknown. Among many possible candidates are interleukin 1, interferon alpha, beta and/or gamma, as well as tumor necrosis factor.

Arguments against interferon as the active mediator of polynucleotide induced resistance lie primarily with (a) the effectiveness of poly A•poly U which is a poor interferon inducer, although this argument is dampened by the recent demonstration by Hovanessian et al., (1982) that although poly A•poly U did not induce interferon detectable in the sera of humans, a protein kinase enzyme, an indicator of interferon action, was increased by the A•U complex; and (b) with the ability of both complexes to induce similar resistance against a variety of bacterial genera. Resistance to the latter has not heretofore been ascribed as being mediated by the interferon pathway. Tumor necrosis factor has been implicated by Parant et al., (1986) as the mediator of non-specific resistance induced by the muramyl dipeptides. No evidence exists as yet as to whether the polynucleotide complexes act in this respect via TNF, or for that matter via interleukin I.

The anionic nature of the polyribonucleotide complexes has been suggested as being responsible for some of their actions. Thus, their adjuvant action on antibody synthesis was implicated in this respect by Diamantstein and Blitstein-Willinger (1975) inasmuch as several other negatively charged polymeric compounds in addition to the polynucleotide complexes stimulated thymidine incorporation into B cells. These included dextran sulphate, poly L-glutamic acid and the polynucleotide complexes as well as others. In addition, the negatively charged maleic acid-divinyl ethers (pyran) have been shown to induce protection of mice against Mengo virus challenge when injected 18 hr before challenge (Merigan and and Finkelstein, 1968). Such resistance lasted for as long as 60 days despite the disappearance of serum interferon after 4-6 days. A number of anionic polymers, pyran co-polymer, polyacrylic acid and poly I•poly C, also were compared for their resistance inducing properties against Listeria monocytogenes infection in mice by Remington and Merigan (1970). While all three induced resistance, the time of initiation and the duration of the effect varied from 14 days for the poly I•poly C to 2 months for the pyran co-polymer. As these authors pointed out, such prolonged protection was inconsistent with an interferon mechanism. Whether or not the protective signal was initiated by the anionic nature of the molecules is also open to question, since none of the polynucleotides alone induced resistance despite their strong anionic charge. The strict requirement for the complexing of the polynucleotides suggests the existence of a "receptor" specific for a structural confirmation peculiar to the double-stranded helical complex rather than the charge alone. Thus, although several strongly polyanionic compounds can act as immunomodulating agents, the charge alone does not explain this activity for all such compounds.

SUMMARY

Attention has been directed to early work documenting the efficacy of polyribonucleotide complexes in inducing nonspecific increase in resistance in several species to multiple viral and bacterial pathogens. Both a strong (poly I·poly C) and a weak (poly A·poly U) inducer of interferon were active and the helical complex of opposite base pairs was required for this effect. Neither homoribopolymer alone was effective. The effector cells and molecular mediators of this effect are unknown. Different host pathways leading to increased resistance may be activated by different compounds of a polyanionic nature.

REFERENCES

Abruzzo LV, Rowley DA (1983). Homeostasis of the antibody response: Immunoregulation by NK cells. Science 222: 581-585.

Baccarini M, Bistoni F, Lohmann-Matthes M-L (1985). In vitro natural cell mediated cytotoxicity against Candida albicans: Macrophage precursors as effector cells. J Immunol 134: 2658-2665.

Braun W, Ishizuka M, Yajima Y, Webb D, Winchurch R (1971). Spectrum and mode of action of poly A·U in the stimulation of immune responses. In Beers RF, Braun W (eds): "Biological effects of polynucleotides," New York: Springer-Verlag, pp. 139-156.

Cheers C, Cone RE (1974). Effect of polyadenine+polyuridine on brucellosis in conventional and congenitally athymic mice. J Immunol 112:1535-1539.

Cone RE (1980). The influence of synthetic homoribopolynucleotide complexes on the immune response. Pharmacol Ther 8:321-337.

Diamantstein T, Blitstein-Willinger E (1975). Relationship between biological activities of polymers. I. Immunogenicity, C3 activation, mitogenicity for B cells and adjuvant properties. Immunology 29:1087-1092.

Fenje P, Postic B (1970). Protection of rabbits against experimental rabies by poly (I:C). Nature 226:171-172.

Field AK, Tytell AA, Lampson GP, Hilleman MR (1967). Inducers of interferon and host resistance. II. Multi-stranded synthetic polynucleotide complexes. Proc Natl Acad Sci USA 58:1004-1010.

Hamilton LD, Babcok VI, Southam CM (1969). Inhibition of Herpes simplex virus by synthetic double-stranded RNA (polyriboadenylic and polyribouridylic acids and polyriboinosinic and polyribocytidylic acids). Proc Natl Acad Sci USA 64:878-883.

Hovanessian AG, Riviere U, Montagnier L, Michelson M, Lacour J, Lacour F (1982). Enhancement of interferon-mediated protein kinase on mouse and human plasma in response to treatment with polyadenylic-polyuridylic acid [poly (A)·poly (U)]. J Ifn Res 2:209-215.

Johnson AG (1979). Modulation of the immune system by synthetic polynucleotides. Springer Sem Immunopathol 2:149-168.

Kende M (1985). Prophylactic and therapeutic efficacy of poly (I,C)-LC against Rift Valley Fever virus infection in mice. J Biol Resp Mod 4:503-511.

Landy M (1956). Increase in resistance following administration of bacterial lipopolysaccharides. Ann New York Acad Sc 66:292-299.

Madraso ED, Cheers C (1978). Polyadenylic acid-polyuridylic acid (poly A:U) and experimental murine brucellosis. I. Effect of single and double stranded polynucleotides on <u>Brucella abortus</u> in vivo and in vitro. Immunology 35:69-76.

Martinez D, Lynch RJ, Meeker JB, Field AK (1980). Macrophage dependence of polyriboinosinic acid-polyribocytidylic acid-induced resistance to Herpes simplex virus infection in mice. Infect Imm 28:147-153.

Merigan TC, Finkelstein MS (1968). Interferon stimulating and in vitro anti-viral effects of various synthetic anionic polymers. Virology 35:363-374.

Morrison DC, Ryan JL (1979). Bacterial endotoxins and host immune responses. Adv Immunol 28:293-450.

Parant M (1987). Muramyl peptides as enhancers of host resistance to bacterial infections. This volume.

Remington JS, Merigan TC (1970). Synthetic polyanions protect mice against intracellular bacterial infections. Nature 226:361-363.

Richmond JY, Hamilton LD (1969). Foot and mouth disease virus inhibition induced in mice by synthetic double-stranded RNA (polyriboinosinic and polyribocytidylic acids). Proc Natl Acad Sci USA 64:81-86.

Rowley D (1956). Rapidly induced changes in the levels of non-specific immunity in laboratory animals. Brit J Exp Path 37:223-228.

Rowley D (1964). Endotoxin induced changes in susceptibility to infections. In Landy M, Braun W (eds): "Bacterial Endotoxins," New Brunswick: Rutgers University Press, pp. 359-372.

Takayama K, Qureshi N, Ribi E, Cantrell JL (1984). Separation and characterization of toxic and non-toxic forms of lipid A's. Rev Infect Dis 6:439-443.

Weinstein MJ, Waitz JA, Came PE (1970). Induction of resistance to bacterial infections of mice with poly I·poly C. Nature 226:170.

Woodhour AF, Friedman A, Tytell AA, Hilleman MR (1969). Hyperpotentiation by synthetic double stranded RNA of antibody responses to influenza virus vaccine in adjuvant 65. Proc Soc Exp Biol Med 131:809-817.

Immunopharmacology of Infectious Diseases: Vaccine Adjuvants and Modulators of Non-Specific Resistance, pages 303–311

EFFECTS OF LOW MOLECULAR WEIGHT IMMUNOMODIFIERS PRODUCED BY MICROORGANISMS ON EXPERIMENTAL TUMORS AND INFECTIONS

Masaaki Ishizuka, Tomio Takeuchi and Hamao Umezawa
Institute for Chemotherapy, Microbial Chemistry Research Foundation, Numazu, Shizuoka, Japan 410-03

The study of low molecular weight enzyme inhibitors produced by microorganisms was initiated by Umezawa, and inhibitors of proteases and enzymes involved in the biosynthesis or metabolism of catechol amines have been found (Umezawa, 1982). This study was extended to the search for low molecular weight immunomodifiers, and we found bestatin, amastatin, arphamenine, forphenicine, forphenicinol, ebelactones, *etc.*, all of which were found to enhance humoral and cellular immunity (Umezawa, 1981). Among these immunomodifiers, bestatin and forphenicinol have been studied in detail. In this paper, we will review the effects of bestatin and forphenicinol on the immune system, experimental tumors, and microbial infections.

BESTATIN

Bestatin was discovered by testing culture filtrates of microorganisms for inhibition of aminopeptidase B (Umezawa et al., 1976)(Fig. 1). It inhibits not only aminopeptidase

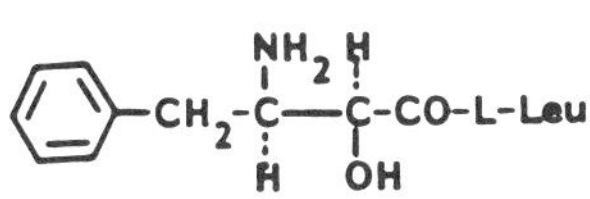

Figure 1. Structure of bestatin.

B but also leucine aminopeptidase (Suda et al., 1976). It is produced by Streptomyces olivoreticuli. We have studied the effect of bestatin on immune responses and on experimental murine tumors and found that bestatin augments immune responses and inhibits tumor growth through activation of host defense mechanisms (Umezawa et al., 1976; Ishizuka et al., 1980; Abe et al., 1984).

Effect on Immune Systems in Mice

Bestatin augmented delayed-type hypersensitivity (DTH) to sheep red blood cells (SRBC) and oxazolone over a wide dose range. In immunosuppressed mice bestatin restored their reduced response to almost normal levels. The administration of a high dose of bestatin, more than 50 mg/kg, increased the number of antibody-forming cells (Ishizuka et al., 1980; Ishizuka et al., 1981). Bestatin also augments the Graft-versus-Host (GVH) reaction in newborn mice, and in irradiated mice (Umezawa et al., 1986). The generation and action of suppressor cells for DTH and antibody formation are inhibited by bestatin in mice and suppressor factors found in cancer patients are also reduced in activity by bestatin treatment. Bestatin stimulates the proliferation of T lymphocytes *in vivo* and *in vitro* (Müller et al., 1979; Ishizuka et al., 1980; Müller et al., 1982).

The supernatant of bestatin-containing macrophage cultures increased the production of interleukin 1 (IL-1), and the drug also enhanced the production of interleukin 2 (IL-2) by Con A in spleen cell cultures (Umezawa et al., 1986). In this case, bestatin alone did not show the effect. This effect of bestatin on IL-2 production has also been observed by Dunlap et al. (1984) and by Kishter et al. (1985).

Effect on Colony-Forming Cells (CFU/c) in Bone Marrow Cell Cultures

Bestatin prevents bone marrow depression induced by cyclophosphamide or mitomycin C in mice. In mice given bestatin the number of bone marrow stem cells increased, as did the number of CFU/c in bone marrow cell cultures (Ishizuka et al., 1981).

Antitumor Effect against Experimental Tumors

Bestatin suppressed tumor growth when the treatment was started on day 8 or day 14 after the inoculation of IMC carcinoma cells (Ishizuka et al., 1980; Ishizuka et al., 1981). Thirty days after the tumor inoculation, antitumor activity of spleen cells taken from mice treated with or without bestatin was examined by the Winn assay. The results indicated that bestatin augments the activity of cytotoxic T cells against IMC carcinoma cells and that of NK cells against YAC-1 cells (Ishizuka et al., 1986). The antitumor effect of bestatin on IMC carcinoma was markedly reduced in athymic mice (Balb/c nu/nu). The administration of bestatin on days 7 to 11 after the tumor inoculation inhibited the growth of myeloid leukemia C1498, and spleen cells taken from these mice inhibited the tumor growth by the Winn assay (Abe et al., 1984).

Bestatin enhanced the antitumor effects of cyclophosphamide and adriamycin against L-1210; 5FU, mitomycin C, and Cis-platinum against Colon 26 adenocarcinoma in mice; and bleomycin against AH66 hepatoma in rats (Abe et al., 1985).

Bestatin suppressed lymph node metastases of P388 leukemia (Tsuruo et al., 1981).

Effect on Infection of *Pseudomonas aeruginosa*

The effect of bestatin on *Pseudomonas* infection was examined in normal and in immunosuppressed mice. Strain No. 12 of *Pseudomonas aeruginosa*, which was isolated from a patient, was used throughout this experiment. The intraperitoneal inoculation of *Pseudomonas* into normal healthy mice (ICR 4 weeks old, female) caused the death of 7 out of 10 within 48 hours after the inoculation, whereas the oral administration of bestatin at 0.8-3.1 mg/kg immediately after the inoculation protected the animals from the infection.

The effect of bestatin on the infection in immunosuppressed mice was also examined. Mice were immunosuppressed with 200 mg/kg of cyclophosphamide given intraperitoneally 4 days before the infection, and some were also given bestatin daily for 4 days before the infection. The intraperitoneal inoculation of *Pseudomonas* caused the death of 7 out of 10 mice treated with cyclophosphamide alone, whereas bestatin (10 μg/mouse) protected 8 of 10 immunosuppressed mice from death.

The effect of bestatin on vaccination with heat-killed *Pseudomonas aeruginosa* was examined in cyclophosphamide-treated mice. Mice were injected with 200 mg/kg of cyclophosphamide intraperitoneally, and 3 days thereafter they were immunized with 1 x 10^7 cells of heat-killed *Pseudomonas aeruginosa* No. 12. After the vaccination, bestatin was given once every 2 days for a total of 3 times; and 14 days thereafter, the mice were inoculated intraperitoneally with 4 x 10^8 cells of *Pseudomonas*. Although 6 out of 10 normal and 3 out of 10 cyclophosphamide-treated mice survived, both groups having been vaccinated, 7 out of 10 of the latter category survived when vaccination was followed by bestatin treatment.

FORPHENICINOL

In the screening for inhibitors of alkaline phosphatase, we discovered forphenicine in culture filtrates of *Streptomyces fulvoviridis* var. *acarbodicus* (Aoyagi et al., 1978). Forphenicine exhibits immuno-enhancing effects through activation of macrophages (Umezawa, 1981). Though, the intraperitoneal injection of forphenicine produced the effect, its oral administration did not.

A derivative which we synthesized and named forphenicinol had only weak activity in inhibiting alkaline phosphatases, but it enhanced immune responses (Ishizuka et al., 1982; Morishima et al., 1982)(Fig. 2).

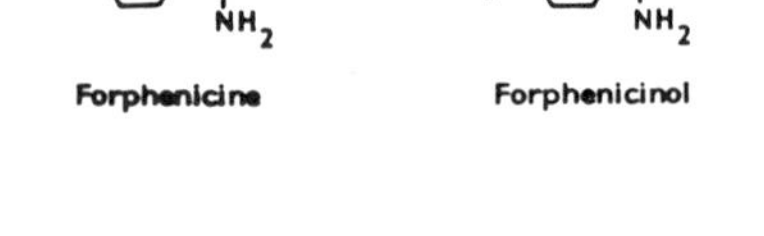

Figure 2. Structures of forphenicine and forphenicinol.

Effect on the Immune System in Mice

Forphenicinol given orally or intraperitoneally at the time of immunization enhanced DTH to SRBC and to oxazolone. It also restored the reduced response of DTH in immunosuppressed mice. Forphenicinol did not show a mitogenic effect on lymphocytes *in vitro* (Ishizuka et al., 1982). The drug given orally promoted phagocytosis of yeasts by peritoneal macrophages and increased the generation of Ia-positive peritoneal macrophages in healthy and L-1210-bearing mice (Okura et al., 1986).

Forphenicinol induced IL-1 production in macrophage cultures. Although it alone could not induce interferon or tumor-necrosis factor (TNF), the oral administration of forphenicinol enhanced the production of γ-interferon and TNF in BCG-sensitized mice (Okura et al., 1986).

Antitumor Effect on Experimental Tumors

Forphenicinol inhibited the growth of murine syngeneic and allogeneic tumors (Ishizuka et al., 1982). It enhanced the antitumor effects of 6-mercaptopurine, aclacinomycin, cyclophosphamide, *etc*. When combined with surgical resection of primary tumors, forphenicinol administration suppressed the growth of recurrent tumors and prolonged the survival period of the mice (Okura et al., 1986). Although forphenicinol was ineffective against mouse leukemia L-1210, in combination with L-1210-vaccine it prolonged the survival period of L-1210-bearing mice, and the increase in the number of Ia-positive macrophages in the peritoneal cavity coincided with the prolongation of the survival period (Okura et al., 1986). The administration of forphenicinol also inhibited the growth of mouse thymoma EL-4 and induced cytotoxic or cytostatic activity against macrophages and splenocytes in EL-4-bearing mice, but not in normal mice (Okura et al., 1986). As reported by Nitta et al. (1985), forphenicinol augmented the concomitant immunity towards tumors in mice. These results suggest that the antitumor activity of forphenicinol may be due to enhancement of concomitant immunity.

Protection against *Pseudomonas aeruginosa* Infection

As reported previously, we found that the administration of forphenicinol exhibited a protective effect against a weak infection of _Pseudomonas aeruginosa_ in mice (Ishizuka et al., 1982). Further study on the protective effect of forphenicinol against _Pseudomonas aeruginosa_ in normal and immunosuppressed mice was performed (Naito et al., 1986) and is described below.

Normal mice (ICR, 6 weeks old, female) were infected with _Pseudomonas aeruginosa_ No. 12, which had been isolated from a patient, by intravenous and intratracheal routes, and then forphenicinol was given orally with various dosage schedules. The administration of forphenicinol increased the survival rate of normal and immunosuppressed mice infected with _Pseudomonas aeruginosa_. The most effective protection by forphenicinol was achieved by the administration one day before the infection in normal mice by both routes. In immunosuppressed mice, made so by cyclophosphamide treatment, the multiple administration of forphenicinol on days 5, 3, and 1 before the infection was also effective in increasing their survival rate markedly.

The effect of orally administered forphenicinol on the growth of _Pseudomonas aeruginosa_ No. 12 in the peritoneal cavity of mice was also examined. The growth was reduced in mice given forphenicinol. Macrophages and polymorphonuclear cells (PMNs) were taken from mice given forphenicinol and their killing effect against _Pseudomonas aeruginosa_ No. 12 was examined _in vitro_. Among these cells, PMNs were markedly bactericidal, whereas macrophages were not. The effect of forphenicinol on induction of the killing activity in PMNs was tested _in vitro_. Although the _in vitro_ treatment with forphenicinol did not activate PMNs, these cells incubated with macrophages which had been pretreated with forphenicinol did show the killing effect. It indicates that forphenicinol-activated macrophages stimulate PMNs to have the killing activity.

CONCLUSION

As described in this paper, the low molecular weight immunomodifiers bestatin and forphenicinol (the former found during the screening for inhibitors of enzymes on cell membranes or surfaces, and the latter, a derivative of forphenicine, found in the same way) bind to cells and induce or enhance the production of cytokines in them; consequently they modulate the immune system. Chemically defined low molecular weight immunomodifiers should have low toxicity and well characterized pharmacological behavior. Since both compounds described in this paper have low toxicity, they should contribute to an increase in the rate of cure of cancer and infections in immunodeficient patients.

REFERENCES

Abe F, Shibuya K, Ashizawa J, Takahashi K, Horinishi H, Matsuda A, Ishizuka M, Takeuchi T, Umezawa H (1985). Enhancement of antitumor effect of cytotoxic agents by bestatin. J Antibiotics 38: 411-413.

Abe F, Shibuya K, Uchida M, Takahashi K, Horinishi H, Matsuda A, Ishizuka M, Takeuchi T, Umezawa H (1984). Effect of bestatin on syngeneic tumors in mice. Gann 75: 89-94.

Aoyagi T, Yamamoto T, Kojiri K, Kojima F, Hamada M, Takeuchi T, Umezawa H (1978). Forphenicine, an inhibitor of alkaline phsophatase produced by actinomycetes. J Antibiotics 31: 244-246.

Dunlap BE, Dunlap SA, Rich DH (1984). Effect of bestatin on in vitro response of murine lymphocytes to T cell stimuli. Scand J Immunol 20: 237-245.

Ishizuka M, Aoyagi T, Takeuchi T, Umezawa H (1981). Activity of bestatin: Enhancement of immune responses and antitumor effect. In Umezawa H (eds): "Small Molecular Weight Immunomodifiers of Microbial Origin - Fundamental and Clinical Studies of Bestatin," Tokyo: Japan Scientific Societies Press, Oxford: Pergamon Press, p 17.

Ishizuka M, Ishizeki S, Masuda T, Momose A, Aoyagi T, Takeuchi T, Umezawa H (1982). Studies on effects of forphenicinol on immune responses. J Antibiotics 35: 1042-1048.

Ishizuka M, Masuda T, Kanbayashi N, Fukasawa S, Takeuchi T, Aoyagi T, Umezawa H (1980). Effect of bestatin on mouse immune system and experimental murine tumors. J Antibiotics 33: 642-652.

Ishizuka M, Masuda T, Kanbayashi N, Watanabe Y, Matsuzaki M, Sawazaki Y, Ohkura A, Takeuchi T, Umezawa H (1982). Antitumor effect of forphenicinol, a low molecular weight immunomodifier, on murine transplantable tumors and microbial infections. J Antibiotics 35: 1049-1054.

Ishizuka M, Masuda T, Mizutani S, Takeuchi T, Umezawa H (1986). Antitumor effector cells in tumor-bearing mice activated by bestatin. In preparation.

Ishizuka M, Sato J, Sugiyama Y, Takeuchi T, Umezawa H (1980). Mitogenic effect of bestatin on lymphocytes. J Antibiotics 33: 653-662.

Kishter S, Hoffman FA, Pizzo PA (1985). Production of and response to interleukin-2 by cultured T cells: Effect of lithium chloride and other putative modulators. J Biol Resp Modif 4: 185-194.

Morishima H, Yoshizawa J, Ushijima R, Takeuchi T, Umezawa H (1982). Synthesis of forphenicinol and forphenicine. J Antibiotics 35: 1500-1506.

Müller WEG, Schuster DK, Zahn RK, Maidhof A, Leyhausen G, Folke D, Koren R, Umezawa H (1982). Properties and specificity of binding sites for the immunomodulator bestatin on the surface of mammalian cells. Intl J Immunopharmacol 4: 393-400.

Müller WEG, Zahn RK, Arendes J, Munsch N, Umezawa H (1979). Activation of DNA metabolism in T-cells by bestatin. Biochem Pharmacol 28: 3131-3137.

Naito K, Arakawa H, Watanabe Y, Okura A, Ishizuka M, Takeuchi T, Umezawa H (1986). Protective effect of forphenicinol, a low molecular weight immunomodifier, against Pseudomonas aeruginosa infection in mice and its mechanisms. Submitted for publication.

Nitta K, Tanaka T, Takeuchi M (1985). Effect of forphenicinol, a small molecular weight immunomodifier, in combination with cyclophosphamide on growth of and immunity to syngeneic murine tumors. Cancer Treatment Rep 69: 285-291.

Okura A, Arakawa H, Yoshinari T, Naito K, Ishizuka M, Takeuchi T, Umezawa H (1986). Effect of forphenicinol on the production of Ia-positive macrophages in mice with or without L1210 leukemia and on the growth of L1210 in immunized mice. J Antibiotics 39: 575-580.

Okura A, Nakadaira M, Naito K, Ishizuka M, Takeuchi T, Umezawa H (1986). Effect of forphenicinol on γ-interferon production in mice sensitized with BCG. J Antibiotics 39: 569-574.

Okura A, Sawazaki Y, Naito K, Ishizuka M, Takeuchi T, Umezawa H (1986). Antitumor effect of forphenicinol, a low molecular weight immunomodifier, in combination with surgery on Meth A fibrosarcoma, Lewis lung carcinoma, and adenocarcinoma 755. J Antibiotics 39: 564-568.

Suda H, Aoyagi T, Takeuchi T, Umezawa H (1976). Inhibition of aminopeptidase B and leucine aminopeptidase by bestatin and its stereoisomer. Arch Biochem Biophys 177: 196-200.

Tsuruo T, Naganuma K, Iida H, Yamori T, Tsukagoshi S, Sakurai Y (1981). Inhibition of lymph node metastasis of P388 leukemia by bestatin in mice. J Antibiotics 34: 1206-1209.

Umezawa H (1981). Small molecular weight immunomodifiers produced by microorganisms: Their screening and discoveries, and the genetics of microbial secondary metabolites. In Umezawa H (eds): "Small Molecular Weight Immunomodifiers of Microbial Origin - Fundamental and Clinical Studies of Bestatin," Tokyo: Japan Scientific Societies Press, Oxford: Pergamon Press, p 1.

Umezawa H (1982). Low molecular weight enzyme inhibitors of microbial origin. In "Annual Review of Microbiol", Vol. 36: Annual Reviews Inc., p 75.

Umezawa H, Aoyagi T, Suda H, Hamada M, Takeuchi T (1976). Bestatin, an inhibitor of aminopeptidase B produced by actinomycetes. J Antibiotics 29: 97-99.

Umezawa H, Ishizuka M, Aoyagi T, Takeuchi T (1976). Enhancement of delayed-type hypersensitivity by bestatin, an inhibitor of aminopeptidase B and leucine aminopeptidase. J Antibiotics 29: 857-859.

Umezawa H, Ishizuka M, Takeuchi T, Abe F, Shibuya K (1986). Bestatin, a low molecular weight immunomodifier produced by microorganisms. J Industrial Microbiol, in press.

Immunopharmacology of Infectious Diseases: Vaccine Adjuvants and Modulators of Non-Specific Resistance, pages 313–324

COMPARATIVE ANALYSIS OF MODULATORS OF NONSPECIFIC RESISTANCE AGAINST MICROBIAL INFECTIONS

Page S. Morahan, Edward R. Leake, Daniel J. Tenney, and Mary Sit
Department of Microbiology and Immunology, The Medical College of Pennsylvania, Philadelphia, Pennsylvania 19129

INTRODUCTION

Since the early 1900's there have been numerous experimental observations and clinical anecdotes that resistance to microbial infections and tumors can be increased nonspecifically. The role of macrophages (MO), natural killer (NK) cells, and granulocytes (PMN) has been well documented. The classic work of Mackaness demonstrated that *Mycobacterium* infection increased the nonspecific antibacterial activity of MO, and it is now known that such "activated" MO also possess antiviral, antiparasitic and antitumor activity. Many of the effects of the mycobacterial infection can now be reproduced by treatment with chemically defined molecules derived from bacteria, such as monophosphoryl lipid A and muramyl dipeptide (see relevant chapters in this Symposium). Dramatic activation of NK cells and MO can also be produced by interferons, interferon inducers and other synthetic compounds (Table 1). It has not yet been possible, however, to modulate nonspecific resistance for consistently beneficial effects; thus interest in immunotherapy has waxed and waned.

NEED FOR COMPARATIVE EVALUATION OF IMMUNOMODULATORS

In contrast to conventional antimicrobial chemotherapy, nonspecific immunomodulation has potential for broad spectrum activity against diverse microorganisms. MO, NK cells and PMN are common components of early nonspecific resistance against microbial infections, and are involved in amplifying specific immune responses later in infection.

TABLE 1. Immunomodulators Under Investigation for Nonspecific Enhancement of Antimicrobial Resistance

Compound	General Structure
	--Microbially derived --
C. parvum	Killed whole cells
MTP-PE	Muramyl tripeptide-phosphatidylethanolamine
MDP	Muramyl dipeptide
MDP-GDP	Lipophylic MDP
MPL	Monophosphoryl lipid A
TDM	Trehalose dimycolate
	--Biologicals--
IFN-B	Murine natural highly purified beta interferon
rIFN-A	Human recombinant alpha A/D interferon
rIFN-G	Murine recombinant gamma interferon
IL-1	Murine recombinant interleukin 1
	--Chemicals--
Pyran	Polydisperse maleic anhydride divinyl ether copolymer
MVE-2	Maleic anhydride divinyl ether copolymer
MA-CDA	Cyclohexyl-1,3-dioxepin maleic anhydride polymer
MA-MP	4-Methyl-2-pentenoyl maleic anydride copolymer
IA-ST	Itaconic acid-styrene copolymer
ABPP	2-amino-5-bromo-6-phenyl-4(3H)-pyrimidinone
AIPP	2-amino-5-iodo-6-phenyl-4(3H)-pyrimidinone
ABMP	2-amino-5-bromo-6-methyl-4(3H)-pyrimidinone
Avridine	Lipoidal amine (CP20,961) in liposomes
LS2616	Quinoline-3-carboxamide
ADA202-718	Ethylene-2,2'-bis(dithiol) bis(ethanol)
Imuthiol	Sodium diethylthiocarbamate
CL246,738	3,6-bis(2-piperidinoethoxy) acridine trihydrochloride
CL259,763	N-{4-[(4-fluorophenyl)-sulfonyl] phenyl} acetamide

Immunodulation and antimicrobial chemotherapy also differ in that the most dramatic effects of immunomodulators are generally observed with prophylactic treatment. Protection for weeks can sometimes be achieved (Morahan 1981). Immunomodulation could be uniquely useful for prophylactic treatment in settings where individuals are likely to be exposed in a certain period to an unknown assortment of infectious agents, e.g. day care centers, schools, chronic care institutions, military operations, immunosuppressive treatments for transplants and cancer.

To be clinically useful in prophylactic or early therapeutic treatment, immunomodulation must be nontoxic, produce resistance to a wide variety of microorganisms, and not cause adverse effects against some infections while increasing resistance to others. Unfortunately, several immunomodulators have been shown to both increase and decrease resistance, depending upon the particular regimen of treatment and microbial infection (Murasko et al. 1983; Schuller and Morahan 1979). Altering only one aspect of drug administration, such as schedule or route, may change protective or ineffective results into disease potentiation (Table 2). Drug vehicles may also provide a problem, as shown by potentiation of Listeria infection by avridine administered in liposomes. There is therefore a need for continued systematic evaluation of immunomodulators against diverse microbial infections, together with more precise delineation of their mechanisms of action on nonspecific immune effector cells and immunoregulatory circuits.

TABLE 2. Enhanced and Decreased Resistance of Immunomodulators Against *L. monocytogenes* Infection.

Regimen				Mortality	Survival
Drug	Dose	Schedule	Route	Dead/Total (%)	MST
Control	-	-	-	19/51 (37%)	10.7
CP	35	-7	ip	0/10 (0%)	>14.0*↑
Pyran	50	-7	ip	4/24 (17%)	13.0*↑
Pyran	50	-1	ip	21/23 (91%)*	5.0*↓
MVE-2	50	-7	ip	0/32 (0%)*	>14.0*↑
MVE-2	50	-1	ip	9/23 (39%)	10.5
Avr/Lipo	50	-7	ip	11/12 (92%)*	4.0*↓
Avr/Lipo	50	-1	ip	21/24 (88%)*	5.0*↓
MDP	4	-7	ip	9/12 (75%)*	6.9*↓
MDP	4	-1	ip	2/13 (15%)	12.5
Imuthiol	25	-7	sc	7/10 (70%)	7.0
Imuthiol	25	-1	sc	2/10 (20%)	10.3
Imuthiol	25	0	sc	8/10 (80%)	6.8*↓
ABPP	250	-2to0	ip	10/10 (100%)*	3.5*↓
ABPP	250	-2to0	p.os	3/10 (30%)	9.6
AIPP	250	-2to0	ip	9/10 (90%)*	4.5*↓
AIPP	250	-2to0	p.os	7/10 (70%)	6.7

CD-1 mice were treated by the indicated doses (mg/kg), routes and days in relation to challenge. Mortality and median survival time (MST) in days were calculated. *Increased (↑) or decreased (↓) resistance, $p < 0.05$

COMPARATIVE EVALUATION OF IMMUNOMODULATORS FOR RESISTANCE

We have investigated several classes of immunomodulators (Table 1) against three systemic (i.p.) microbial infections for which different aspects of nonspecific resistance mechanisms are important-- herpes simplex virus type 2 (HSV-2), encephalomyocarditis (EMC), and Listeria monocytogenes (Morahan et al., 1984; Dempsey and Morahan, 1985). MO are involved in the early limitation of L. monocytogenes, as well as in the subsequent Listeria specific T cell-mediated elimination of bacteria. Early production of interferon by MO and other cells appears to be a major component of resistance to EMC, with complete elimination of virus involving specific antiviral antibody. Activated MO and NK cells appear early after infection with HSV, and extensive investigation in vitro supports a role for MO later in infection as amplifiers of specific T cell and antibody dependent cytotoxic antiviral effects.

Barrier raised female CD-1 (Charles River Laboratories, Kingston, RI) mice were randomized, housed in microisolator cages and maintained free of common endogenous inapparent viral infections that can either increase or decrease the apparent effects of immunomodulators (Dempsey et al., 1986). Immunomodulators with known antimicrobial activity were included in each experiment, as were negative vehicle treatment controls. Mortality data within each experiment were analyzed by the Chi square test, and survival data by the Mann Whitney U test. Only the lowest doses tested of drugs that showed activity are shown in Tables 2-4.

Single prophylactic systemic treatment with either C. parvum or MVE-2, used as positive controls in HSV-2 and EMC virus infections, afforded almost complete protection from mortality, as we and others have previously documented (Morahan, 1981; Morahan et al., 1986). Several other synthetic immunomodulators, which are reported to be interferon inducers and MO activators, were equally effective on prophylactic administration (Li et al., 1985; Wang et al., 1985; Niblack et al., 1979). Acridine trihydrochloride CL246,738 was received courtesy of Dr. Durr, Lederle Laboratories, Pearl River, NY, the pyrimidinones courtesy of Dr. Renis, Upjohn, Kalamazoo, MI, and avridine in liposomes from Dr. Hoffman, Pfizer Research Laboratories, Groton, CT. The pyrimidinones and CL246,738 were active with oral or parenteral administration, and single admnistration of ABPP was as effective as repeated administration. Repeated treatment with the quinoline-3-carboxamide NK cell inducer, LS2616 (Kalland et al., 1985), received courtesy of Dr. Stahlhandske, Aktiebolaget Leo, Helsingborg, Sweden, was moderately effective against EMC virus, but not against HSV-2.

Our initial quantitative evaluation of the efficacy of the three types of IFN revealed that all three IFNs were at least partially effective against both viruses. Generally, repeated therapeutic treatment with 10,000 units was required for signficant activity against EMC virus for beta

Table 3. Immunomodulators protective against EMC virus

Regimen					Mortality	Survival
Drug	Dose	Schedule	Route	Vehicle	Dead/Total (%)	MST
			-- Microbial Products --			
CP	35	-7	i.p.	PBS	0/12 (0%)*	>14.0*
CP	35	-1	i.p.	PBS	4/12 (25%)*	11.0*
MPL	4	-7	i.p.	Squal	14/20 (70%)	7.2
TDM	4	-7	i.p.	Squal	12/19 (63%)*	7.9*
MPL+TDM	4+4	-7	i.p.	Squal	11/20 (55%)*	8.8*
MDP	4	-1to+2	i.p.	PBS	12/20 (60%)	11.0*
			-- Chemicals --			
MVE-2	50	-1	i.p.	PBS	0/10 (0%)*	>14.0*
Avridine	50	-1	i.p.	1%CMC	0/10 (0%)*	>14.0*
ABPP	200	-7	i.p.	1%CMC	6/10 (60%)	8.3*
ABPP	100	-1	i.p.	1%CMC	1/10 (10%)*	>14.0*
ABPP	200	-1	p.os	1%CMC	2/10 (20%)*	>14.0*
CL246,738	200	-1	p.os	1%CMC	0/15 (0%)*	>14.0*
LS2616	160	-4to+14	H_2O	H_2O	6/10 (60%)*	8.8*
LS2616	160	-4to+3	H_2O	H_2O	4/10 (40%)*	9.1*
			-- Biologicals --			
IFN-A	2400	0to+6	i.p.	PBS/B	4/10 (40%)*	9.8*
IFN-B	10000	0to+6	i.p.	PBS/B	6/12 (50%)*	10.5*
IFN-G	760	0to+6	i.p.	PBS/B	5/10 (50%)*	8.7*

CD-1 mice were treated by the indicated doses (mg/kg or units for IFNs) and schedule (days, BID for IFNs) in relation to challenge with ca. 4 LD_{50} of EMC. CMC = carboxymethylcellulose, Squal = 2% squalene, PBS/B = PBS + 0.2% bovine serum albumin. Experimental mortality and MST (days) were compared with the various naive and vehicle control groups (not shown for brevity), which averaged 87.8% $\pm$2.1 mortality and 5.4$\pm$0.2 days MST in the 15 experiments.
*Increased resistance, $p < 0.05$

IFN (received courtesy of Dr. Murasko, Philadelphia, PA) or alpha A/D rIFN (received courtesy of Dr. Sorter, Hoffman-La Roche Inc, Nutley, NJ), while less gamma rIFN (received courtesy of Dr. Shepard, Genetech, Inc., South San Francisco, CA) appeared to be effective. Alpha A/D rIFN and gamma rIFN were more effective against HSV-2 than beta IFN. The results suggest that the IFNs may produce antiviral activity by different mechanisms, involving both direct IFN mediated effects as well as immunomodulatory effects on NK cells and MO. Differences in distribution of the IFNs also may be involved since the pharmacokinetics of the IFNs vary considerably. Repeated administration of IL-1, a major product of MO, had a slight effect against HSV-2 infection; more investigation is clearly warranted for MO products such as IL-1 and tumor necrosis factor.

TABLE 4. Immunomodulators Protective Against HSV-2

Regimen					Mortality	Survival
Drug	Dose	Schedule	Route	Vehicle	Dead/Total(%)	MST
			-- Microbial Products --			
CP	35	-7	i.p.	PBS	3/11 (27%)*	18.4*
CP	35	-1	i.p.	PBS	9/12 (75%)	13.4
			-- Chemicals --			
MVE-2	50	-1	i.p.	PBS	0/11 (0%)*	>21.0*
Avridine	50	-1	i.p.	1%CMC	0/12 (0%)*	>21.0*
ABPP	200	-1	i.p.	1%CMC	3/10 (30%)*	17.1*
ABPP	250	-2to0	i.p.	PBS	0/9 (0%)*	>21.0*
ABPP	100	-3to-1	i.p.	1%CMC	4/10 (40%)*	17.1*
ABPP	200	-3to-1	p.os	1%CMC	3/9 (33%)*	16.8*
ABMP	250	-2to0	i.p.	PBS	1/10 (10%)*	19.8*
AIPP	250	-2to0	i.p.	PBS	0/9 (0%)*	>21.0*
CL246,738	50	-1	p.os	1%CMC	1/10 (10%)*	18.9*
			-- Biologicals --			
IFN-A	<300	0to+8	i.p.	PBS/B	2/10 (20%)*	19.8*
IFN-B	10000	0to+6	i.p.	PBS/B	13/24 (54%)	16.3*
IFN-G	760	0to+8	i.p.	PBS/B	2/10 (20%)*	18.8*
IL-1	3000	0to+8	i.p.	PBS	4/9 (44%)	15.7

CD-1 mice were treated as indicated in Table 3 and challenged with ca. 5000 PFU. Mortality in the various naive and vehicle control groups in the 14 experiments averaged 81.8% $\pm$3.3, with an average MST of 11.8$\pm$0.5 days. *Increased resistance, $p < 0.05$

Treatment of mice with the microbial products or analogs produced modest antiviral activity against EMC virus. Optimum activity of the detoxified monophosphoryl lipid A (Ribi, 1984) required combination with trehalose dimycolate. This is similar to its reported activity against influenza virus infection (Masihi et al., 1986). Whether combining MPL with MDP would be effective remains to be determined. Considerable investigation was performed with MTP-PE (received courtesy of Dr. Dietrich, Ciba-Geigy Ltd, Basel, Switzerland), including a variety of vehicles, free MTP-PE or MTP-PE encapsulated in liposomes (Table 5). Marginal protective effects were observed in some experiments; however, they were not consistently observed. This contrasts with the partial protection found with other HSV models using certain MTP-PE regimens (Koff et al., 1985; Gangemi, personal communication). MTP-PE can also produce partial protection against influenza virus infection (Dietrich et al., 1983; Six, Gangemi, personal communications). The reduction in mortality with MTP-PE, MPL+TDM, and MDP, however, does not appear to be as profound as with MVE-2, CP, or some synthetic agents (Tables 2-4). Other synthetic agents, which are reported to activate macrophages or have other immunomodulatory activity, failed to provide antimicrobial efficacy by the doses and regimens tested (Table 5; Kuus et al., 1985; Renoux et al., 1986; Wang et al., 1986; Hiestand and Strasser, 1985; Audibert et al., 1985). It is of course possible that other regimens may be found that are effective.

The issue of variability in effectiveness of the analogs of microbial structures, and lack of effect of some synthetic immunomodulatory agents, is an important problem to solve. Several important variables are listed in Table 6. For example, the genetic background of the mouse may determine which immunologic effector mechanisms are most active against a given virus infection; in the CD-1 mouse which has low NK cell activity, macrophage activation appears to be more important than NK cell activity (Morahan et al., 1986), while in the C57Bl/6 mouse genetic resistance to the virus correlates closely with NK cell activity and interferon production. Another important variable that is increasingly being recognized is inapparent infection of mice with viruses such as mouse hepatitis virus that can increase antiviral resistance, presumably through macrophage activation and interferon production (Dempsey et al., 1986). Stress is a variable that has been little studied; it has been well established that immunomodulation and the neuroendocrine axis are interconnected (Johnson, 1985). Finally, limited structure activity relationships have been performed with immunodulators in regard to induction of nonspecific resistance; such studies should help indicate potential mechanisms of action, and choices of combination therapies suitable for diverse microbial pathogenesis patterns and resistance mechanisms.

TABLE 5. Ineffective Immunomodulator Regimens.

Drug	Dose	Schedule /Route	Comments
MPL/TDM	8+8	-7, s.c.	EMC
	8+8	-7, i.p.	HSV,veh.effect
MA-CDA	50	-1, i.p.	EMC & HSV
MA-MP	50	-1, i.p.	EMC & HSV
IA-ST	50	-1, i.p.	EMC & HSV
Imuthiol	25	-7or-1, i.p.	EMC, Listeria
		-7,-1,0or0to+8, s.c.	HSV
IL-1	30to3000	+2 hr, i.p.	EMC
ADA202-718	25	-1, p.os	EMC & HSV
		i.p.	HSV
CL259,763	400or200	-1, p.os	EMC & HSV
LS2616	160	-4to-1,+6or+21, H_2O	HSV
		0to+21, H_2O	HSV
		-4to-1or+6, p.os.	HSV
ABPP or AIPP	200	-7,-1or-2to0, i.p.	Listeria
MDP	4or0.1	-1to+2, or +1, i.p.	EMC, Listeria
MDP-GDP	4to0.1	-2to+2, i.p.	EMC
MTP-PE	4to0.1	-7,-2to0,+2 or intermittent,i.p., i.v.,p.os	EMC, HSV, Listeria
Avr/Lipo	50	-7or-1, i.p.	Listeria

Useful correlations of effector cell augmentation and therapeutic activity of immunomodulators against several tumors have recently been developed (Talmadge and Chirigos, 1986). These have allowed determination of their probable mechanisms of antitumor activity. Such systematic studies of antimicrobial action have been performed for relatively few immunomodulators (Morahan, 1979). For some of the compounds and regimens with marked antimicrobial activity, we have evaluated the role that monocytes, NK cells and tissue MO may play in the enhanced resistance by defining resistance in CD-1 mice selectively depleted of cells by treatment with

TABLE 6. Reasons for Variability in Assays for Antimicrobial Efficacy of Immunomodulators

<u>Microorganism</u>
-Strain, passage history and virulence characteristics
-Pathogenesis of infection, route of infection, etc.
<u>Mouse</u>
-Genetic background
-Age, developmental state of immune system, etc.
-Sex
-Inapparent infections
-Stress, as affected by shipping, randomization, numbers per cage, handling, etc.
<u>Immunomodulator</u>
-Mechanisms of action, as affected by pleiotropic effects on heterogeneous cell populations, immunoregulatory circuits and genetic background
-Pharmacokinetics, as affected by molecule, vehicle, liposomes, route, schedule, etc.
-Vehicle effects
-Endotoxin contamination
-Combination with other immunomodulators or conventional antimicrobial therapy

^{89}Sr (Morahan et al., 1986). We have recently shown that circulating monocytes and NK cell activity can be markedly reduced by ^{89}Sr treatment without affecting tissue MO, or natural resistance to EMC, HSV-2 or Listeria. Moreover, there is no change in enhanced resistance induced by immunomodulators such as MVE-2, <u>C. parvum</u> and avridine in liposomes (Morahan et al., 1986). These results suggest that the antimicrobial action of these immunomodulators may occur through tissue MO activation. Whether the activity of the pyrimidinones, CL246,748 or the various IFNs occurs via NK cell or tissue MO activation or direct antiviral activity remains to be determined in this depletion model. Until the mechanisms of antimicrobial action are determined systematically for a variety of agents, in infections involving a spectrum of host resistance parameters, we will be unable to realize the full potential of immunotherapy against infectious diseases.

SUMMARY

Three immunomodulators, pyran, MVE-2 and *C. parvum*, provided significant protection with prophylactic administration against the three infections tested. Several synthetic immunomodulators were very effective with prophylactic administration against both EMC and HSV-2 viral infections; these included CL246,738, the pyrimidinones, and avridine in liposomes. Recombinant alpha and gamma IFNs and natural beta IFN were effective on repeated therapeutic treatment against both EMC and HSV-2; alpha and gamma IFN were significantly more effective than beta IFN, and were more effective against HSV-2 than EMC. The efficacy of IFNs against Listeria needs to be evaluated. Certain immunomodulator regimens were protective against viral infections but enhanced Listeria infection; this is troubling for clinical potential. It points out the need for more systematic comparative investigation of immunotherapy in a variety of infection models. At the same time, the fact that a given drug regimen can inhibit or enhance an infectious disease process provides an experimental tool to better define pathogenesis and resistance mechanisms important in different microbial processes.

ACKNOWLEDGEMENTS

This research has been supported by contract N00014-82-K-0669 from the Office of Naval Research, grant CA35961 from the National Cancer Institute and contract DAMD17-86-C-6117 from the US Army Medical Research and Development Command.

REFERENCES

Audibert F, LeClerq C, Chedid L (1985). Muramyl peptides as immunpharmacological response modifiers. In "Biological Response Modifiers," New York: Academic Press, p 307-327.

Dempsey WL, Morahan PS (1985). Immune mechanisms of host resistance to viruses and assessment of immunotoxicologic effects. In Dean JA, Munson AE, Luster MI (eds): "Immunotoxicology and Immunopharmacology," New York: Raven Press, p 55-68.

Dempsey WL, Smith AL, Morahan PS (1986). Effects of inapparent murine hepatitis virus infection on macrophages and host resistance. J Leuk Biol 39:559-566.

Dietrich FM, Lukas B, Schmidtruppin KH (1983). Prophylactic and therapeutic effects of MTP-PE, a synthetic muramyl peptide, in experimental virus infections. 13th International Congress of Chemotherapy.

Hiestand PC, Strasser M (1985). Immunomodulatory properties of ethylene-2,2'-bis(dithio)bis(ethanol) and related compounds in vivo. Int J Immunopharm 7:141-151.

Kalland T, Alm G, Stalhandske T (1985). Augmentation of mouse natural killer cell activity by LS 2616, a new immunomodulator. J Immunol 134:3956-3961.

Kuus K, Ottenbrite RM, Kaplan AM (1985). In situ activation of murine peritoneal macrophages by cyclohexyl-1,3-dioxepin and 4-methyl-2-pentenoyl maleic anhydride copolymers. J Biol Res Mod 4:56-59.

Johnson HM (1985). Neuroendocrine hormones and the immune system. In "Biological Response Modifiers," New York: Academic Press, p 245-263.

Li LH, Wallace TL, Richard KA, Tracey DE (1985). Mechanism of antitumor action of pyrimidinones in the treatment of B16 melanoma and P388 leukemia. Cancer Res 45:532-538.

Masihi KN, Lange W, Brehmer W, Ribi E (1986). Immunobiological properties of nontoxic lipid A: enhancement of nonspecific resistance of muramyl dipeptide in combination with trehalose dimycolate against viral infection and adjuvant effects. J Immunopharmacol, in press.

Morahan PS (1981). Anionic polymers and polysaccharides: Overview of interferon inducing ability, antitumor activity and mechanisms of action. In Hersh EM, Chirigos MA, Mastrangelo MJ (eds), "Augmenting Agents in Cancer Therapy," New York (Raven Press), p 105 192.

Morahan PS, Bradley SG, Munson AE, Duke S, Fromtling RA, Marciano-Cabral F (1984). Immunotoxic effects of diethylstilbestrol on host resistance: comparison with cyclophosphamide. J Leuk Biol 35:329-341.

Morahan PS, Dempsey WL, Volkman A, Connor J (1986). Antimicrobial activity of various immunomodulators: independence from normal levels of circulating monocytes and natural killer cells. Infec Immun 51:87-93.

Murasko DM, Fresa K, Mark R (1983). Enhancement or inhibition of tumor growth by interferon: dependence on treatment protocol. Int J Cancer 32:751-757.

Niblack JF, Otterness JG, Hemsworth GR, Wolff JS, Hoffman WW, Kraska AR (1979). CP-20,961: a structurally novel synthetic adjuvant. J Reticuloend Soc 26:655-666.

Renoux M, Giroud JP, Florentin I, Guillaumin JM, Degenne D, Renoux G (1986). Early changes in immune parameters induced by an acute non-antigenic inflammation in mouse: influence of imuthiol. Int J Immunoph 8:107-117.
Ribi EJ (1984). Beneficial effects of the endotoxin molecule. J Biol Resp Mod 3:1-9.
Schuller GB, Morahan PS (1979). Mechanisms of immunomodulator induced enhancement of Friend leukemia virus disease. J Nat Cancer Inst 62:1257-1260.
Talmadge JE, Chirigos MA (1985). Comparison of immunomodulatory and immunotherapeutic properties of biologic response modifiers. Springer Semin Immunopathol 8:429-443.
Wang BS, Lumanglas AL, Ruszala-Mallon VM, Durr FE (1985). Induction of tumor-inhibitory macrophages with a novel synthetic immunomodulator, 3,6-bis(2-piperidinoethoxy) acridine trihydrochloride (CL 246,738). J Immunol 135:679-683.
Wang BS, Ruszala-Mallon V, Wallace RE, Citarella RV, Lin Y, Durr FE (1986). Modulation of the immune response to tumors by a novel synthetic compound, N-[4-[(4-fluorophenyl)sulfonyl]phenyl] acetamide (CL 259,763). Cancer Immunol Immunoth, in press.
Wing EJ, Boehmer S (1984). Dissociative effects of a novel immunomodulating agent (CP-20,961) on host defenses in mice. J Immunopharm 6:339-358.

Immunopharmacology of Infectious Diseases: Vaccine Adjuvants and Modulators of Non-Specific Resistance, pages 325–335

THE IMMUNOMODULATORY PROPERTIES OF CHINESE MEDICINAL MATERIALS

K.N. Leung and H.W. Yeung

Department of Biochemistry and Chinese Medicinal Research Center, The Chinese University of Hong Kong, Shatin, N.T., Hong Kong.

ABSTRACT

A considerable number of Chinese medicinal herbs have been found to have immunomodulatory activities. They work either by strengthening and reinforcing the immune system or act as modifiers and regulators which inhibit immune responses. In this paper, the effect of two Chinese medicinal plants (Ginseng and Tian-hua-fen) on both the non-specific and specific components of the immune system will be discussed. These plants may be considered as prototypes of Chinese medicinal materials with immunomodulatory properties as their active principles have been purified, characterized and then properly evaluated by modern immunologic techniques.

INTRODUCTION

Although traditional Chinese medicine was practised by the Chinese people since ancient times, however, most of the Chinese medicinal materials have not yet been thoroughly investigated and validated by modern scientific methods. The efficacy of these natural products is primarily based on centuries-old empirical observations and clinical experience. To many Western scientists, the Chinese medicinal materials are being viewed with scepticism as they are generally available in bulky crude forms and are freshly made into concoctions for oral administration according to prescriptions. In recent years, there is an increasing interest in the search of potential drugs that are capable of modulating immune responses with less serious side effects. Since the therapeutic principles of traditional Chinese medicine concern not only the elimination of pathogenic factors but also the reinforcement of resistance to disease, it is conspicuous that many Chinese medicinal drugs are indeed capable of elevating or modulating human immune functions. Although many commonly used Chinese medicinal plants are known to have immunomodulatory activities (Table 1), nevertheless, there are few reports which are devoted to the systematic studies of the immunopharmacology of Chinese medicinal materials. In this paper, the immunomodulatory properties of two widely used Chinese medicinal plants (Ginseng and Tian-hua-fen) will be described. The active principles of these plants have been purified and characterized and they work either by stimulating the immune system non-specifically or act as potent inhibitors which suppress immune responses.

IMMUNOMODULATORY PROPERTIES OF GINSENG

The ginseng plant of the Araliaceae family is one of the most popular natural tonics used in Oriental countries for thousands of years. Traditional Chinese medicine regarded ginseng as a medicinal material that can replenish vital energy and improve body strength. Commercial ginsengs are of two main species: Panax ginseng C.A. Meyer is the source of Chinese or Korean ginseng while Panax quinquefolium is the source of American ginseng. Among the major chemical constituents of ginseng, the saponins (which are called panaxosides by the Russian and ginsenosides by the Japanese) are the pharmacologically active components and have been the targets of research for many years. A recent report showed that at least 30 different tetracyclic dammarane-type of ginsenosides have so far been isolated from Panax ginseng (Shoji, 1985) and that ginsenosides of various abundance have been found in ginseng root as well as in the aerial organs of the ginseng plant.

Ginseng extracts or ginsenosides were found to display a broad spectrum of pharmacological activities on various body systems (Ng and Yeung, 1986). Ginseng has shown to stimulate and regulate the central nervous system, particularly the cerebral cortex in experimental animals. It has sedative and tranquilizing effects, and is known to

TABLE 1. COMMONLY USED CHINESE HERBS WITH KNOWN IMMUNOMODULATORY PROPERTIES

SCIENTIFIC NAME	COMMON NAME	MAJOR ACTIONS	ACTIVE PRINCIPLES
I. IMMUNOSTIMULANTS:			
Panax ginseng (Araliaceae)	Ginseng (人參)	tonic; promotes mental stability	gensenosides
Astragalus membranaceus (Leguminosae)	Huang-chi (黃耆)	tonic; diuretic anti-pyretic	polysaccharides
Angelica sinensis (Umbelliferae)	Tang-kuei (當歸)	tonic; sedative stimulates blood circulation	?
Ganoderma lucidum (Basidiomycetes)	Ling-chih (靈芝)	nourishing tonic improves body resistance	?
II. IMMUNOSUPPRESSANTS:			
Trichosanthes kirilowii (Cucurbitaceae)	Tian-hua-fen (天花粉)	abortifacient stabilizes pulmonary and intestinal functions	simple protein (trichosanthin)
Glycyrrhiza uralensis (Leguminosae)	Licorice (甘草)	relaxant anti-allergic relieves intoxication	glycyrrhizic acid glycopeptide/ glycoprotein (Lx)
Tripterygium wilfordii (Celastraceae)	Lei-gong-teng (雷公藤)	anti-inflammatory relieves intoxication	tripterine
Lysimachia christinae (Primulaceae)	Desmodii herba (金錢草)	diuretic promotes biliary secretion	?

antagonize fatigue, both physically and mentally. Moreover, ginseng is a cardiotonic and can normalize blood pressure. There is experimental evidence showing that ginseng has a general stimulatory and regulatory effect on the endocrine system, involving the pituitary, thyroid and adrenal glands. Ginseng can influence metabolism by increasing the biosynthesis of DNA, RNA and proteins. It also facilitates energy metabolism and promotes animal growth. It is important to realize that the pharmacological actions of ginseng usually vary with the different physiological states of the organism and may be biphasic in nature. For instance, ginseng can increase blood pressure in case of hypotension or shock but restores normal blood pressure in case of hypertension.

In recent years, there is increasing evidence which suggests that ginseng has an immunomodulatory effect and that administration of ginsenosides not only able to increase the non-specific resistance of the organism but could also modulate the specific immune responses as well. Many research groups have demonstrated that ginseng has significant protective action against a wide variety of harmful physical, chemical or biological stimuli, such as shock, drug-induced inflammation, exposure to cold, heat, radiation and infectious agents. Moreover, ginseng was found to exhibit anti-tumour and anti-microbial activities (Ng and Yeung, 1986). It has been reported that ginseng was able to strengthen the immune functions of cancer patients (Wang, 1981) and that mice treated with ginseng could tolerate infection with a large number of microorganisms (Wang, 1980).

There has been many studies of the effect of ginseng on the non-specific immune mechanisms. Wang et al. (1985) have shown that oral or intraperitoneal administration of ginseng saponins not only increased the phagocytosis of the reticuloendothelial system in normal mice but also in mice bearing the sarcoma S-180. Similarly, subcutaneous injection of ginsenosides into mice (1 mg/mouse for 7 successive days) also enhanced the in vitro phagocytic activity of the mouse peritoneal exudate cells (Bao and Yang, 1984). Singh et al. (1984), on the other hand, had shown that ginseng extracts could augment mouse endogeneous natural killer (NK) activity and exhibited a synergistic effect in the induction of interferon by an interferon inducer of fungal origin (6-MFA). Moreover, oral administration of ginseng saponins could also raise the serum complement content in guinea pigs (Wang et al., 1985).

The effect of ginseng saponins on the cellular and humoral immunity have also been investigated. Bao and Yang (1984) showed that in vivo administration of ginsenosides (1 mg/mouse for 7 successive days) or exposure of splenocytes to ginsenosides in vitro (1 μg/ml) significantly enhanced the lymphocyte transformation reaction in response to stimulation with T or B cell mitogens. There is a number of reports on the immunostimulatory effect of ginseng on the humoral immune response. Li et al. (1980) have shown that ginseng can enhance specific antibody production in guinea pigs immunized with influenza vaccine and in rats immunized with diphtheria toxoid. Other investigators have demonstrated that ginseng extracts or ginsenosides were capable of enhancing the plaque-forming cell response and the level of circulating antibody to sheep red blood cells (SRBC) in mice (Singh et al., 1984; Wang et al., 1985). The enhancing effect of ginsenosides on humoral antibody formation appears to be dependent on the number of immunizations and the dose of antigen used. Significant elevation of the primary antibody response was seen when a suboptimal dose of antigen was used for immunization whereas a slight enhancement was observed when an optimal dose of antigen was used (Bao and Yang, 1984). Likewise, ginsenosides were found to have no enhancing effect on the secondary antibody response to a high dose of antigen. The immunomodulatory effect of ginseng on specific cell-mediated immune (CMI) response was less clear and conflicting results had been reported. Our earlier work had shown that ginseng saponins selectively suppressed the delayed type hypersensitivity (DTH) response to influenza virus when administered to the mice before but not after viral sensitization (Yeung et al., 1982). This selective immunosuppressive effect of ginsenosides could be attributed to their steroid-like structure. In contrast, Singh et al. (1984) had reported that the CMI response to the Semliki forest virus antigen, as measured by the migration inhibition test, was increased by administration of ginseng extract in vivo. The reason for the discrepancy of these findings is unknown, perhaps this might be due to the differences in the T cell parameter being measured, the dose and route of drug administration and the purity of the preparation being used. Thus the effect of ginseng on specific cellular immunity remains to be determined.

The underlying mechanism(s) by which ginseng could exert its influence on cells of the immune system has not been resolved. A recent report had shown that in vivo administration of ginsenosides could elevate the splenic intracellular cAMP level before antigen stimulation while the level of cGMP was raised after antigen stimulation (Bao and Yang, 1984). Based on the in vitro models of B cell differentiation into antibody-forming cells and T cell differentiation into cytotoxic T cells, it is known that cAMP facilitates some stages of antigen-independent differentiation of T and B lymphocytes from precursor cells and inhibits other stages such as lymphocyte proliferation whereas cGMP has just the opposite effects (Plaut et al., 1980). Thus it is conceivable that by affecting the levels of cyclic nucleotides in the cells of the immune system, ginsenosides could exert their modulatory effects on various types of immune reactivities. Whether other mechanisms are also involved in the immunomodulatory effect of ginseng clearly needs further investigation.

IMMUNOSUPPRESSIVE ACTIVITIES OF TIAN-HUA-FEN

Tian-hua-fen, the root tuber of the Chinese medicinal plant Trichosanthes kirilowii Maxim of the Cucurbitaceae family, has traditionally been used as an abortifacient drug for centuries in China. Since it is also known to have anti-pyretic, mucolytic and anti-inflammatory activities, it has been recommended for the treatment of cough, dry mouth, furuncle and carbuncle. A pharmacologically active component, named trichosanthin, was isolated and purified from the crude extract of Tian-hua-fen. It was shown to be a 24,000 dalton basic protein and its chemical structure has recently been elucidated (Wang, 1985). Trichosanthin was shown to be effective in terminating early pregnancy and inducing mid-term abortion in laboratory animals and humans (Chang et al., 1979; Liu et al., 1981; 1985; Jin, 1985). The abortifacient activity of trichosanthin has been attributed to its selective and direct destruction of the syncytiotrophoblasts of the placental villi and this leads to tissue necrosis and eventually abortion (Anon, 1976). In addition to its abortifacient action, trichosanthin was also shown to inhibit the abnormal growth of trophoblast cells, both *in vivo* (Yao, 1978) and *in vitro* (Tsao *et al*., 1986). In view of the importance of trichosanthin as a natural-occurring abortifacient plant protein and its clinical use in inducing mid-term abortion and in the treatment of ectopic pregnancy, hydatidiform mole and choriocarcinoma in China, we have recently initiated studies on the immunomodulatory properties of this plant protein and the results are briefly summarized as follows.

In vitro studies have shown that trichosanthin can markedly inhibit the proliferative response of mouse splenocytes to stimulation with T cell mitogens such as Con A and PHA or with B cell mitogens such as LPS and dextran sulfate. Suppression occurred in a dose-dependent manner and complete abrogation of mitogen responsiveness was observed at a concentration of 50 - 100 μg/ml of the protein, a concentration that did not result in any significant loss of cell viability. Similar results were also reported by Yeh *et al*. (1986) who found that the suppression of Con A response by trichosanthin was not limited to the triggering period since the protein also depressed the initiated Con A response of mouse splenocytes and suppression was not relieved by addition of exogeneous lymphokines. Moreover, we have found that the *in vitro* generation of a primary alloreactive cytotoxic T cell response and the production of interleukin 2 (IL-2) by Con A activated mouse splenocytes *in vitro* were also significantly suppressed in the presence of trichosanthin. In consistent with the *in vitro* observation, we found that single injection of non-toxic microgram amount of trichosanthin into mice could reduce the capacity of their splenocytes to liberate IL-2 in response to Con A stimulation *in vitro*. Similarly, trichosanthin administrated *in vivo* not only resulted in a significant depression of the DTH response but also suppressed the primary humoral antibody response to SRBC. Taken these together, it is clear that trichosanthin could effectively suppress the T and B cell responses both *in vitro* and *in vivo*.

The effect of trichosanthin on cells that are involved in non-specific immunity has also been examined. Although single injection of trichosanthin *per se* did not appear to affect the number of resident peritoneal macrophages, however, the migration of monocytes into the peritoneal cavity as a result of thioglycollate-elicited acute inflammation was markedly suppressed by in vivo treatment of mice with the protein. In addition, the effector functions of macrophages such as the phagocytic and cytostatic activities were markedly depressed by in vitro exposure to trichosanthin. In contrast, similar in vitro treatment did not inhibit the effector phase of NK-mediated cytolysis. Likewise, the in vivo activation of NK cells was not appreciably affected by pretreatment of mice with trichosanthin. Thus, although trichosanthin appears to modulate a variety of immune reactivities, its suppressive effect is not totally non-selective. The available evidence so far suggests that NK cells may not be the primary target for trichosanthin as both the in vivo induction and the in vitro effector function of this cell type were not significantly altered in the presence of the protein, whereas similar conditions were markedly suppressive for other immune reactivities.

The mechanism(s) of immunodepression caused by trichosanthin has not been resolved. Immunosuppression cannot be attributed to the direct lymphocytotoxic effect of trichosanthin as exposure of mouse splenocytes to a high concentration (100 μg/ml) of the protein for at least 48 hours did not lead to any significant loss of cell viability. In addition, the observed suppression is unlikely to be due to a time-shift in the kinetic parameter of an immune response since it was found that the kinetics of the immune responses such as the mitogen-induced lymphocyte transformation in vitro and the DTH and humoral antibody response to SRBC in vivo were not appreciably affected by treatment with trichosanthin. More recently, using computer analysis Zheng and Wang (1986) have reported that there exists a remarkable sequence homology between trichosanthin and the subunit A of Ricin D. Due to this sequence homology and with the fact that trichosanthin is a protein synthesis inhibitor in a cell-free lysate system (Xiong et al., 1980), it could be speculated that the observed immunomodulatory properties of trichosanthin might be due to its inhibitory action on protein synthesis on cells of the immune system. Selectivity of the action of trichosanthin could well be due to the differences in the affinity and amount of specific surface receptors, the efficiency of transportation and internalization of the protein into the cell interior as well as some other intrinsic inherent properties. Although protein synthesis inhibition could account for the immunomodulatory effect of trichosanthin, it has yet to be formally established that this mechanism is the only or the major one involved in the immunosuppression observed.

CONCLUDING REMARKS

Today the traditional Chinese medicine is still used as a practical medical treatment by hundreds of millions of Chinese people especially for diseases which are chronic or degenerative in nature. Since many of the Chinese medicinal materials exert their effects by augmenting or restoring the organism's defense mechanisms, it is hoped that by studying the immunomodulatory properties of Chinese medicinal materials, it may be possible to identify and obtain natural immunomodulators for clinical testing and immunotherapy with minimal side effects. In general, medicinal herbs are known to promote immunity in several ways. They may booster NK activity, increase the phagocytic function of macrophages, induce interferon production or augment the specific cellular and humoral immune responses. In recent years, a number of Chinese herbs with strong clinical evidence have been studied for their immunomodulatory activities. However, many of these studies were performed using total crude extracts or a very heterogeneous mixture of compounds and the active ingredients having the immunomodulatory effect have not been identified. Therefore, a formidable task at present is to isolate and identify unequivocally the effective elements from the Chinese medicinal materials so as to assure uniformity in response to drugs and minimize drug interactions. However, many Chinese medicinal materials have complex components and attempts to isolate the active constituents may often lead to a loss of biological or pharmacological activities as many Chinese medicinal materials are effective only when they are used as compound drugs or in a complex prescription formula. Despite this fact, the elucidation of the immunomodulatory properties of Chinese medicinal materials does open a way to increase our understanding of the action mechanism of these drugs and enables us to verify their true efficacy on a deeper scientific level with a view to improve their therapeutic value for the better health care of mankind.

REFERENCES

Anonymous (1976). Studies on the mechanisms of abortion induction by trichosanthin. Scientia Sinica 19:811-827 (in Chinese).

Bao T, Yang KC (1984). Studies on the effect of ginseng flower total saponins on the murine immune responses and the elucidation of action mechanism. Chinese J Integrated Traditional and Western Med 4:172-175 (in Chinese).

Chang MC, Saksena SK, Lau IF, Wang YH (1979). Induction of mid-term abortion by trichosanthin in laboratory animals. Contraception 19:175-184.

Li XC, Chen TH, Wang LN (1980). Effect of ginseng on specific humoral immune response. Jilin Chinese Medicine and Materia Medica 1:67-71 (in Chinese).

Liu GW, Lau T, Lau FY, Ming TH, Sun PL (1981). Inhibition of early pregnancy by combined trichosanthin in laboratory animals. Reprod Contraception 1:20-24.

Liu GW, Liu FY, Li YJ et al. (1985). A summary of 402 cases of termination of early pregnancy with crystalline preparations of trichosanthin. In CHang HM, Yeung HW, Tso WW, Koo A (eds): "Advances in Chinese Medicinal Materials Research," Singapore: World Scientific Publ. Co., p 327-333

Jin YC (1985). Clinical study of trichosanthin. In Chang HM, Yeung HW, Tso WW, Koo A (eds): "Advances in Chinese Medicinal Materials Research," Singapore: World Scientific Publ. Co., p 319-326.

Ng TB, Yeung HW (1986). Scientific basis of the therapeutic effects of ginseng. In Steiner RP (ed): "Folk Medicine: The Art and the Science," Washington: American Chemical Society, p 139-151.

Plaut M, Marone G, Thomas LL, Lichtenstein LM (1980). Cyclic nucleotides in immune responses and allergy. In Hamet P, Sands H (eds): "Advances in Cyclic Nucleotide Research," New York: Raven Press, Vol. 12, p 161-172.

Shoji J (1985). Recent advances in the chemical studies of ginseng. In Chang HM, Yeung HW, Tso WW, Koo A (eds): "Advances in Chinese Medicinal Materials Research," Singapore: World Scientific Publ. Co., p 455-469.

Singh VK, Agarwal SS, Gupta BM (1984). Immunomodulatory activity of Panax ginseng extract. Proceedings of the 4th International Ginseng Symposium, Korea, p 225-232.

Tsao SW, Yan YT, Yeung HW (1986). Selective killing of choriocarcinoma cells in vitro by trichosanthin, a plant protein purified from root tubers of the Chinese medicinal herb, Trichosanthes kirilowii. Toxicon (in press).

Wang BX (1980). Progress of pharmacological studies of ginseng. Acta Pharmaceutica Sinica 15: 312-320 (in Chinese).

Wang BX, Cui JC, Liu AJ (1985). The effect of ginseng on immune responses. In Chang HM, Yeung HW, Tso WW, Koo A (eds): "Advances in Chinese Medicinal Materials Research," Singapore: World Scientific Publ. Co., p 519-527.

Wang JY (1981). Clinical observation of ginseng on the tumour patients. Jilin Medicine 2: 15-17 (in Chinese).

Wang Y (1985). Chemistry of trichosanthin, a new biologically active plant protein. In Chang HM, Yeung HW, Tso WW, Koo A (eds): " Advances in Chinese Medicinal Materials Research," Singapore: World Scientific Publ. Co., p 289-295.

Xiong YZ, Chu K, Tso JK, Yao KW, Chang K, Hsu CY (1980). A preliminary study of the injurious mechanism of trichosanthin. Acta Biol Exp Sinica 13: 470-471 (in Chinese, abstract in English).

Yao JF (1978). The analysis of 106 cases of malignant trophoblastic tumours treated by combination of Chinese and Western medicine. Jiangsu Med 6: 5-7 (in Chinese).

Yeh M, Chi YY, Shen RZ, Lin GM (1986). The study of in vivo and in vitro responses to trichosanthin in mouse. Acta Biol Exp Sinica 19: 81-90 (in Chinese, abstract in English).

Yeung HW, Cheung K, Leung KN (1982). Immunopharmacology of Chinese medicine 1, Ginseng induced immunosuppression in virus-infected mice. Amer J Chinese Med 10: 44-54.

Zheng XY, Wang YH (1986). The sequence homology of trichosanthin and ricin A chain. Nature (in press).

Immunopharmacology of Infectious Diseases: Vaccine Adjuvants and Modulators of Non-Specific Resistance, pages 337–349

Immunotherapy in the Treatment of Infectious Diseases

John W. Hadden

Program of Immunopharmacology, University of of South Florida Medical College, 12901 N. 30th Street, Tampa, Florida 33612

It is an honor for me to give the final overview talk in this interesting meeting. The many excellent papers presented attest to the current interest in the immunopharmacology of this area. In my talk I would like to highlight certain points in a "broad brush" rather than a detailed review manner.

The treatment of infections with immunostimulating drugs is broadly termed a "prohost" approach since the therapy is designed to increase host defense rather than directly kill the pathogen. The origins of the approach go far back into history with attempts through tonics, as in Chinese traditional herbal medicines, to strengthen the host ("stimulate the yin"). At the turn of the century it was Metchnikoff who advocated stimulating the phagocytes to enhance host resistance. Much of recent vaccine development and its success derive from efforts to specifically prepare the host for expected pathogen challenge. In recent years a number of reviews (Hadden, et al., 1976; Werner, 1979; Friedman & Specter, 1982; Hadden, et al., 1985) have summarized the many experimental works which support the concept that nonspecific immunostimulants have usefullness in both the prevention and treatment of infectious diseases. No doubt, the relatively recent development of a broad understanding of the role of the immune system in defense against infectious disease (see Nahmias and O'Reilly, 1981 for review) and the great success in the last half century of the development of effective antimicrobial chemotherapy have retarded the development of antiinfectious immunotherapy. Despite the relation health security of the western world, it is to be remembered that infectious scourges, particularly parasitic, still plague the world's population. Certainly, the epidemic of the acquired immunodeficiency syndrome (AIDS) reminds us of our vulnerability.

The current concepts of the prohost approach derive from the knowledge that when specific host defense mechanisms are impaired, infection results and the type of infection depends on the nature of the immune defect. The definitions of specific and general defects of the immune system have become increasingly clear in recent years and rather then being a relatively rare event, cellular immunodeficiency is common in a variety of situations including the neonatal period, in protein-calorie and vitamin deficiencies, in parasitic, bacterial and viral diseases, in cancer, in aging, as well as in AIDS. Large segments of the world's population are, as a result, at risk and in many cases, to pathogens for which we have no available specific antimicrobial chemotherapy.

The notion of treating a failing immune system is a relatively new concept; however, in the same way that we, as physicians, treat a failing heart, liver or respiratory system it seems reasonable to treat the defective immune system. It now seems reasonable not only to do so in individuals who are immunodepressed and infected but also to do so immunoprophylactically in those immunodepressed but not infected to prevent infection. A large experience has accumulated to show that a variety of crude bacterial and fungal products will enhance defense against particularly viral pathogens. The increasing repertoire of chemically defined biologicals and drugs having relative specificity for one or another effector cell of the immune system makes the approach to rather specific manipulation of successful experimental and clinical experiences have been presented in this meeting. Highlighted have been those biologicals and drugs which have been most effective or insightful in their application.

Since antibody-mediated mechanisms are generally preserved in secondary immunodeficiency and vaccine and adjuvant applications have focused on these mechanisms, cellular immune responses involving thymus-dependent (T) lymphocytes, macrophages and natural killer cells have been emphasized. It is to be noted, however, that recent advances in vaccine development using synthetic adjuvants like MDP coupled to genetically engineered epitopes offers the prospect of conferring specific resistance, cellular or humoral immunity or both, in the protection against a variety of diseases hertofore unapproached by vaccines (e.g., hepatitis B and malaria) (see Chedid, 1985 for review). Also the development of monoclonal antibodies, particularly human-human monoclonals, offers great potential in the future for adoptive neutralizing serotherapy in the treatment of infectious diseases. These two approaches make it likely that vaccination and antibody-mediated mechanisms are also to contribute to future prohost therapies.

It is useful to remember that the infectious consequences of agammaglobulinemia, that is the lack of ability to make antibodies, involve principally high grade pyogenic pathogens (e.g., streptococcus, staphylococci and pneumococci) which affect the respiratory tract. Our ability to manage these infections with gammaglobulin therapy and antibiotics make it possible for these patients to live into adulthood.

In contrast the lack of T cell-mediated immunity, as occurs in AIDS, opens the door to a much larger spectrum of lethal pathogens for which we often lack effective antimicrobial therapy. Central to the therapy of these diseases is the reconstitution of cellular immune mechanisms. Bone marrow and thymus transplantation represents two efforts which in their place have been useful yet, overall, represent not generally applicable or feasible approaches to treatment. Attempts to replace the humoral role of the thymus have focused on the thymic hormones. A series of proteins have been extracted from the thymus and used in immunoreconstitutive therapy in man and animals with a variety of diseases (see Goldstein, 1984 for review).

Chemically defined thymic hormones in the form of thymosin α_1, thymopoietin, and thymulin (FTS) and two mixed preparations, thymosin fraction V and thymostimulin (TP-1), have been used in large numbers of patients with congenital and acquired cellular immune deficiencies. Rather impressive effects of the administration of the crude thymic extract thymosin fraction V and thymosin α_1, have been observed in chemotherapy-treated immunosuppressed mice to prevent the susceptibility to pathogen challenge (Ishitzuka, et al., 1983). Table I summarizes some of the infectious disease applications in which these hormones have been employed.

Table I

Thymic Hormones	Levamisole
Acute Encephalitis	Brucellosis
SSPE	Meliodosis
Varicella-Zoster	Tuberculosis
CMV	Leprosy
Herpes Keratitis	Aphthous Stomatitis
Recurrent Herpes I	Mcocutaneous candidiasis
	Aspergillosis
	Recurrent Herpes 1 & 2
	Herpes Zoster
Isoprinosine	**Interferon**
Influenza	Laryngeal Warts
Rhinovirus	Chondyloma Acuminatum
Recurrent Herpes 2	Hepatitis B
Acute Viral Encephalitis	Herpes Zoster
SSPE	Herpes Simplex
Hepatitis A & B	CMV
Warts	Rhinovirus
Varicella	
Measles	

In addition to the thymic hormones, interleukins I & II (IL-1 & IL-2) regulate T cell function and development. Based upon recent observations (Hadden, et al., 1981) that interleukin 2 acts to promote immature thymocyte maturation, therapy with IL-2 may be an important adjunct to thymic hormone therapy in T cell deficient individuals.

A number of drugs are thymomimetic in their action (Hadden, 1985). Isoprinosine and NPT 15392 are good examples of those acting directly to induce prothymocyte differentiation and promote T cell functions including interleukin II production. Their immunopharmacologies have been reviewed elsewhere (O'Neill, et al., 1984; Simon, et al., 1983). Isoprinosine has seen the widest clinical experience in viral disease including herpes, virus infections, influenza, and measles-associated subacute sclerosing panencephalitis and its effects are likely due to prohost action (see Table I). Levamisole and other sulphur containing compounds are indirectly thymomimetic through their ability to promote in vivo the a appearance of a thymic hormone-like substance (Renoux, 1978). Diethyldithiocarbamate (DTC-imuithiol) is a sulphur compared sharing a similar immunopharmacology with levamisole presumably through the same mechanisms (Renoux, Renoux, 1984). Levamisole has had extensive application in a variety of infections in man and animals (see Table I).

In addition to therapy directed at reconstituting or promoting T cell function, therapy directed at nonspecific components of the system, like macrophages and natural killer cells, has also seen attention. The interferons activate both these populations of cells and have been used in treatment of a number of viral infections in animals and humans (see Table I).

A number of other agents directly activate macrophages for bactericidal activity including lymphokines (MAF's), endotoxins, tuftsin and muramyl dipeptides. Treatment of animals particularly before pathogen challenge by these agents has been shown to increase host resistance particularly to facultative intracellular bacterial pathogens and parasites. Other agents like isoprinosine, levamisole, aximexon, and NPT 15392 potentiate their effects and may be effective in promoting macrophage mediated resistance.

Natural killer cells are thought to be a primary defense against virus challenge and stimulation of these cells with IL-2 or interferon increases their function. This action can be mimicked and/or potentiated by drugs like isoprinosine, NPT 15392, and cyclomunine and by interferon inducers like pyran copolymer (MVE-2) and pyrimidinoles and in a number of settings enhanced resistance to viral challenge has been demonstrated. One of the relationships which emerges from comparing agents which promote T cell-mediated immunity to those which promote nonspecific resistance at the level of the macrophage or natural killer cell is that while exceptions exist, the former are, generally immunotherapeutic while the latter are immunoprophylactic (Table II). The number of circumstances in which immunoprophylactic agents may find usefulness in clinical medicine may seem limited

Table 2, Agents with Activity in Animal Models of Bacterial, Viral, and Fungal Challenge

Immunoprophylactic	Immunotherapeutic
Interferon	Interferon
Interferon Inducers	Thymic Hormones
MDP and Analogs	Levamisole
RES Expanders - Glycans	Isoprinosine

since seldom can an infection be diagnosed prior to clinical symptoms let alone prior to exposure. By way of a possible example, it is important to note that a large number of individuals with cancer who have been treated aggressively with chemotherapy are prone to infection. Prophylactic immunorestorative treatment of these patients might significantly reduce their morbidity and mortality. Another population at risk for infection are the elderly. Where individuals in this population can be identified as immunologically compromised and at high risk, immunoprophylactic therapy might be applicable. In other settings, immunologic reconstitution of aged animals has seen benefit in terms reduced incidence of malignancy and increased longevity (Bruley-Rosset, et al., 1979). In order for us to understand more clearly the therapeutic and immunoprophylactic potential of these biologicals and drugs we need more experience in the clinical setting. We need more specific information about the immune defects attendant to certain infections in order to address our therapies more specifically to correct these defects. Figure 1 summarizes the actions of the various immunomodulators under discussion on their various target cells. Such a schema emphasizes the potential for immunotherapy to be relatively specific in its application depending on the nature of the hosts immune defect and, or course, on the nature of the central mechanism of resistance to a particular pathogen. It also emphasizes the potential for using combinations of agents in therapy and it is notable that a number of experimental examples attest to the synergistic effects of combinations of both drugs and biologicals. To exemplify these relationships Table III lists some examples of synergistic effects of interferons with other agents. It may be that use of immunoprophylactic agents in combination with immunotherapeutic agents will enhance the therapeutic potential of the former. It also is likely that where

Figure 1 Immunorestorative & Immunomodulation Therapies

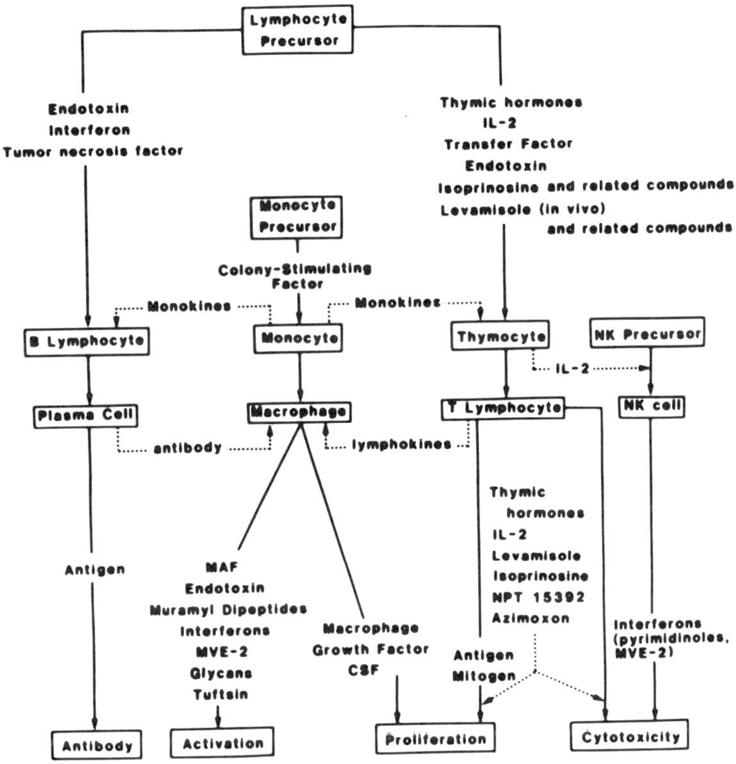

antimicrobial therapy exists but is relatively ineffective, e.g., monocutaneous candidiasis, lepromatous leprosy and drug-resistant tuberculosis, the combination of antimicrobial therapy and immunotherapy may be effective.

Before concluding, I thought it useful to review the status of the immunotherapy of AIDS and the AIDS-related complex (ARC) (see Hadden, 1986 for more complete summary and references). AIDS and its related syndromes have in common the presence of an immunosuppressive retrovirus (HTLV III, LAV, HIV) which infect both T cells and macrophages and produces dysfunction and ultimately death of the cells in the case of the T cells. The mechanisms of effective eradication of the virus are not known. We do

Table III, Summary of Immunotherapy Trials in AIDS and ARC

Thymic Hormones	ARC	AIDS
Thymosin FrV	$\uparrow$IR 6/20 at 60mg (no CR)	-
Thymosin α_1	NR in 10	
Thymopentin	NR in 6 (sub Q)	NR in 7
	$\uparrow$IR 4/6 (IV infusion) ($\uparrow$ CR)	
Thymulin	-	NR in 4
TP-1	$\uparrow$IR 5/7 (no CR)	-
THF	$\uparrow$IR 5/7 (no CR)	$\uparrow$IR & CR in 1
Interleukin II		
Jurkat		NR 5
Buffy Coat		NR 12
Buffy Coat		NR 7
rHuIL-2	NR 6	NR 3
rHuIL-2 (infusion)		$\uparrow$IR 59
Drug		
Imreg	$\uparrow$IR 21/33	
DLE		NR 3
Glucan	$\uparrow$IR in ?/13	NR 6
Azimexon		$\pm\uparrow$IR ?/70
Levamisole		NR 5
Imuthiol (DTC)	$\uparrow$IR 3/6	
Isoprinosine	$\uparrow$IR 20 CR	
"	$\uparrow$IR 157 CR	
"		$\uparrow$IR 40/48

IR = Immune Response; NR = No Response; CR = Clincial Resp.

know that, while perhaps 1,000,000 people are seropositive in the United States, only 20,000 have contracted AIDS. Those that are seropositive are thought to sustain the presence of latent, potentially activatable virus. What mechanisms keep the virus in check are not clear since most of the antibodies detected in these patients are only poorly neutralizing. With viral activation progressive cellular immunodeficiency develops such that peripheral T cells are depleted and all forms of the expression delayed type hypersensitivity are compromised. Concommitant destruction of both the epithelial and lymphoid component of the thymus occurs with a failure to reconstitute the peripherial T cell system. The therapeutic strategies in this disease have focused on molecular and cellular reconstitution of the T cell system alone or in conjunction with antiviral therapy. The antiviral strategies are summarized elsewhere (Wormser, 1986). It is of note that interferon treatment of the Kaposi's Sarcoma in AIDS patients has produced a 20-40% complete and partial response rate yet has not reversed significantly the cellular immune defects. I will summarize here the other immunotherapeutic approaches.

Table IV, Interferon - Synergistic Interactions

αIFN + β IFN; α IFN + γ IFN
IFN + Chemotherapy
IFN + Immunomodulators (Isoprinosine, cimetidine, etc.)
IFN + IL-2
IFN + TNF
IFN + MDP/LPS/Liposomes
IFN + Monoclonal Antibody (Imaging)

Bone marrow and thymus transplants and lymphocyte infusions have been attempted in a number of AIDS patients without obvious clinical benefit nor enduring reconstitution. A recent example reported by Fauci and coworkers at the Paris AIDS meeting suggests that such efforts in conjunction with antiviral therapy may be more successful.

Thymosin (α_1 & fraction V) have been employed in 30 ARC patients. In a small subgroup of 6 responders treated with 60mg/day of fraction V several parameters of immune response improved. Clinical responses were not observed; however, it was noted that none of these 6 progressed to AIDS. Thymopentin by infusion but not by bolus injection improved lymphoproliferative responses in 6 ARC patients again without clinical data. Both TP-1 and thymic humoral factor (THF) have increased cellular immune parameters in 5 of 7 ARC patients without evidence of clinical response. Neither thymulin nor thymopentin benefitted AIDS patients; however, THF apparently benefitted one AIDS patient both clinically and immunologically. The immunotherapeutic effects of these thymic hormone preparations are evident in these studies with the ARC patients; however, the magnitude and duration of the effects are not such as to indicate major reversal of the immune deficiency. Nonetheless, controlled trials in ARC patients are needed to determine whether symptoms are reduced and conversion of ARC to AIDS is delayed or reduced.

Interleukin II has been used in crude (buffy coat) purified (Jurkat), and cloned (rHu-IL-2) form using a variety of doses. While virtually no significant effects were observed in the first 27 patients, Lane & Fauci have recently presented in Paris (June, 1986) that 59 patients treated with very high doses of cloned IL-2 by continuous infusion showed immune improvement as evidenced by increased lymphocyte counts (1500 → 4000) and decreased virus recovery. This form of therapy, while cumbersome and expensive, deserves exploration, particularly in combination with antiviral and/or thymic hormone therapy. While dialyzed leukocyte extract (DLE) has seen no effect, a similar extract (Imreg) has shown increased DTH responses in several patients with AIDS & ARC. Further immunological and clinical information is awaited on this material. Soluble glucan has been employed in several ARC patients with evidence of induction of IL-1 (thus fever); however, no positive responses in AIDS were observed. Azimexon and levamisole have both been adjudged not to be useful in AIDS and both showed unacceptable toxicity. Imuthiol (DTC) has not shown the same toxicity as levamisole and has been reported to increase immune response in 3 of 6 ARC patients and also in other unreported cases of AIDS and ARC (Renoux, personal communication).

Isoprinosine has been employed in more than 177 patients with ARC in multicenter controlled trials. Increased T11 and T4 number and NK cell activity have been observed. Bekesi, et al. (1986) also observed in 20 ARC patients decreased antigen-antibody complexes and spontaneous Ig production by B lymphocytes. Wallace & Bekesi (1986) reported decreased symptom scores and conversion to AIDS in one group of ARC patients. Further information on clinical responses from the multicenter study is awaited. Initial AIDS data are encouraging. Both DTC and isoprinosine have recently been shown to inhibit HTLV III expression in vitro (i.e., reverse transcriptase, P15 & P41 proteins) (Pompidou, et al., 1986). Of the chemically defined, orally active drugs both Imuthiol and isoprinosine seem to be the most active and interesting. Their use in combination with antiviral agents and the biologicals seem warranted.

These immunotherapy trials in AIDS and ARC make it clear that the therapeutic window for treatment is restricted to the less ill ARC patients and that reconstitution in AIDS itself will require heroic measures like bone marrow and/or thymus reconstitution under antiviral protection. We personally are working on more complex molecular strategies using combinations of thymic hormones and the thymomimetic drugs with interleukin II to attempt reconstitution of the athymic nude mouse. If functional T cells can be generated by this means, the use of the therapies which are effective in AIDS in conjunction with antiviral therapy should provide a better strategy. It is important to realize that even if we fail to develop effective reconstitution therapy in AIDS we may be able to employ immunotherapy to more effectively manage their infections. For example, antiviral therapy (CMV, hepatitis, herpes, EBV, etc.) oriented toward boosting natural killer cells may be benefitted by synergistic combinations of interferon, IL-2, isoprinosine, NPT 15392, and others. Similarly antimicrobial therapy (Mycobacterium avium, candida, etc.) oriented toward boosting macrophage microbicidal function in the absence of T cells may be benefitted by synergistic combinations of lymphokines (including interferon), muramyl dipeptides, detoxified monophosphoryl lipid A, liposomes, and others. We have much to learn about immunotherapy from these unfortunate patients. The spin-offs from the effort may have great impact on the progress of this field in general as it relates to nonAIDS related infections.

In conclusion, the immunotherapy of microbial diseases, particularly viral infections for which no effective chemotherapy exists and bacterial, fungal, or parasitic infections for which antimicrobial therapy is ineffective or poorly effective is at the same time an old and a new approach. The increasing sophistication of the science of immune regulation, i.e. immunopharmacology, implies that such therapies in the future will have unparalleled efficacy and safety. A new era of clinical immunomodulation is clearly emerging.

REFERENCES

Bekesi G, Wallace J, Tsang P, Roboz J (1986). Normalization of immunoregulatory T helper and T suppressor sublineage and cell mediated immunity by isoprinosine in preclinical homosexual males: An in vivo study. Cancer Detect Prev 9 (in press).

Bruley-Rosset M, Florentin I, Kiger N, Schulta J, Mathe G (1979). Restoration of impaired immune functions of aged animals by chronic bestatin treatment. Immunol 38:75.

Chedid L (1986). Use of muramyl peptides in synthetic and semisynthetic vaccines. In Chedid L, Hadden JW, Spreafico F, Dukor P, Willoughby D (eds): "Advances in Immunopharmacology 3," Oxford: Pergamon Press, p 329.

Friedman H, Specter S (1982). Immunotherapy and immunoregulation. In Came PE, Caliguiri LA (eds): "Chemotherapy of Viral Infection," Berlin: Springer Verlag, p 313.

Goldstein AL (1984). "Thymic Hormones and Lymphokines." New York: Plenum Press.

Hadden JW, Lopez C, O'Reilly RJ, Hadden EM (1976). Levamisole and inosiplex: Antiviral agents with immunopotentiating action. NY Acad Sci 284:139.

Hadden JW (1984). Perspectives on the immunotherapy of aids. In Selikoff IJ, Teirstein AS, Hirschman SZ (eds): "Acquired Immune Deficiency Syndrome," New York: Annals of New York Academy of Sciences, p 76.

Hadden JW (1985). Thymomimetic drugs. In Miescher P, Bolis L, Ghione M (eds): "Symposium on Immunopharmacology," Serono Symposium, New York: Raven Press, Vol 23, p 183.

Hadden JW (1985). Immunostimulation therapy in the treatment of infectious diseases. In Hadden JW, Sorice F, Touraine J-L (eds): "Immunotherapy and Viral Diseases," EOS special issue, Rome: Sigma Tau, Vol 5, p 51.

Hadden JW (1986). Current status of the immunotherapy of aids and the aids-related complex. In Wormser G (ed): "Acquired Immunodeficiency Syndrome," New Jersey: Noyes Publications (in press).

Hadden JW, Specter S, Galy A, Touraine J-L, Hadden EM (1986). Thymic hormones, interleukins, endotoxin and thymomimetic drugs in T lymphocyte ontogeny. In Chedid L, Hadden JW, Spreafico F, Dukor P, Willoughby D (eds): "Advances in Immunopharmacology 3," Oxford: Pergamon Press, p 487.

Ishitsuka H, Umeda V, Sakamoto A, Yagi Y (1983). Protective activity of thymosin α_1 against tumor progression in immunosuppressed mice. In Klein T, Specter S, Friedman H, Szentivanyi A (eds): "Biological Response Modifiers in Human Oncology and Immunology," New York: Plenum Press, Vol 166, p 89.

Nahmias AJ, O'Reilly RJ (1981). "Comprehensive Immunology: Immunology of Human Infection Part 1 and 2," New York: Plenum Press.

O'Neill G, Ginsberg T, Hadden JW (1984). Immunopharmacology of the hypoxanthine containing compounds isoprinosine and NPT 15392. In Kende M, Gainer J, Chirigos M (eds): "UFDA Conference on Immunomodulation in Veterinary Medicine," New York: Alan R. Liss, p 525.

Pompidou A, Delsauz MC, Talvi L, Mace B, Coutance F, Falkenrodt A, Lang JM (1985). Isoprinosine and imuthiol, two potentially active compounds in patients with aids-related complex symptoms. Cancer Res (suppl) 45:46715.

Renoux G (1978). Modulation of immunity by levamisole. Phar Ther 2:397.

Renoux G, Renoux M (1984). Diethyldithiocarbamate (DTC): A biological augmenting agent specific for T cells. In Fenichel RL, Chirigos M (eds): "Immune Modulation Agents and Their Mechanisms," New York: Marcel Dekker, p 7.

Simon LN, Hoehler FK, McKenzie DT, Hadden JW (1983). Isoprinosine and NPT 15392: Immunomodulation and cancer. In Klein T, Specter S, Friedman H, Szentivanyi A (eds): "Biological Response Modifiers in Human Oncology and Immunology," New York: Plenum Press, Vol 166, p 241.

Tsang KY, Fudenberg H (1984). Restoration of immune responses in aging animal models. In Cooper EL (ed): "Stress, Immunity, and Aging," New York: Marcel Dekker, p 257.

Wallace JI, Bekesi JG (1986). A double-blind clinical trial of the effects of inosine pranobex in immunodepressed patients with prolonged generalized lymphadenopathy. Clin Immunol Immunopath 39:179.

Werner GH (1979). Immunopotentiating substances with antiviral activity. Phar Ther 6:235.

Wormser G (1986). "Acquired Immunodeficiency Syndrome," New Jersey: Noyes Publications.

Index